IPS
Textbook of
Undergraduate Psychiatry

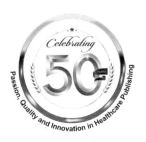

IPS
Textbook of
Undergraduate Psychiatry

Indian Psychiatric Society Publication

Editors

PK Singh MD
Professor and Head
Department of Psychiatry
Patna Medical College
Patna, Bihar, India

Om Prakash Singh MD
Professor
Department of Psychiatry
West Bengal Medical Education Service
Kolkata, West Bengal, India

Vinay Kumar MD
Consultant Psychiatrist
Manoved Mind Hospital and Research Center
Patna, Bihar, India

Assistant Editor

Vijendra Nath Jha
Assistant Professor
Department of Psychiatry
Darbhanga Medical College
Darbhanga, Bihar, India

Foreword

AK Agarwal
Past President
Indian Psychiatric Society

JAYPEE BROTHERS MEDICAL PUBLISHERS
The Health Sciences Publisher
New Delhi | London

Jaypee Brothers Medical Publishers (P) Ltd.

Headquarters
Jaypee Brothers Medical Publishers (P) Ltd
4838/24, Ansari Road, Daryaganj
New Delhi 110 002, India
Phone: +91-11-43574357
Fax: +91-11-43574314
Email: jaypee@jaypeebrothers.com

Overseas Office
J.P. Medical Ltd
83 Victoria Street, London
SW1H 0HW (UK)
Phone: +44 20 3170 8910
Fax: +44 (0)20 3008 6180
Email: info@jpmedpub.com

Website: www.jaypeebrothers.com
Website: www.jaypeedigital.com

Inquiries for bulk sales may be solicited at: jaypee@jaypeebrothers.com

IPS Textbook of Undergraduate Psychiatry

First Edition: **2021**

ISBN: 978-93-5270-423-1

Printed at: Samrat Offset Pvt. Ltd.

Contributors

Aarthi Ganesh
Schizophrenia Research Foundation (SCARF)
Chennai, Tamil Nadu, India

Abhinav Tandon
Consultant Psychiatrist
Dr AKT Neuropsychiatric Center
Allahabad, Uttar Pradesh, India

Aditi Singh
Assistant Professor
Department of Psychiatry
Ramaiah Medical College and Hospitals
Bengaluru, Karnataka, India

Ajit Avasthi
Former Professor and Head
Department of Psychiatry
Postgraduate Institute of
Medical Education and Research
Chandigarh, India

Ajit V Bhide
Senior Consultant and Head
Department of Psychiatry
Formerly Head and Preceptor, Family Medicine
St Martha's Hospital
Bengaluru, Karnataka, India

Akhilesh Sharma
Associate Professor
Department of Psychiatry
Postgraduate Institute of
Medical Education and Research
Chandigarh, India

Amit Khanna
Clinical Fellow Psychiatry
HDUHB, NHS Wales, UK
Assistant Professor, IHBAS
New Delhi, India

Amlan Kusum Jana
Associate Professor
Department of Psychiatry
KPC Medical College
Kolkata, West Bengal, India

Ananya Mahapatra
Assistant Professor
Department of Psychiatry
Dr Ram Manohar Lohia Hospital and
Postgraduate Institute of Medical
Education and Research
New Delhi, India

Atul Ambekar
Professor
National Drug Dependence Treatment Center
All India Institute of Medical Sciences
New Delhi, India

Avinash DeSousa
Research Associate and
Consultant Psychiatrist
Department of Psychiatry
Lokmanya Tilak Municipal
Medical College
Mumbai, Maharashtra, India

Baxi Neeraj Prasad Sinha
Consultant Psychiatrist and Clinical Director
(Teesside AMH)
Tees, Esk and Wear Valleys NHS Foundation Trust
Wessex House, Falcon Court
Stockton-on-Tees
England, UK

Damodharan Dinakaran
Assistant Professor
Department of Psychiatry
National Institute of Mental Health and
Neurosciences (NIMHANS)
Bengaluru, Karnataka, India

Deeksha Elwadhi
Trust Doctor, St Ann's Hospital
BEH Mental Health Trust
London, England, UK

Ganesan Venkatasubramanian
Professor
Department of Psychiatry
National Institute of Mental Health and
Neurosciences (NIMHANS)
Bengaluru, Karnataka, India

K John Vijay Sagar
Professor and Head
Department of Child and
Adolescent Psychiatry
National Institute of Mental Health and
Neurosciences (NIMHANS)
Bengaluru, Karnataka, India

Lakshmi Vijayakumar
Founder Sneha
Head
Department of Psychiatry
Voluntary Health Services
Chennai, Tamil Nadu, India

Malay Kumar Ghosal
Professor and Head
Department of Psychiatry
Medical College
Kolkata, West Bengal, India

MS Bhatia
Director-Professor and Head
Department of Psychiatry
University College of Medical Sciences and
Guru Teg Bahadur Hospital
New Delhi, India

N Prasanna Kumar
Associate Professor
Department of Psychiatry
Andhra Medical College
Visakhapatnam, Andhra Pradesh, India

Naren P Rao
Additional Professor
Department of Psychiatry
National Institute of Mental Health and
Neurosciences (NIMHANS)
Bengaluru, Karnataka, India

Neelanjana Paul
Associate Professor and Head
Department of Psychiatry
ICARE Institute of Medical Sciences and Research
Haldia, West Bengal, India

Nilesh Shah
Professor and Head
Department of Psychiatry
LTM Medical College and General Hospital
Mumbai, Maharashtra, India

Nishant Goyal
Associate Professor
Department of Psychiatry
I/C, fMRI Centre and KS Mani Centre for
Cognitive Neurosciences and Erna Hoch
Centre for Child and Adolescent Psychiatry
I/C, Academic Section
Central Institute of Psychiatry
Ranchi, Jharkhand, India

Niska Sinha
Assistant Professor
Department of Psychiatry
Indira Gandhi Institute of Medical Sciences
Patna, Bihar, India

Nitin Gupta
Senior Consultant, Neuropsychiatrist and
Therapist
Gupta Mind Healing and
Counselling Center
Chandigarh, India

NN Raju
Professor
Department of Psychiatry
King George Hospital
Visakhapatnam, Andhra Pradesh, India

Om Prakash
Associate Professor of Psychiatry
Consultant in Adult and Geriatric Psychiatry
Department of Psychiatry
Institute of Human Behavior and
Allied Sciences (IHBAS)
New Delhi, India

Om Prakash Singh
Professor
Department of Psychiatry
West Bengal Medical Education Service
Kolkata, West Bengal, India

Piyali Mandal
Associate Professor
National Drug Dependence Treatment Center
All India Institute of Medical Sciences
New Delhi, India

PK Dalal
Professor and Head
Department of Psychiatry
King George's Medical University
Lucknow, Uttar Pradesh, India

PK Singh
Professor and Head
Department of Psychiatry
Patna Medical College
Patna, Bihar, India

Pragya Lodha
Research Associate and Clinical
Psychologist
Desousa Foundation
Mumbai, Maharashtra, India

PSVN Sharma
Professor
Department of Psychiatry
Kasturba Medical College, Manipal
Manipal Academy of Higher Education
Manipal, Karnataka, India

R Srinivasa Murthy
Mental Health Consultant
SVYM Palliative Care
Mysuru, Karnataka, India

R Thara
Vice Chairman
Schizophrenia Research Foundation (SCARF)
Chennai, Tamil Nadu, India

Rajesh Kumar
Professor and Head
Department of Psychiatry
Indira Gandhi Institute of Medical Sciences
Patna, Bihar, India

Rajesh Sagar
Professor
Department of Psychiatry
All India Institutes of Medical Sciences
New Delhi, India

Ravi Gupta
Certified Sleep Physician (World Sleep Federation)
Additional Professor
Department of Psychiatry
All India Institute of Medical Sciences
Rishikesh, Uttarakhand, India

RC Jiloha
Professor
Department of Psychiatry
Hamdard Institute of Medical Sciences and Research
New Delhi, India

Rohit Verma
Associate Professor
Department of Psychiatry
All India Institute of Medical Sciences
New Delhi, India

S Nambi
Professor and Head
Department of Psychiatry
Sri Balaji Medical College and Hospital
Chennai, Tamil Nadu, India

Samir Kumar Praharaj
Professor and Head
Department of Psychiatry
Kasturba Medical College, Manipal
Manipal Academy of Higher Education
Manipal, Karnataka, India

Sandeep Grover
Professor
Department of Psychiatry
Postgraduate Institute of Medical
Education and Research
Chandigarh, India

Santosh K Chaturvedi
Senior Professor
Department of Psychiatry
National Institute of Mental Health and
Neurosciences (NIMHANS)
Bengaluru, Karnataka, India

Satish C Girimaji
Senior Professor
Department of Child and Adolescent Psychiatry
and Dean (Behavioral Sciences)
National Institute of Mental Health and
Neurosciences (NIMHANS)
Bengaluru, Karnataka, India

Savita Malhotra
Former Dean
Professor and Head
Department of Psychiatry
Postgraduate Institute of Medical
Education and Research
Chandigarh, India

Shivananda Manohar
Assistant Professor
Department of Psychiatry
JSS Medical College and Hospital
JSS Academy of Higher Education and Research
Mysuru, Karnataka, India

Shreemit Maheshwari
Assistant Professor
Amaltas Institute of Medical Sciences
Dewas, Madhya Pradesh, India

Shubhangi R Parkar
Professor and Head
Department of Psychiatry
Chief: Bombay Drug Deaddiction Center
Convener, MCI Nodal Center
GS Medical College and KEM Hospital
Mumbai, Maharashtra, India

SK Kar
Associate Professor
Department of Psychiatry
King George's Medical University
Lucknow, Uttar Pradesh, India

Sucharita Mondal
Assistant Professor
Department of Psychiatry
All India Institute of Medical Sciences
Raipur, Chhattisgarh, India

Suhas Chandran
Assistant Professor
Department of Psychiatry
St John's Medical College Hospital
Bengaluru, Karnataka, India

Sushmita Bhattacharya
Senior Resident
Department of Psychiatry
Kalpana Chawla Government Medical College
Karnal, Haryana, India

Swaminath G
Former Professor and Head
Department of Psychiatry
Dr BR Ambedkar Medical College
Bengaluru, Karnataka, India

Swapnajeet Sahoo
Assistant Professor
Department of Psychiatry
Postgraduate Institute of
Medical Education and Research
Chandigarh, India

TS Sathyanarayana Rao
Professor
Department of Psychiatry
JSS Medical College and Hospital
JSS Academy of Higher Education and Research
Mysuru, Karnataka, India

Vanteemar S Sreeraj
Assistant Professor
Department of Psychiatry
National Institute of Mental Health and
Neurosciences (NIMHANS)
Bengaluru, Karnataka, India

Varghese P Punnoose
Professor and Head
Department of Psychiatry
Government Medical College
Kottayam, Kerala, India

Vidya KL
Geriatric Mental Health
King George Medical University
Lucknow, Uttar Pradesh, India

Vijaya Raghavan
Consultant Psychiatrist
Schizophrenia Research Foundation
Chennai, Tamil Nadu, India

Vinayak Vijayakumar
Consultant Psychiatrist
Department of Psychiatry
Voluntary Health Services
Chennai, Tamil Nadu, India

Vinod K Sinha
Professor (Retd.)
Department of Psychiatry
Central Institute of Psychiatry
Ranchi, Jharkhand, India

YC Janardhan Reddy
Professor and Head
Department of Psychiatry
OCD Clinic
National Institute of Mental Health and
Neurosciences (NIMHANS)
Bengaluru, Karnataka, India

Indian Psychiatric Society

Plot 43, Sector: 55
Gurugram, Haryana, India
PIN: 122003

The need of an authentic book on Psychiatry that meets the requirements of undergraduate students of India and by extension that of the South Asian subcontinent, has long been felt. A book of this nature, by offering minimum essential knowledge of psychiatry, will prepare the average medical graduate to deal with mental health problems at the primary care level which is of immense significance for the delivery of mental healthcare services in a country like ours, as India is woefully short of psychiatrists. The Indian Psychiatric Society has always emphasized the need for psychiatric training and has written and represented to the competent authorities.

We are proud of our successive publication committees led by Dr Vinay Kumar and Professor PK Singh who are part of the editorial team of this book along with Honorary Editor of Indian Journal of Psychiatry Professor Om Prakash Singh for taking up the responsibility of preparing this multiauthor textbook of psychiatry. We are sure, the book will empower undergraduate medical students to treat common psychiatric illnesses. At the same time, we would advise our postgraduate teachers to recommend this as first book for newly admitted postgraduate students.

We express sincere gratitude to all the editors for their commitment and hard work without which it was difficult to produce a quality textbook like this. We congratulate all the authors for their brilliantly written chapters and express our sincere thanks to them. We also thank internationally acclaimed medical publishers M/s Jaypee Brothers Medical Publishers (P) Ltd, New Delhi, India, for partnering with us in our academic endeavors.

This book must find a place in the satchels of all medical students and shelves of libraries of all medical colleges in India.

Long live Indian Psychiatric Society.

Mrugesh Vaishnav
President, IPS

PK Dalal
President-elect, IPS

Vinay Kumar
Hon General Secretary, IPS

Foreword

Psychiatry has taken long strides during the last few decades. The mental health issue has been found to be common in our population and the national mental health survey found that nearly 10.6% of our population suffers from mental illnesses. The treatment gap between needs and services is huge and nearly 85% goes untreated or poorly treated. Current undergraduate education does not prepare them for this challenge. Medical Council of India has provided a detailed curriculum for psychiatry for undergraduate education. A department of Psychiatry has become essential part of medical colleges in India. There is a welcome news that All India Institute of Medical Sciences, Rishikesh, Uttarakhand has a full paper in psychiatry in final MBBS examinations. There are a large number of textbooks on undergraduate education in psychiatry from the west. Most of our students did not feel comfortable with these books. Many Indian psychiatrists have tried to fulfill this need in the past. Unfortunately, most of these were not accepted by the student community.

This book is being produced by the Indian Psychiatric Society after considering every aspect of what is expected from such a book. This is a multiauthor book. Most of the authors are experts in the field and provide text that is rooted in the reality of this country. There are 32 chapters and every area has been comprehensively covered. I have gone through some chapters and I found them easy-to-read. This book is a path-breaking venture and I hope it will be accepted by the medical students of India. No venture can be perfect, but it will go on maturing with time.

AK Agarwal
Past President, Indian Psychiatric Society
Professor and Head (Rtd.)
Department of Psychiatry
King George's Medical University (KGMU)
Lucknow, Uttar Pradesh, India

Preface

If the discipline of psychiatry is to be strengthened, it has to begin from the level of under-graduate medical education. Every medical graduate must be able to function as a basic psychiatrist just as he is expected to function as a basic physician and a basic surgeon, which is implicitly ingrained in his medical degree, MBBS making him a Bachelor of Medicine and Bachelor of Surgery. Empowering him in addition to become a basic psychiatrist, will also ensure delivery of comprehensive health care to all patients by our medical graduates. That would be inclusive of mental health, in addition to general physical health care. It is with this perspective that we decided to bring out a textbook of psychiatry for undergraduate medical students under the auspices of Indian Psychiatric Society. Other than the three of us, we have received valuable inputs, guidance and advice from our esteemed colleagues, Dr NN Raju and Dr RK Chadda, in giving shape and substance to this textbook.

This book has tried to cover the whole length of breadth of the field of psychiatry, though at the beginner's level, but through the power of the pen of acknowledged leaders of the field. It is said that if you have to learn the basics, learn it from the masters. In tune with that spirit, this book begins with a discussion of the nature of mind, which is very unconventional, but in the opinion of the editors a very crucial component. Unless we know what mind is, how can we know what mental disorders are? Further, it goes on to discuss the basic principles of psychosocial sciences and biological sciences as related to psychiatry. Book further progresses on to discuss the concepts of mental health and mental disorders, classification and clinical evaluation, communication skills, and further goes on to discuss the established psychiatric syndromes. At the end, it touches upon community psychiatry, forensic psychiatry, cultural psychiatry and also the history and future of psychiatry. Throughout the book, editors have endeavored to enforce simplicity, lucidity and precision of language; keeping only mainstream, consensual opinions to avoid controversy; presenting a blend of research evidence and Indian experience; relying mostly on only one system of classification but keeping the content of chapters not bound to it; factual information has been kept at a level to serve the twin goals of meeting the needs of undergraduate medical students as well as being used as a primer by the postgraduate psychiatry students; unity and interdependence of physical and mental health has also been emphasized wherever appropriate. We have kept the perspective that sooner or later the discipline of psychiatry will be granted the stature of independent subject at the undergraduate level. We hope that this book shall stand the trial of time and enlightened readership.

PK Singh
Om Prakash Singh
Vinay Kumar

Acknowledgments

The task of introducing the book will not be complete unless we express our sincere thanks to all the esteemed authors who have so painstakingly contributed such beautifully written authoritative chapters, despite their extremely busy schedules and other great responsibilities. We also express our sincere thanks and heartfelt appreciation to Shri Jitendar P Vij (Group Chairman), Mr Ankit Vij (Managing Director), and Ms Chetna Malhotra Vohra (Associate Director–Content Strategy) of M/s Jaypee Brothers Medical Publishers (P) Ltd, New Delhi, India, for accepting to bring out a book of psychiatry, meant primarily for the undergraduate medical students under the aegis of our national professional body, the Indian Psychiatric Society. They deserve all praise for their artisanship and professionalism. We will also like to place on record our deep appreciation for constant support, encouragement and persistent supervision by all the top leadership of Indian Psychiatric Society, the President, the President-elect and the Honorary General Secretary. We will also like to express our appreciation and thanks to all the members of the Successive Publication Subcommittees for their help and guidance. Finally, most respectfully, we will like to say a big 'thank you' to Professor AK Agarwal for having agreed to write the foreword of this book. He has been a constant source of encouragement and affection to all of us and a pioneer in the field of psychiatry teaching. Hopefully, this book will be welcomed and warmly received by students and teachers both and shall lead to a quantum jump in the standards of undergraduate psychiatry teaching in India. We also hope that this book will prove a gateway book for those who intend to specialize in the discipline of psychiatry. Long live IPS and its traditions.

PK Singh
Om Prakash Singh
Vinay Kumar

Contents

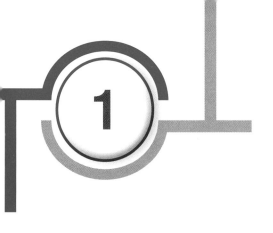

Nature of Mind: Real or Virtual

PK Singh

INTRODUCTION

Human mind has always remained engaged in pursuing a question as to "What is Mind." This primary and perpetual question has remained unanswered despite a continuous pursuit by seekers of knowledge and truth of all classes and creed across all ages of history. It is primary because it is the mind itself, which enables this question to be asked, after appearance of a highly developed mind at some point of time during the course of evolution, which is endowed with faculty of self-awareness in addition to the faculty of general awareness. It is primary also because our total existence is primarily mental in character. All other attributes are secondary. It is perpetual because it has remained unanswered despite several millennia of relentless pursuit by mankind from the first philosophers to the tech-age super-scientists. There is no prospect of finding the answer in near future. This question has vexed all classes of people, the seer, the sages, the learned, and the laity, all alike. Therefore, understandably the postulated answers have been equally varied.

THE PARADOX

One of the biggest paradoxes of life is that our only instrument of knowledge, the mind, is not structured to know itself in the same manner, as it is empowered to know the "objective world." To be able to discover the true nature of mind appears to be outside the cognitive jurisdiction of mind itself, though it appears empowered to experience, observe, and uncover the mysteries of material world around.

There is an analogous parallel here with brain. The stimuli, which produce pain on touching the peripheral organs, do not produce pain when brought directly in contact with substance of brain. The corollary of all this is that we have to make-do with the inferred interpretations of mind, at least for the time being. Mind is not available to be experienced objectively in the same manner, as the material entities are experienced through sensory organs in the external three-dimensional space.

ORIGIN OF THE QUESTION

The origin of the question as to, what is mind—is from the veritable mind itself. Inbuilt curiosity and structured quest for knowledge are the forces, which lead to asking questions about oneself. Conscious experience is the primary source, which leads to realization of a dichotomy in the way the body is experienced and the way the mental events are experienced. There appears to be a qualitative difference between the somatic and the psychic dimensions.

On the basis of everyday common life experience, it appears that physical world is primary and its mental experience is secondary. However, when we try to analyze it logically, it turns out that our mental experiences are primary and the physical world that it represents is secondary. This is so because what is available to us to experience is the mental representation of the external world and the impressions that the external world has cast upon the mental dimension of our existence. The way we experience the external world is not exactly how the external world in all probability is. *It is the mental edition of the external world.* This mental edition must necessarily be different for different organisms that are capable of conscious experience and also, for the same reason, different for each individual.

A very blatant example would be the difference in the mental editions of external world of organisms having color vision and those who do not have it. One would have a chromatic image and the other would have an achromatic image for the same segment of the external world. In that sense, all our experiences are virtual in nature relative to the unique and individual-specific organization of our brain. Two more examples regarding virtuality of experience are from the world of illusions. The illusion of white color emerging out of a mixture of seven colors and the experience of continuous motion getting synthesized within our own minds out of a series of discontinuous frames presented to the person at more than certain critical speed are other commonplace examples, which suggest that what we experience at the conscious level are creations of our own mind.

MIND AND THE BODY

Mind and the body, as we experience it, continue to exist and function as independent but in a seamlessly integrated manner. They are also interdependent. They are qualitatively different and seem to work by different set of rules. Mind can only be experienced subjectively by the individual himself, while body is available for objective scrutiny by both the self and others. Mind is private while body is public. Body is made of material units, while mind apparently is nonmaterial, as far we are able to understand at the moment. Therefore, body displays properties of weight, volume, and other physicochemical characteristics, which mind does not. Mind on the other hand has property of consciousness, of being aware of self and the outside world, has certain degree of freedom from the dictates of space and time, and is able to create a symbolic representational noumenal world, which is completely private in nature.

JUSTIFICATION OF PURSUIT

The irrepressible human urge to know one's true self and realize fuller potentials, provides ultimate justification for such pursuits. To be able to more rationally understand the issues related to mental health and mental disorders provides another strongly humane reason to justify such pursuits. Any venture that proposes to discuss the disorders of mind must also discuss the nature of mind. Textbooks of Psychiatry mostly deal only with disorders of mind, but surprisingly hardly ever discuss the nature of mind. Only by inclusion of this topic in the mainstream of mental health sciences, we can hope to make any headway on this path, facilitated by collective wisdom. The issue of validity of psychiatric entities is always in question. It can substantively improve only if we develop better understanding and insight into the phenomena of mind.

CONCEPTS/DEFINITIONS OF MIND

Oldest scriptures/literatures from all cultures and religion show evidence that man has always tried to know about his inner self. This inner self has been the mind or manas and the soul. But, all of them—the seers, the philosophers, and the scientists—do not seem to be talking about the same thing, when they refer to mind or manas. It has been variously defined by people who pursue different paths of enquiry.

The mind is defined as the sum of the cognitive abilities that enable consciousness, perception, memory, thinking, imagination, and judgment. It may also be defined as the conscious and unconscious mental activity of a person (*Yogapedia*).

According to the *Vedas*, the mind represents the air element in the body. It forms part of the subtle body. According to the *Upanishads*, the subtle parts of food become the mind in the body and nourish it.

The mind is a set of cognitive faculties including consciousness, perception, thinking, judgment, language, and memory. It is usually defined as the faculty of an entity's thoughts and consciousness. It holds the power of imagination, recognition, and appreciation, and is responsible for processing feelings and emotions, resulting in attitudes and actions (Wikipedia).

The school of materialism asserts that nothing exists except matter. Mind is just an epiphenomenon of matter according to them. This view is also known as epiphenomenalism. They do not consider mind as immaterial stuff but rather as a very special kind of material stuff. Such phenomena as sensations, perceptions, and thoughts consist in the various qualities and relations of the atoms. They are only complex forms of matter in motion. The philosophy of idealism or psychical monism defines mind as an independent and immaterial reality. It denies the existence of matter and reduces it to being of secondary importance, and holds mind to be the primary reality.

According to the philosophy of neutral monism, whatever exists in nature is neither material nor mental but some neutral substance out of which both material and mental substances are formed. Every human being consists of two different substances namely mind and body. Mind is defined as a substance, which has no spatial location. It is referred to as the locus or center or owner of thoughts, feelings, and sense-experiences. On the other hand, body is the locus of all the physiological changes.

Plato was the first western philosopher to declare that mind is an immaterial entity, separate and distinct from the body, and able to exist without it. Plato held that the mind (psyche) is incharge of the body and directs its movements. Plato believed in the subsistence of both material entities and immaterial entities.

The most definitive statement of dualism is found in the philosophy of Descartes according to whom mind and matter are two separate and distinct sorts of substances, absolutely opposed in their natures and each capable of existing entirely independent of the other. The chief notion in Descartes was the primacy of consciousness, i.e., the mind knows itself more immediately and directly than it can know anything else. Mind knows external world, i.e., matter only through the impressions of the external world casts upon it in the form of sensation and perception. According to Descartes, all philosophy begins with the individual's mind and he makes his first argument in the words "I think, therefore I am" (cogito ergo sum).

There are many more theories and approaches to examine the issue of mind, but none of them seem to be able to show a path that can lead to a universally and uniformly applicable theory to resolve the enigma of mind.

REAL OR VIRTUAL

Whether mind is virtual or real cannot be answered in a categorical yes or no format. All logic leads to the conclusion, in the opinion of the author, that mind is a virtual reality. It is virtual as well as real. It is virtual by its nature because the way we understand our mind is through our experiences only, which are, as we have seen, creations of our own apparatus of consciousness and therefore virtual. It is real because it is the most immediately accessible experiential knowledge; such experiences make real differences in our lives through pain and pleasure, anxieties and fear, pursuit and planning, and even actions that can lead to survival or death.

Therefore, there cannot be anything that is more real than such mental experiences of ours as far as our lives are concerned. Veritably, it has a reality quotient that is undeniable, substantial, and tangible, because our reality originates from our own existence. Reality can be assessed only in terms of the effects that it produces. In the present instance of mental dimension of man, it has got effects, which range from sustenance of life to causation of death.

LIMITS OF SCIENCE

Science is guided by empirical observation, which is the ultimate source of its validity. Observations are made through sensory channels or its extensions and amplifications. Anything that is beyond the limits of the receptive capacity of our senses cannot be brought within the ambit of scientific analysis.

As such, human sensory channels are receptive to a very narrow range of ambient influences present, when seen on a cosmic scale. It is further limited by its complete inability to objectively observe the workings and events of mind.

RELATIONSHIP WITH MATTER

Mind–matter interaction keeps happening all the time—continuously and seamlessly. In fact, it is at the core of our existence. Every time a sense-impression is formed or a voluntary act or speech is initiated, there is conversion of the mental into the material and vice-versa; all this happening seamlessly and effortlessly. But, the dimension of mind–matter interaction becomes much more complex when we come to know that matter itself exists in different forms and types.

The matter with which we are familiar with and the matter, which matters most in our everyday life, is not the only type of matter that exists in the universe. This commonplace matter, known as baryonic matter, may exist in different states, such as solid, liquid, gas, and plasma states. This is what we are mostly familiar with. But science is just beginning to understand that matter of other types also exists in the universe, which is qualitatively different. There is evidence for dark matter, evidence for shadow matter or mirror matter, and evidence for antimatter. There may be many more yet to be discovered types of matter. Dark matter is a hypothetical form of matter that is thought to account for approximately 85% of the matter in the universe. Mirror matter, also called shadow matter, is a hypothetical counterpart to ordinary baryonic matter that we are familiar with. Antimatter is defined as a form of matter that is constituted by similar particles but with opposite properties. A related mysterious hypothesis is that of dark energy. Dark energy is an unknown form of energy, which is hypothesized to permeate all of space, tending to accelerate the expansion of the universe.

Since these various forms of matter and energy would surely have some interactive relationship with the ordinary baryonic matter that we are made of, it is quite logical to hypothesize that they will have some role to play in the emergence and actions of the dimension that we recognize as mind.

PARAPSYCHOLOGY

The discipline of parapsychology provides opportunity to study paranormal phenomena and experiences, which are different from abnormal experiences. Paranormal refers to parallel experiences, which are real experiences but not through mainstream channels of conscious experience. Whereas, abnormal refers to experiences of such kinds that are not real even though they appear to be experienced through mainstream channels of conscious experience. These fall in the domain of psychiatry. Parapsychology refers to supposedly scientific study of behavior and experience, which manifest independent of or without subservience to the known laws of space, time, and causality.

Parapsychology is divided into two main branches—(1) extra-sensory perception (ESP), which is the study of communications ostensibly without the known sensory organs and, (2) psychokinesis (PK) or the study of physical events that apparently occur without involvement of any recognized motor organs.

The kind of phenomena that are studied in parapsychology are telepathy, precognition, retrocognition, reincarnation, clairvoyance, near-death experience, mystical experiences, pre-death visions, experience of apparitions and mediumship, out of body experiences, etc.

Even though the predictability and replicability of such events and experiences are low compared to other natural events, which are studied by the methods of science, many personal life experiences and a few verified reports do suggest that they are possibly valid events and experiences because of their sheer undeniable definitiveness. May be we have to invent better methodologies to understand and validate them. To demonstrate the validity of such events and experiences, we will have to show that these influences of mental nature can traverse to materially discontinuous entities, across the span of space and time without the supportive substrate of intervening matter. Any such observation shall be of great theoretical importance, because it will provide support for the premise that mind and matter are sovereign entities and can exist independent of each other. That means the mind can exist in a disembodied form and format also.

CONCLUSION

In our pursuit to unravel the enigma of mind, we are still on the voyage. The end of voyage is not within our sight, the distance is not known to us. This distance can be traversed only through the relay race of life and carried forward by each generation of committed explorers. Mind is our only instrument of knowledge, which has limitations engineered into its design by the Divine. It allows experience only of the personal consciousness but does not allow objective evaluation of consciousness of other selves.

As of now, our conscious experience is the only and the primary resource that opens the windows for us to the world of phenomena. It is this very source, which generates the question, and also provides the answer about the nature and workings of mind. In fact, each of us lives within his own cognitive island, though we remain receptive and responsive to much larger part of the cosmic universe. Beyond this island, there are other sovereign worlds also. Even if we are able to ask the right kind of questions related to the mystery of mind and are able to find the right place and method to look for it, I would consider that we have made some progress.

The take home messages of this chapter are very few. The first one is that mind has to be treated as a virtual reality. It appears as if it is virtual, but behaves as if it is real. However, it merits to remain one of the primary pursuits in our quest of knowledge. The impressions of the external world that we experience within our minds are our first window to the universe of truths. All theories will have to account for and be inclusive of this "Primary Human Truth." The purpose of this chapter shall be deemed to have been fulfilled, if it succeeds in sensitizing the minds of future generation to endeavor to answer some of the vital questions related to the phenomena of mind.

TAKE-HOME MESSAGES

- "What is Mind"—is a primary and perpetual question, which has remained unanswered till date despite having been pursued continuously since earliest times by both the intellectual elite and the laity.
- The biggest paradox, which is also a stumbling block, is that our very instrument of knowledge, the mind, is not structured to know itself. It is not possible to objectively observe the mind.
- Mind and the body, as we experience it, continue to exist and function as independent as well as interdependent entities but in a seamlessly integrated manner.
- The mind is defined by *Yogapedia* as the sum of the cognitive abilities that enable consciousness, perception, memory, thinking, imagination, and judgment. It may also be defined as the conscious and unconscious mental activity of a person.
- It is important to understand the "order" of mind to be better able to understand the "disorders" of mind.
- Whether mind is virtual or real cannot be answered in a categorical yes or no format. In the opinion of the author, mind is a virtual reality. It is virtual as well as real. It is virtual because it seems to be a construct of our own consciousness and it is real because it matters most in our everyday lives inclusive of all our pains and pleasures, as well as our decisions to continue to exist or otherwise.

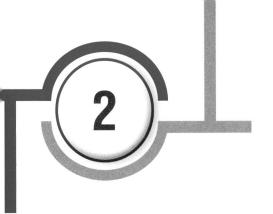

2. Basic Biological Sciences for Psychiatry

Rohit Verma, Vanteemar S Sreeraj, Damodharan Dinakaran, Ganesan Venkatasubramanian

INTRODUCTION

Brain is the most important organ of body from the perspectives of the discipline of psychiatry. Brain is understood as an organ made up of gray and white matter composed of discrete nerve cells (neurons), dendrites, axons, synapses (connections between neurons), receptors, neural circuits, and supporting cells. Mind on the other hand had been conceptualized as subjective entity composed of perceptions, emotions, thoughts, memory, consciousness, and information processing that is difficult to measure. Modern neuroscience has provided a new understanding of the brain by opening up possibilities for unifying the two concepts. Brain is now understood as a continually changing plastic organ, in its structure as well as its function. We now know that these plastic changes are generated in neuronal pathways modulating neurotransmitter release and leading to activation of genes and synthesis of new proteins, receptors and other membrane components to finally bring about a morphological and physiological change in the circuit activity. Thus, the dynamic state of brain observed at the biochemical, physiological and anatomical levels, culminates into information processing, perception, cognition, emotion, or behavior as a continuum.

Research in psychiatric disorders has led to substantial advances and emergence of critical insights on the pathogenesis of various psychiatric disorders. These exciting advances have generated immense scope for identifying biomarkers for psychiatric disorders through several novel research strategies. This chapter attempts a select overview of some of fundamental principles of biological sciences, more specifically neurobiology, and related research techniques in psychiatry.

NEUROANATOMY

Human nervous system is divided into central and peripheral systems. Central nervous system (CNS) consists of brain and spinal cord while peripheral nervous system (PNS) is made of peripheral nerves and ganglia. Human brain is organized structurally into cerebrum, cerebellum, midbrain, pons, and medulla oblongata. Thalamus, hypothalamus, midbrain, pons, and medulla contain host of nuclei important in regulating key functions of the body. Cerebral cortex is in turn subdivided into bilateral frontal, temporal, parietal, and occipital lobes. Differentiation into gray and white matter represents organization of neuronal cell bodies and the axonal tracts, respectively. Human brain has evolved in a manner that it has proportionately a larger cerebral cortex area that helps a person to specialize in various functions like language, emotion, cognition, socialization, etc. making it unique relative to the brain of animals. The spinal cord is a tubular bundle of nervous tissue extending from the medulla oblongata to the lumbosacral region of the vertebral column. The primary function is transmission of nerve signals from the motor cortex to the peripheral body organs and carries the afferent fibers of the sensory neurons to the sensory cortex. The spinal cord contains reflex arcs that can independently control central pattern generators and reflexes. The PNS is divided into somatic and autonomic nervous system (ANS). The somatic nervous system contains "afferent" neurons that carry sensory information from the peripheral sense organs to the CNS, and "efferent" neurons that provide motor instructions to the muscles. ANS is divided into sympathetic and parasympathetic systems, which are important for regulating the body's organ functions such as breathing, circulation, digestion, salivation, etc. Autonomic nerves also contain afferent and efferent fibers.

Macroorganization of Brain

At the organ level, various brain regions have a sort of specificity attached to them in terms of a tendency for certain functions to be preferentially localized to one hemispheric region. These regions may serve a particular role within the pathways of the nervous system. Common sensory functions like vision, hearing, and touch are organized in occipital, temporal, and parietal lobes, respectively. Taste and smell functions involve various nuclei and tracts.

Human consciousness is attributed to the coordinated activity of cerebral cortex along with wakefulness promoting reticular activating system of the brainstem. Memory is divided into explicit and implicit types. Explicit memory operations are largely hippocampus based while implicit memory is striatal based. Executive functions like working memory, planning, and judgment are primarily handled by prefrontal cortex (specifically the left dorsolateral prefrontal cortex). Human emotions involve organized functioning of limbic system, dorsal anterior cingulate cortex, and medial prefrontal cortex. Reward processing involves dopamine projections from midbrain to nucleus accumbens. Human motivation has been attributed to the mesocortical circuit, again involving dopaminergic transmission.

Microorganization of Brain

The brain consists primarily of two types of cells—neurons and glia. There are about 80 billion neurons and 100 billion glial cells. Neurons play the primary role in brain functioning, while glial cells aid in the facilitation of neuronal activity. Neurons are the structural and functional units of nervous system. Neurons consist of a soma (or cell body), which contains the nucleus; dendrites, which are processes that extend from the cell body and receive signals from other neurons; and axon, which extends from the cell body and transmits signals to other neurons. In 1906, Professor Cajal was awarded the prestigious Noble prize in physiology and medicine for his work, "the neuron doctrine" that states "each nerve cell is a totally autonomous physiological canton and they communicate by contiguity and not continuity." The basic kinds of connections between neurons are chemical synapses and electrical gap junctions. At synapses, the axons of one neuron generally contact the dendrite or cell body of another neuron. Here the plasma membrane of the signal-passing neuron (the presynaptic neuron) comes into close apposition with the membrane of the target (postsynaptic) cell. There are extensive arrays of a molecular machinery that link the presynaptic and postsynaptic neurons and carry out the signaling process. At these synapses, neurotransmitters are released for interneuronal communications, which are a major site for action of various psychotropic agents. Alternatively, adjacent neurons may connect directly to each other via gap junctions allowing various molecules, ions, and electrical impulses to pass directly through, from one cell to another. Neural networks are formed by connection of neurons to each other.

Neuroglia plays an important supportive role in maintaining the signaling abilities of neuron though they themselves do not participate in synaptic transmission directly. Glial cells are of three types namely astrocytes, oligodendrocytes, and microglia. Astrocytes maintain the chemical environment of the neuron. Oligodendrocytes help in myelination of axons in CNS while their counterparts in periphery are called Schwann cells. Microglia acts as brain scavenger that removes cellular breakdown products following normal turnover or injury.

Neuron consists of three parts—the soma or cell body, dendrites, and axon. The soma is the body of the neuron containing the nucleus. The axon and dendrites are filaments that extrude from soma. Dendrites are shorter filaments that branch profusely, getting thinner with each branching. Axon is the larger filament that leaves the soma at a swelling called the axon hillock and can extend for long distances. Usually, dendrites via the dendritic spine receive signals from other neurons and then transmit these signals through the axon to other neurons.

Each neuron is enclosed by a plasma membrane, a bilayer of lipid molecules with many types of protein structures embedded in it. These structures may form ion channels that permit specific types of electrically charged ions to flow across them and ion pumps that actively transport ions from one side of the membrane to the other. Voltage-gated ion channels can remain in open or closed states depending on the voltage difference across the membrane. Chemically gated ion channels switch between open and closed states by interactions with chemicals that diffuse through the extracellular fluid. The ion channels and ion pumps help in producing a voltage difference across the membrane providing a basis for electrical signal transmission between different parts of the membrane.

Neural Transmission

The key to neural function is the synaptic signaling process, known as neuro-transmission, which is partly electrical and partly chemical. The fundamental process that triggers the release of neurotransmitters is the action potential, a propagating electrical signal that is generated by virtue of the electrically excitable membrane of the neuron. As a result of this process, signaling molecules called neurotransmitters are released by the axon terminal of the presynaptic neuron, which bind to and activate the receptors on the dendrites of the postsynaptic neuron. In retrograde neurotransmission, dendrites of the postsynaptic neuron release retrograde neurotransmitters (e.g., endocannabinoids) that bind and activate the receptors located on the axon terminal of the presynaptic neuron, mainly at GABAergic and glutamatergic synapses.

Once the neurotransmitters are released in the synaptic cleft to attach to the postsynaptic receptors predominantly, some of them also bind to receptors on the presynaptic neuron. These receptors are called autoreceptors and they give a feedback to the presynaptic neuron to maintain the optimal concentration of neurotransmitters in the synapse. Neurotransmitters are metabolized/deactivated by enzymes in the synaptic cleft once their action is completed. Presynaptic neurons also contain channels called transporters which reuptake the neurotransmitters from synapse back to the presynaptic terminals. Antidepressant blocks these transporters and increases serotonin concentration in synaptic cleft.

Neurotransmission can also occur through electrical synapses through gap junctions, which allow direct connection between neurons leading to rapid transmission of signals through spreading of action potential, which move only in one direction due to the rectifying channels.

Glial cells are not merely passive supporters of neuronal function but are involved in integrating information and providing modulatory feedback to neurons. Gap-junctional communication between astrocytes and neurons has resurfaced as a second pathway for intercellular communication between glia and certain types of neurons. Slow interactions between astrocytes and neurons can regulate the establishment of both chemical and electrical connectivity, and such connections can subsequently be used for relatively rapid reciprocal communication between glia and neurons. Glial cells use a different code from neurons, consisting of elevations of their internal free calcium level that can be initiated by the action of a variety of neurotransmitters and neuronal activities.

The receptors after receiving signals from first messengers/neurotransmitters translate it to intraneuronal second messengers. Second messenger system handles the intracellular signal transmission.

Second Messenger System

Extracellular factors are termed as "first messengers" in the transmission of biological information. After the extracellular factors (such as neurotransmitters) cause transmission of signals to the receptors on the postsynaptic neurons, the receptor generates changes in the intracellular compartment through second messenger molecules present inside the cell. They trigger a cascade of physiological changes such as proliferation, differentiation, migration, survival, and apoptosis leading to signal transduction **(Table 2.1)**.

Table 2.1: Common second messengers.		
Types	*Properties*	*Examples*
Hydrophobic molecules	Water-insoluble molecules that are membrane-associated and diffuse from the plasma membrane into the intermembrane space where they can reach and regulate membrane-associated effector proteins	Diacylglycerol (DAG), and phosphatidylinositol (PI)
Hydrophilic molecules	Water-soluble molecules that are located within the cytosol	Cyclic nucleotides (e.g., cyclic adenosine monophosphate, or cAMP, and cyclic guanosine monophosphate, or cGMP), ions (e.g., Ca^{2+}), or phospholipid-derived molecules (e.g., inositol triphosphate or IP3)
Gases	These can diffuse both through cytosol and across cellular membranes	Nitric oxide (NO), carbon monoxide (CO), and hydrogen sulfide (H_2S)

Usually, a ligand (containing first messenger) binds to a membrane-spanning receptor molecule causing a conformational change in the receptor, which affects the activity of the receptor, eventually leading to contact with another membrane-bound protein—the "primary effector". The primary effector then creates a signal that can diffuse within the cell. This signal is carried by the "second (or secondary) messenger". The secondary messenger may then activate a "secondary effector" leading to signal transduction, which occurs at required time periods localized to specific regions of cell by utilizing specific enzymes or ion channels that promote synthesis/release/breakdown of second messenger molecules.

The calcium ion (Ca^{2+}) plays an important role in the rapid responses of neurons. During resting state, cytoplasmic levels of Ca^{2+} are low in neurons and energy is spent to pump these ions out of the cell. The ions are normally bound or stored in intracellular components (such as the endoplasmic reticulum) and can be released during signal transduction. When activated, the enzyme phospholipase C produces DAG and IP3, which increases calcium ion permeability of the membrane. Active G-proteins facilitate calcium entry into the cell by opening of calcium channels leading to a rapid increase in cytoplasmic Ca^{2+} concentration causing a cascade of intracellular changes and activities. In addition, calcium and DAG together activate protein kinase C that phosphorylates other molecules (such as activation of cAMP), leading to altered cellular activity. This leads to nuclear signaling and promotes nuclear synthesis by the activation of transcription factors through molecules such as cAMP response element binding protein (CREB). Lithium is found to alter the second messenger systems to act as a mood stabilizer.

Neurodevelopmental Process

There are nearly 80 billion neurons in human brain, 99% of which are present at birth along with other supportive cells such as glial cells. The process of development of neurons occurs in stages beginning in utero and unlike previously believed, continues throughout adult life although limited. Factors playing a role in the entire process include both genes as well as environment.

Neurogenesis

During embryonic development, the mammalian nervous system is derived from the neural tube, which contains neural stem cell (NSC) that will later generate neurons. A threshold amount of NSCs is required to initiate neurogenesis. These early stem cells are called neuroepithelial cells (NECs) that later change into as radial glial cells (RGCs) becoming elongated with radial morphology. RGCs are the primary stem cells of CNS and reside in the embryonic ventricular zone lying adjacent to the ventricular system of the neural tube. RGCs proliferate and divide directly into daughter neurons or indirectly into a subclass of neuronal progenitors called intermediate neuronal precursors (INPs), which will divide one or more additional times to produce neurons. Neurogenesis also occurs in adulthood, although to a much lower extent. Prominently, it occurs at only two brain regions—the subventricular zone (SVZ) of striatum and the dentate gyrus of hippocampus.

Migration

Newly born neurons migrate long distances to reach their final destinations, maturing, and generating neural circuitry through the growth of axons and dendrites. Neurons migrate along glial cells scaffolding with the leading tip of the axon being led by a growth cone. Neurons generate in specific tissue compartment or "neurogenic niche" determined by their parent stem cells. The whole process usually takes place over a fairly long period of time from a neurodevelopmental standpoint but is most active in utero to the first year of life and is nearly complete by the time a child is 3 years old.

Differentiation

Various molecular and genetic factors determine the rate and type of neurons generated (excitatory or inhibitory). Although it nearly completes by the age of 3, differentiation continues at some level throughout life. Differentiation is sensitive to changes in neurochemistry or may occur in response to chemical signals that are influenced by microenvironmental cues, which are signals/stimuli that occur in a specific, localized area of the brain. The microenvironmental cues may be composed of experiences or events that alter these chemicals or microenvironmental signals during development and can impact the way neurons differentiate, thus altering functional capacity. Differentiation is sensitive to these microenvironmental cues based on their pattern, intensity, and timing. These microenvironmental cues may be in various forms such as increase of the mother's heart rate in utero or changes in stress hormones in the infant.

Arborization

This is the process of branching out of dendritic networks from the neuron allowing the neuron to receive, process, and integrate complex patterns of activity that will, in turn, determine its activity. Neurons die when they are not connected to active neural networks. A pregnant mother's own neurochemistry can affect the fetus' neural differentiation.

Synaptogenesis

As discussed earlier, a given set of neurons are connected to each other. Synaptogenesis is the process by which developing neurons make connections with one another and form neuronal communication at synapses. These connections are not random but are guided by genetic and environmental cues. The strength and survival of these connections are based on their use with the principle of "cells that fire together, wire together". Patterned repetitive experiences during the first years of life refine and sculpt these connections. The more a connection is used, the stronger it becomes.

Myelination

There is creation of more efficient electrochemical transduction down the neuron as specialized glial cells wrap around the axons enabling them for more rapid and complex functioning and allows for more smooth, regulated functioning. It begins at birth and continues through adolescence. Myelination is regionally specific based upon development, i.e., related to the part of the brain that is developing at the time.

Synaptic Sculpting (Pruning)

Pruning is the process of constantly changing synaptic connections. These connections are use-dependent and are constantly being made and broken. The more neurons are used, the closer they grow together. As neurons grow closer together, the connections become more efficient. Neurons that are not actively used with sufficient activity die.

Apoptosis

It is the process of programmed death of neurons. Not all neurons that are born are needed. Death of neurons occurs when there is a lack of adequate connection to an active neural network. Thus, one may refer to brain as the "use it or lose it" organ.

Neurodevelopmental Basis of Psychiatric Disorders

Schizophrenia is a chronic, severe mental illness leading to impaired overall functioning capacity of the individual. Illness is characterized by delusions, hallucinations, disorganized behavior, cognitive deficits, and negative symptoms. Recent advances in the last two decades have shed light in understanding the structural and functional brain pathology associated with this illness. Reduced hippocampal volume, enlarged lateral ventricles, and hypofrontality have been consistently shown to be associated with schizophrenia. Gray matter volume reduction in bilateral insula, inferior frontal gyrus, anterior cingulate, and superior temporal gyrus was seen to be associated with the expression of above cluster of symptoms. Especially, individuals with schizophrenia are noted to have prominent auditory verbal hallucinations (AVH) and it is associated with gray matter volume reduction in left superior temporal gyrus and right superior temporal gyrus, which are areas for speech/phonological perception and processing in healthy individuals.

Bipolar disorder is a mood disorder, where individuals experience extreme mood states (mania and depression) that adversely affect the productivity and lead to disability. In bipolar disorder, the key areas of emotional regulation namely, amygdala and anterior paralimbic cortex play a role and inhibitory control exerted by dorsolateral and ventrolateral prefrontal cortex upon these areas is reportedly dysfunctional. Though there is an overlap of areas involved in schizophrenia and bipolar disorder, there are subtle differences. Individuals with bipolar illness have less gray matter reduction than schizophrenia patients in those overlapping areas and have been repeatedly shown to be associated with gray matter reduction in cerebellar region.

Depression, a mood disorder, is the leading cause of disability as per a recent World Health Organization (WHO) report. Multiple reports have suggested a reduction in hippocampal volume, which correlated with prolonged stress in patients with depression. Also, anterior cingulate cortex, a part of prefrontal cortex involved in emotional regulation, has reduced volume in patients with depression. Individuals who had experienced repeated episodes of depression have increased risk for developing cognitive decline and dementia given the repetitive insults to hippocampus.

Amygdala, with its primary role in fear conditioning and processing of aversive stimuli have been consistently implicated in the development of anxiety spectrum disorders and persistence of depressive symptoms. Obsessive-compulsive disorder involves occurrence of distressing repetitive thoughts, images that leads to significant anxiety which in turn leads the individual to perform neutralizing acts/rituals which maintains the illness vicious. Dysfunctional orbitofrontal cortex and caudate nucleus are implicated in the genesis and maintenance of obsessions and compulsions. Altered activity of cortico-striato-thalamo-cortical circuit/loop has been postulated as the mechanism underlying this illness.

Substance use and addiction are major health concerns in both developing and developed nations affecting especially the adolescent and young adult population. Abnormalities in reward pathway and neurotransmitter dopamine are implicated in the etiopathogenesis of substance addiction and related gambling and other behavioral addictions. Dopamine projections arising from the ventral tegmental part of midbrain and ending in nucleus accumbens, a part of ventral striatum, called the reward pathway is primarily implicated by several lines of evidence in addictive disorders. Other dopamine projections to cortical areas (mesocortical projection) play key role in motivation, reward processing, comparative, and hedonic evaluation.

NEUROCHEMISTRY

Neurotransmitters are broadly divided into small molecule transmitters [glutamate, gamma-aminobutyric acid (GABA), dopamine, histamine, serotonin, epinephrine, norepinephrine, and acetyl choline] and neuropeptide large molecule transmitters (enkephalin, substance P, vasopressin, oxytocin, and cholecystokinin). Other transmitters include enkephalin, neurosteroids, and gaseous transmitters like nitric oxide.

Chemical neurotransmission implicated in neuropsychiatric disorders involves monoamines, amino acids, and neuropeptides which form the major bulk of neurotransmitters in the brain. Recently there are emerging importance of other neurotransmitters like nucleotides, eicosanoids, gases, and anandamides. Apart from neurotransmitters, which flow from one neuron to the other, we have other molecules called neuromodulators and neurohormones. Neuromodulators alter the way a neuron responds to neurotransmitter over a longer time period. Neurohormones are the ones released into bloodstream before reaching the target neuronal system.

- *Monoamines*: It consists of serotonin, dopamine, norepinephrine, histamine, adrenaline, and melatonin. They have a crucial role in sleep and arousal, emotive, and cognitive functions of brain. Disturbances in monoamines are observed in most of the psychiatric conditions. Serotonin, norepinephrine, and, to smaller extent, dopamine are found to be depleted in depression and anxiety disorders. Dopamine is increased in mesolimbic pathways and reduced in mesocortical pathways in schizophrenia. In substance dependence, dopamine is flooded by the addictive drugs in reward circuit in brain. This causes increased feeling of pleasure leading to repeated use of the substances. Histamine regulates the biological functions of sleep and appetite by its actions at hypothalamus. Drugs acting on acetylcholine system have a major role to play in conditions like dementia, Parkinsonism, and tobacco dependence.
- *Amino acids* GABA, glutamate and glycine containing neurons innervate virtually every neuron in the CNS and form the core part of neurochemical system in the brain. GABA is an inhibitory neurotransmitter and its depletion can give rise to anxiety disorders. Increase in GABA activity relieves anxiety while also having sedative and antiepileptic effects. Glutamate is the excitatory neurotransmitter, which acts through its N-methyl-D-aspartate (NMDA) and AMPA (α-amino-3-hydroxy-5-methyl-4-isoxazolepropionic acid) receptors. These receptors are implicated in neuroplasticity but excess glutamatergic activity results in

neuronal damage termed as "excitatory neurotoxicity". This is implicated in impaired cognition in post-traumatic head injury and neurodegenerative disorders like Alzheimer's dementia. Glycine is an essential component in NMDA activation system, where it acts as an excitatory neurotransmitter while being an inhibitory neurotransmitter in other regions. Excitatory-inhibitory imbalance has been implicated in many psychiatric conditions like schizophrenia, mood disorders, and substance use disorders.

- *Peptides*: More than 100 neuropeptides are present in the neuronal system. They integrate the neurotransmitter, endocrinal, immunological, autonomic, and behavioral systems. Corticotropic-releasing factor and urocortins are a principal element in stress and its responses. Peptides like thyrotropin-releasing hormone, oxytocin, and vasopressin are released from neurons into the vascular tissue to act at end organs in regulating endocrinal and complex behavioral responses. Monomamines are modulated by peptides like neurotensin, neuropeptide y, substance P, and cholecystokinin and hence have wider implications in psychotic and mood disorders. They determine the genetic variability and a greater understanding is hoped to assist in individualizing psychotropic drug response as part of pharmacogenomics.

- *Neurotropic factors*: These are the polypeptide growth factors influencing the proliferation, differentiation, and degeneration of cells of the CNS. Abnormalities in factors like neurotropic growth factor, brain-derived neurotropic factor, and neurotropin-3 and 4 as a family could lead to disruption in brain growth

and maturity in different developmental phases of life. The neuronal response to injury is also compromised in states of neurotropic dysfunction. These could have an etiological role in neurodevelopmental disorders and neurodegenerative disorders.

NEUROPHYSIOLOGY

The functioning of the nervous system is multifaceted and after incorporating various processes results into a complex array of behaviors, emotion, and cognition. In neurons, action potentials play a central role in cell-to-cell communication by providing for—or, with regard to saltatory conduction, assisting—the propagation of signals along the neuron's axon toward synaptic boutons situated at the ends of an axon; these signals can then connect with other neurons at synapses. Action potentials in neurons are also known as "nerve impulses" or "spikes", and the temporal sequence of action potentials generated by a neuron is called its "spike train". A neuron that emits an action potential, or nerve impulse, is often termed as "firing". An action potential occurs when the membrane potential of a specific neuronal location rapidly rises and falls.

Action potentials are produced by voltage-gated ion channels embedded in a plasma membrane of the neuron. When the membrane potential of the neuron is near the (negative) resting potential (–70 mV), these channels remain closed. But they rapidly open when the potential difference reaches a precisely defined threshold voltage, depolarization occurs. After the channels open, an inward flow of sodium ions changes the electrochemical gradient, which in turn produces a further rise in the membrane potential. The further potential increase leads to opening of more sodium channels proceeding explosively until all the available sodium channels are open, resulting in a large upsurge in the membrane potential. The rapid influx of sodium ions causes the polarity of the plasma membrane to reverse, and the sodium channels then rapidly inactivate and close restricting further sodium entry into the cell. Potassium channels are meanwhile activated due to the increasing membrane potential, leading to an outward flow of potassium ions, returning the electrochemical gradient to the resting state (repolarization). Before achieving stable resting state, there is a state of after hyperpolarization achieved with a transient negative shift of the membrane potential due to the slow closing of the potassium channels. The sodium ions are actively transported out of the plasma membrane and potassium inside the cell using the Na-K ATPase restoring the resting potential. The depolarization at a location causes adjacent locations to similarly depolarize and thus the action potential travels in an axon. The action potential travels in one direction only, to the axon terminal where it signals other neurons.

Action potentials are most commonly initiated by excitatory postsynaptic potentials (EPSPs) from a presynaptic neuron. Typically, neurotransmitter molecules are released by the presynaptic neuron, which then binds to postsynaptic receptors leading to opening of various types of ion channels. The ion channels cause changes in local membrane permeability and membrane potential. The synapse generates excitatory signals if the neurotransmitter binding depolarizes the membrane and is inhibitory if the binding decreases the voltage (hyperpolarizes the membrane). The change thus produced (depolarization or hyperpolarization of the membrane) propagates passively to nearby regions of the membrane. The stimulus effect decays exponentially over time and distance traveled. Some fraction of a depolarization may reach the axon hillock and may cause sufficient membrane depolarization to provoke a new action potential. Usually, the excitatory potentials from several synapses work together at nearly the same time to provoke a new action potential. Their joint efforts can be thwarted; however, by the counteracting inhibitory postsynaptic potentials (IPSPs).

Neural Plasticity

Earlier it was believed that once the development and maturation halt in early critical phase of childhood, brain becomes static and remains unchanged. But, now it is known that brain is flexible and can be altered even in adulthood. Neuroplasticity, also known as brain plasticity and neural plasticity, refers to the ability of the brain to make adaptive changes in the structure and function of the CNS. Plasticity thus not only refers to the increase in the numerical count of the neurons by neurogenesis; but also, to the changes in connectivity, morphology, and biochemical substrates which often happens in response to learning, experience, and focal stimulation. Neuroplasticity can be observed at multiple scales, from microscopic changes in individual neurons to larger-scale changes such as cortical remapping in response to injury. Such neuroplastic effects can be secondary to a variety of external and internal factors such as environmental stimuli, behavior, thought, and emotions. It has implications in development, learning, memory, and recovery from brain damage.

Synaptic plasticity denotes changes in the connections between neurons, whereas nonsynaptic plasticity refers to changes in the intrinsic excitability of neurons. Synaptic plasticity is the ability of synapse to strengthen or weaken over time, dependent upon increase or decrease in the activity. Synaptic plasticity can be achieved by altering the number of neurotransmitter receptors located on a synapse, changes in the quantity of neurotransmitters released into a synapse and changes in how effectively cells respond to those neurotransmitters. Postsynaptic calcium release regulates synaptic plasticity in both excitatory and inhibitory synapses.

Synaptic plasticity may occur for short-term (lasting milliseconds to a few minutes) or long-term (lasting minutes to hours). Short-term plasticity can occur either as synaptic enhancement or depression and either strengthen or weaken a synapse. Short-term synaptic enhancement results from an increased availability of neurotransmitters from the presynaptic terminal. Synaptic enhancement is classified based on the duration of action as neural facilitation, synaptic augmentation. Synaptic fatigue or depression can arise as a result of depletion of the readily releasable vesicles in the presynaptic terminal or from postsynaptic feedback activation of presynaptic receptors.

Long-term post-tetanic potentiation plasticity involves excitatory synapses lasting minutes or more. It can occur as long-term depression (LTD) or long-term potentiation (LTP) involving majorly the NMDA receptors. LTD is induced by a minimum level of postsynaptic depolarization and simultaneous increase in the intracellular calcium concentration at the postsynaptic neuron. Prolonged periods of low-frequency stimulation at the presynaptic neuron will result into LTD. LTP results in an increase in synaptic response following potentiating pulses of electrical stimuli (high frequency) sustaining above the baseline response level for longer period. The long-term persistence of synaptic effects may be attributable to

growth of pre- and postsynaptic structures such as axonal bouton, dendritic spine, and postsynaptic density.

Kindling is a phenomenon observed in animal models, wherein repeated subthreshold leads to sensitization of the brain which manifests in the form of increase in duration, severity, and/or frequency of the full response. Affective disorders and substance use disorders are akin to kindling; however, animal models have not yet demonstrated it.

Evoked Potentials

The regular electroencephalography (EEG) recordings are made when a person is engaged continuously in the same activity like rest, sleep, or cognitive task. Changes in the electrical activity can be provoked by repeated brief sensory or cognitive stimuli. Each stimulus generates small amplitude electrical changes that are recorded and the electrical events from these repeated stimuli are mathematically averaged to receive evoked potentials (EPs). For example, a subject is made to hear repeated beeps of sounds. The electrical activity after each beep is recorded. This will occur over the ongoing background EEG activity. By averaging repeated electrical signals, the random ongoing background noise is eliminated and only the signals evoked by the stimuli remain. This signal comprises of electrical activity generated from the peripheral sensory nerves like cochlear nerve in case of auditory signaling till the sensory and processing circuits in the brain. Term "evoked potential (EP)" is used for recordings from some part of CNS.

The *early part of EP* provides information regarding processing of sensory stimuli. It will be helpful in distinguishing sensory loss due to medical or psychogenic causes.

For example, the early part of EP would be deranged, if a person is having deafness due to cochlear degeneration whereas they might be intact in dissociative blindness. These initial EPs arising out of cochlear nerves arise 1–3 ms after the stimuli. The signal arising from brainstem presents 0–20 ms.

Mid-latency EP (50–250 ms) and *late EPs* follow early EPs and are termed as *event related potentials (ERP)*. Mid-latency EPs are generated from medial geniculate bodies, inferior colliculus and primary auditory cortex for auditory stimuli. The waves are designated by polarity (P for positive and N for negative waves) and time latency. Hence, P50 means a positive wave arising 50 ms after the stimuli. P50 is implicated in sensory gating phenomenon. Our brain at higher cortices automatically filters out irrelevant information coming from the environment thus prevents overloading of information. In patients with schizophrenia, P50 is found to be abnormal. This abnormal sensory gating could be one of the pathophysiological processes in hallucinations where one perceiving voices in absence of an external sensory stimulation.

Late latency EPs—most well-known among these is P300 with *odd-ball paradigm*. They suggest anomalies in the higher order information processing systems like attention, working memory, error detection, and automatic detection of mismatch. P300 is observed with smaller amplitudes in patients with schizophrenia and are related to the level of psychotic symptoms at certain point of time.

Similar to ERP when EPs are recorded using magnetic recordings they are termed as *evoked-related field* (ERF).

Neurophysiological Tools

This functional aspect of the brain is complex and can be evaluated using different physiological tools. It includes direct evaluation of the electrical and metabolic activities of brain or through indirect assessment of sensory, motor, or autonomic activities. These evaluations might not have found utility in routine clinical evaluations in psychiatric illnesses but have profound contributions in understanding their pathophysiology. A variety of electro-physiological instrument are now available to evaluate the neuronal physiology such as electroencephalogram (EEG), magnetoencephalogram (MEG), quantitative EEG (qEEG), and polysomnography. Electro-physiological techniques have a high temporal resolution with the events (i.e., can detect changes in terms of milliseconds) but usually lacks the spatial resolution (difficult to distinguish signals from different subcortical regions). Unlike them, imaging techniques give a good spatial data though temporality gets compromised. Neuroimaging studies have been exponentially growing in past few decades. They provide both structural and functional data using techniques such as computed tomography (CT), magnetic resonance imaging (MRI), magnetic resonance spectroscopy (MRS), diffusion tract imaging (DTI), functional MRI (fMRI), functional near-infrared spectroscopy (fNIRS), positron emission tomography (PET), and single photon emission CT (SPECT). Recent emergence of neuromodulatory techniques like transcranial magnetic stimulation (TMS) and transcranial electrical stimulation (TES) is also found to be of use in assessing the neurophysiological status of brain.

Psychoneuroendocrine Axis

Hypothalamo-pituitary-adrenal axis (HPA axis) is the key mediator in translating available environmental information into hormonal signals that work by fine tuning of the steroidal hormone release in response to stressful situations. Neurons of paraventricular nucleus (PVN) in hypothalamus secrete corticotropin releasing hormone (CRH), which binds to the anterior pituitary cell receptors and promotes release of adrenocorticotropic hormone (ACTH). Adrenal glands respond to ACTH by increasing the synthesis and release of steroidal hormones which are neuroplastic factors effecting the adaptive changes in brain by exerting their influence on the intracellular glucocorticoid and mineralocorticoid receptors. Glucocorticoids have negative feedback influence on PVN in hypothalamus and hippocampus.

Hormonal dysregulation in the form of either increases or decreases in cortisol secretion with aberrant HPA axis for prolonged duration had been shown to be neurotoxic especially to hippocampal volume. Aberrant HPA axis and hormonal dysregulation in response to stress had been consistently reported in patients with schizophrenia. Evidence from animal models suggests exposure to excess steroidal hormones in the developing brain might lead to development of symptoms suggesting psychosis. Stressful environmental factors that lead to persistent activation of maternal HPA axis during antenatal period exposes the fetal brain to steroidal hormones thereby making the brain vulnerable to development of psychosis during later age as postulated by the neurodevelopmental model of schizophrenia.

Though men and women are equally affected by schizophrenia, there is a trend for slightly delayed onset of symptoms and a better response to antipsychotic medications with less negative symptoms in women. Women also experience a perimenopausal onset of symptoms. Effects of sex hormones especially estrogen in providing such a protective effect in women had been postulated by researchers. Oxytocin, initially conceptualized as a hormone behind mother-child bonding, has been recently conceptualized to play a critical role in prosocial behavior of human beings. It is postulated to play a key role behind the social cognitive deficits noted in schizophrenia, social phobia, and autism spectrum disorders and therefore newer treatment options targeting oxytocin synthesis and release are being considered for these illnesses.

In more than half of patients with depression, it has been noted that there is an increased secretion of cortisol throughout the 24-hour period. Also, there is impairment in the negative feedback mechanism, where the available excess steroids fail to diminish the secretion of CRH which further leads to uncontrolled cortisol production as shown during chronic stress. Dexamethasone when given orally overnight suppresses the secretion of steroid hormones in normal individuals famously known as the dexamethasone suppression test (DST). In patients with depression, it is a consistent finding that DST is abnormal.

Psychoneuroimmune Axis

Similar to endocrine system, immune system is also closely linked to brain and behavior. Stress is known to affect immune functioning partly mediated by endocrinal system. Symptoms of inflammatory conditions like fatigue, lack of energy, reduced appetite, and reduced ability to feel pleasure overlaps with depressive disorders. Chronic inflammatory conditions like HIV/AIDS, multiple sclerosis, and medical conditions impacting immune systems like diabetes, carcinomas, and cardiovascular diseases have a high comorbidity of depression associated with increase in interleukins, chemokines, and C-reactive proteins. Evidences are accumulating regarding the role of inflammatory biomarkers in the etiopathogenesis of schizophrenia and bipolar disorders.

GENETICS

Chromosomes are thread-like structure of nucleic acids and protein found in the nucleus, carrying genetic information in form of genes. Gene is the basic unit of heredity, made up of DNA, and acts as instructions to make the product a cell may synthesize (monomer or a nucleic acid). An allele is one of a pair of genes appearing at a particular location on a particular chromosome and controls the same characteristic (phenotype). By phenotype one refers to the set of observable characteristics of an individual resulting from the interaction of its genotype with the environment. Endophenotype is a genetic epidemiology term, which is used to separate behavioral symptoms into more homogeneous and stable phenotypes with a clear genetic connection. Single nucleotide polymorphism (SNP) represents a difference in a single DNA building block, called a nucleotide. Candidate gene studies deal with the associations between genetic variation within prespecified genes of interest and phenotypes or disease states. Linkage gene studies reflect upon the genetic linkage, which is the tendency of DNA sequences that are close together on a chromosome to be inherited together during the meiosis phase of sexual reproduction. Genome-wide association studies (GWASs) also known as whole genome association study (WGA study, or WGAS) scan the entire genome for common genetic variation primarily with focusing on SNP.

Human genome project came up with nearly 24,000 human genes and about 30–50% of them are expressed across different parts of brain. Though the comprehensive etiopathological basis of psychiatric disorders is not yet elucidated, several studies indicate most of the severe mental disorders are to a great extent influenced by genetic inheritance. Genetic epidemiology and gene mapping are two broad ways of evaluation of genes to a condition. Family studies and twin studies form the genetic epidemiology. Studying the families has shown higher aggregation of psychiatric disorders in families of affected individuals and higher concordance rates among monozygotic twins than dizygotic twins. These types of early genetic epidemiological studies built a strong ground for presence of genetic susceptibility. Genetic mapping implicates the genetic loci on chromosomes causing the condition. It uses two basic approaches of linkage analysis (look at the known loci which are transmitted together across generations more often than not) and association studies (attempts at evaluating the frequency of presence of risk allele in affected individuals). The linkage analysis is conducted by sampling the genetic markers from the multigenerational families where pedigree analysis is done. The other way is by studying the genotypes in affected sibling pairs.

The gene mapping techniques use known DNA sequences on chromosomes, which are called genetic markers. Microsatellite markers, also termed simple sequence length polymorphisms (SSLPs) or simple tandem repeats (STR), have variation in 2–4 base pair length variations. SNPs have variations in one base pair.

The efforts to identify specific genetic loci for specific psychiatric conditions have been largely unsuccessful. This is primarily due to complex etiological mechanism. Psychiatric conditions do not follow simple Mendelian inheritance pattern. Simple non-Mendelian patterns include incomplete penetrance, genetic anticipation, genomic imprinting, mosaicism, and extranuclear inheritance. Complex patterns like locus heterogeneity (different genes for same phenotype in different person), polygenic inheritance (multiple risk genes cumulatively add to the risk of phenotypic expression), and epigenetic factors (environmental factors like activities, stressors, drugs, toxins, etc. influence the genetic expression) are more likely to be involved in behavioral disorders. Multifactorial causation by intertwining of genetic as well as environmental (by nongenetic mechanisms) factors is commonly observed in mental disorders.

Heterogeneity of psychiatric disorders adds another major source of complexity. It is unlikely that a single gene can explain the symptom manifestations of a whole disorder. Intermediate phenotypes could be the link between high-level disease syndrome and low-level genetic variations. Hence, concept of endophenotypes has emerged, which are measurable microscopic/internal phenotypes like neurophysiological, biochemical, endocrinological, neuroanatomical, cognitive, or neuropsychological factors.

Recent proposals for critical shifts in research paradigms, for example, proposal of Research Domain Criteria (RDoC), hopefully might help addressing some of these issues.

Recent technological and computational advances along with newer insights on genome, in the context of big data sets comprising of samples involving patients, unaffected relatives, and healthy controls, have facilitated GWASs. Given the availability of SNP chips, detailed analyses of gene risk factors are feasible through current studies. With the introduction of new technologies such as whole genome SNP chips, a more comprehensive evaluation of genetic risk factors for psychiatric disorders is now possible. Researchers are optimistic that next-generation sequencing (NGS) technology along with the insights derived from the previous genetic studies can potentially unravel the missing heritability in psychiatric disorders.

Nature versus Nurture

Genetic basis of behavioral conditions does not mean they alone will influence the pathogenesis. Current concept in psychiatry holds a mid-path approach viewing that along with the nature (genes/neuronal wiring), the environmental factors (life experiences/learning) play an equally important role. Although genes contain all the information an organism uses to function, the environment plays an important role in determining the ultimate phenotypes an organism displays. The phrase "nature and nurture" refers to this complementary relationship. The relative contributions may vary across disorders.

Despite most of major mental disorders having genetic basis, onset is usually during adolescence. Conditions like schizophrenia deteriorate over time. Hence, the issue of it being a neurodevelopmental versus neurodegenerative disorder has often been discussed. Individuals born with genetic vulnerability show early developmental impairments in the form of higher frequency of minor physical anomalies, low general intelligence, and impaired social cognition. Over and above this vulnerability, a second hit can happen as prenatal and perinatal insults and a third hit may occur at childhood/adolescence/early adulthood. The cumulative effect may lead to the onset of the illness, which usually coincides with the period of maturation of brain. Thus, neurodevelopmental model suggests none of the hit alone would be sufficient enough to herald the pathogenesis of illness. The alternative hypothesis of neurodegeneration suggests schizophrenia to be a progressive disorder with neuronal loss and gliosis, degenerative atopic changes, and neurocognitive deterioration happening over the course of illness. Both the models have merits and demerits and none alone can explain the pathogenesis in entirety.

CONCLUSION

Several facets of basic biological sciences and related research techniques are summarized in this chapter. With expanding scope of these cutting-edge techniques based on the foundations of these fundamental sciences, one is very hopeful that novel and translational insights will be available in the near future to enhance our understanding of psychiatric disorders. It will also enhance our understanding of the phenomena of mind and the biological basis of different faculties of mental functioning.

TAKE-HOME MESSAGES

- Brain is the sheet-anchor of mind but not a synonym for mind. The two are qualitatively different.

- Neuroanatomy, neurophysiology, neuro-chemistry, along with neuroendocrine and neuroimmune dimensions of study are of great relevance for understanding the biologic basis of different mental functions.

- Neurons are the structural and functional units of brain, which carry out all the key functions in conjunction with the seminal supportive role being played by the neuroglia.

- Study of various aspects of the synaptic chemical neurotransmission as well as the second messenger system is very important.

- Neurogenesis is nearly complete at the time of birth, but some neurogenesis continues even during adulthood, which provides the basis for neuroplasticity.

- Structural and functional scan studies, EEG, qEEG, EPs, and MEG are some of the methods of studying brain structure and function.

- Genetic factors interacting with environ-mental influences lead to the emergence of final phenotype/endophenotype.

- Nervous tissue works in very close association with endocrine and immune systems both in health and disease.

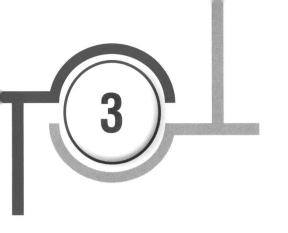

Basic Psychosocial Sciences for Psychiatry

Ajit Avasthi, Swapnajeet Sahoo

INTRODUCTION

The term "psychosocial" refers to the psychic and the social dimensions of human beings. The Psychosocial Sciences include all those disciplines of knowledge, which deliberate upon both normal and abnormal functioning of these two dimensions. Psychology and Sociology are two such principal disciplines.

In simpler terms, psychology is the study of human behavior and thinking process. It includes the study and understanding of basic mental processes, such as perception, memory, attention, motivation, etc. Over the years, psychology has been divided into several branches like cognitive psychology, developmental psychology, experimental/behavioral psychology, forensic psychology, etc., but the basic principles of psychology in all these branches remain the same. Psychological modes of treatments have now become an important and integral part of management of most psychiatric disorders. These methods are widely practiced all over the world.

Similarly, sociology is the science, which studies society, social factors, and individual or group's relationship with the society and social institutions. It also tries to explore the relationship between society and mental health. The psychosocial dimension of mental health has to be understood as distinct and different from the biomedical dimension of human beings. However, they all function in unison and with seamless coherence.

Both psychology and sociology are two vast subjects, which have a wide range of principles and applications. Some of the principles of psychology and sociology are of great relevance to the field of psychiatry. In this chapter, we will be discussing some of these basic principles. For simplicity, we have divided the chapter into three parts—*(1) basic psychological sciences, (2) basic sociological sciences, and (3) how these two interact with each other*.

BASIC PSYCHOLOGICAL SCIENCES RELATED TO PSYCHIATRY

In this section, we will discuss the principles of *learning, perception, attention, memory, emotions, motivation, attachment, personality, intelligence, awareness, language, and defense mechanisms*. All these principles are of great relevance to the field of psychiatry. Understanding of these principles helps us in understanding of the healthy mind as well as the mind in states of disorder. Over the years, it has been found that these principles of psychology are not just hypothesis or theories but have been proven on basis of scientific experiments too. Now coming to each one of the above-mentioned principles individually in brief.

Learning

It is defined as a relatively lasting change in behavior that occurs as a result of previous experience. It implies that there occurs an acquisition of the response and retention of the response, which further becomes a part of an organism's behavior repertoire. There are several views about the importance of learning in shaping of one's mental faculties. However, now it is well established that both innate abilities and acquired experiences affect learning and have their effect on mental processes. There are three basic schools of thought regarding types of learning. They are behavioral learning, observational learning, and cognitive learning.

Behavioral Learning

The behavioral learning is based upon the principles of conditioning. Conditioning is a broad term to describe a form of learning involving the formation, consolidation, or weakening of a relationship between a stimulus and a response. There are two types of conditioning for which there is experimental evidence—classical conditioning and operant conditioning.

Classical conditioning is the process by which an organism learns to respond in a particular way to a stimulus that previously did not produce that response, i.e. the stimulus, which was once "neutral" (the conditioned stimulus or CS) becomes response producing when it is paired with another stimulus (the unconditioned stimulus or US) and results in elicitation of a characteristic response (the conditioned response or CR). Previously, the US is used to elicit a usual unconditioned response or the UCR but after classical conditioning, CS gives rise to CR, which is almost similar to UCR. It was first explained by the Russian Physiologist Ivan Pavlov.

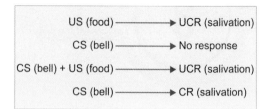

Fig. 3.1: Classical conditioning (Pavlovian experiment). (CR: conditioned response; CS: conditioned stimulus; UCR: unconditioned response; US: unconditioned stimulus)

The process of classical conditioning is illustrated in **Figure 3.1**.

Some modifications of this type of conditioning have been done to find out the strength of association. Delay conditioning in which the CS is presented for a short duration prior to the onset of the US and continues until the termination of the US, resulting in the formation of a strong CS–US association. Trace conditioning, in which there is a delay between the offset CS and the onset of the US (the bell comes on and goes off before the food is presented), results in less effective association of CS–US. Extinction in classical conditioning occurs, if the CS is presented alone (without the US) for repeated trials (bell without the food), resulting in decrease in the strength of the CS–US association and finally returning back to the original (preconditioning) situation. These principles have been established in the origin of anxiety disorders, particularly in phobias, and behavior therapies based on the classical conditioning are well-established psychological treatment for the same, thus, justifying the importance of learning in psychiatric disorders.

Operant conditioning is a learning process that involves changing the probability of a response by manipulating the consequence of that response. It follows the law of effect given by Thorndike, which states that

Table 3.1: Examples of operant conditioning.

	Stimulus applied (+)	Stimulus withdrawn (−)
Increased behavior (reinforcement)	Positive reinforcement: Giving a child chocolate for eating his vegetables curry	Negative reinforcement: Allowing a child to leave the table for finishing his vegetables curry
Decreased behavior (punishment)	Positive punishment: Scolding a child for not eating vegetables curry	Negative punishment: Putting a child in a closed room or keep him standing outside room for an hour for not eating vegetables curry

responses followed by satisfaction are more likely to be repeated while those followed by unpleasant feelings are less likely to be repeated. The operant conditioning came to the limelight after the work of BF Skinner. It is different from classical conditioning, as it is dependent on voluntary actions performed by the individual/organism. If the reward is a positive outcome (such as chocolate), the process is referred to as positive reinforcement, and if the reward is the removal or prevention of an unpleasant outcome, the process is called negative reinforcement. It should be kept in mind that both positive and negative reinforcements lead to an increase in the probability that the voluntary action will be performed. This is totally opposite to punishment in which the outcome of a voluntary action is unpleasant, such as infliction of pain/electric shock. These outcomes lead to a decrease in the probability of the occurrence of such voluntary actions. This is explained in **Table 3.1.**

Observational Learning

While the above two types of conditioning could explain many aspects of learning, individuals can also learn without direct reinforcement or punishment. This has been proved by Albert Bandura by a series of experiments that learning can indeed occur by observation alone and such learning is called observational learning. Example is children learn to play with a specific toy or a game by just observing others playing the same and even at times from just observing from a video or television program. Such type of learning involves the components of attention (the individual focuses on a behavior), retention (the individual retains the behavior in his memory), production process (the individual has the ability to perform the behavior), and motivation (a situation arises wherein the learnt behavior is perceived as useful for the individual), leading to a successful observational learning.

Cognitive Learning

Some forms of learning do not require either conditioning or observation such as studying a book chapter, understanding the concepts therein, and reaching new realizations about the topic and finding its relation to previous acquired knowledge. Such type of learning requires a degree of conscious awareness on the part of the individual, and is known as cognitive learning.

Perception

It is related to the functioning of the sensory systems and how information from the external world is received and inferred. Perception is an active process, which involves the reception and interpretation of the information gathered from the different sensory organs of the body. It is dependent on two processes, i.e., "bottom-up" processing (information is processed from external environment stimuli to higher order areas in the brain) and "top-down" modulation (reverse of bottom-up processing) by the higher mental functions. The psychological construct of an individual can modulate the sense of perception (influenced by factors like knowledge and expectations). Thereby, sensory events are inferred based on a mixture of what occurs in the external world and on prevailing internal psychological constructs. When a perception is centered on what is predicted, it is termed as a perceptual set. It has been seen that an individual's personality and experience influence his/her perceptual set, e.g., anxious individuals tend to respond more quickly to a threat-related material than nonanxious individuals.

Other important aspects of perception in psychology are attention and object constancy. The importance of attention in perception can be understood by the way people specifically and selectively attend to the diverse facets of the environment and isolate out the others. For example, even in a congested noisy chamber, people can listen and attend to a single speaker by shifting their attention to the concerned speaker. Similarly, when we identify a stimulus that is significant to us, our attention shifts (when someone calls out our name in a crowd, we attend to it). Object constancy refers to one's ability to perceive objects as unchanged, despite alterations in variables like proximity, brightness, etc. (e.g., one can perceive the direction of a sound as constant even while engaged in movements of head).

The importance of perception in psychiatry lies in the fact that perceptual deceptions and distortions in the form of illusions and hallucinations form a very important set of symptoms-cluster and

may lead further to formation of secondary delusions.

Attention

Attention can be defined as the focusing of mental efforts on specific sensory or mental events. In simpler words, it is the selective awareness or focus on a specific stimulus or content of consciousness. At a given time, our brain has a limited processing capacity and attention is therefore selective, governing the degree to which different stimuli in our environment are perceived at that time. Attention may be caused to be aroused in several ways. It may be by conscious individual choice, by the imperatives of social communication or as a response to an unanticipated stimulus. It is different in different individuals and many factors play a role in attention processing. For example, babies have an inborn ability and preference to attend to specific instances of visual or auditory stimulation, which are essential for survival and emotional gratification, while adults are able to relate their attention to the uniqueness, complexity, and novelty value of the stimulus. As circumstances become gradually more familiar or are found similar to circumstances previously experienced by an individual, he becomes less attentive because of reduced novelty value of the situation. "Attention span" is a related concept, which refers to the amount of time that a person is able to attend to continuously on a task without being distracted. More recent theories of attention have explained how individuals are able to conduct more than one task at a time due to the phenomenon of habituation and practice. For example, when one is initially learning to drive a car, one is unable to attend to other stimuli like music in the car. But with practice, driving becomes habitual and one is able to enjoy the music in the car or even hold a conversation with another person, while continuing to attend simultaneously to the task of driving on the road. Most of the psychiatric disorders, including depression, mania, and schizophrenia, have abnormalities in attention processing as a core feature of their symptomatology.

Memory

Memory is the capacity to store and later recall earlier learned facts and practices. The brain's capacity to store and later recollect previous mental contents is one of the most fascinating and complex human behaviors. The memory process occurs in three stages—encoding (registration), storage (retention), and retrieval (recall). As the name implies, in first process, stimuli/information is received by the brain, followed by its storage in specific areas of the brain. In the retrieval stage, memory permits the earlier learned facts to be recalled back into consciousness. Memory can be further classified into three types—immediate, recent, and remote memory. Immediate memory lasts for seconds, e.g., repeating what one has just heard. Recent memory covers a period of minutes to days; while remote memory comprises of data that has been stored for longer periods of time, extending from days to a lifetime. When converting material for long-term memory, the brain uses meaningfulness as a chief determinant for encoding. The more the meaning of any information is particularized, the more likely it will be better recalled later. Items are frequently shifted back and forth from one type of memory to the other type. Retrieval of memory can be divided into two types—declarative and nondeclarative systems. The declarative/explicit memory deals with information available to consciousness for

declaration. It has been further subdivided to semantic (factual memory) and episodic (specific autobiographical events). The nondeclarative/implicit/procedural memory deals with such information, which does not require conscious thoughts (e.g., walking and driving) and are also known as motor skills.

The failure in the recovery of data from either memory can be the consequence of several factors including interference, decay, or storage problems. Emotive factors, such as anxiety, too contribute to memory failure in some conditions. For example, excessive anxiety during examinations can cause a pupil to fail to recall the answers irrespective of the fact that he may have well memorized. Amnesia, a limited or total loss of memory, might be caused by injury to the brain, stroke, brain infections, etc.

Emotions

Emotions have been defined by Strickland as "reactions which can be both psychological and physical, subjectively experienced as strong feelings, many of which prepare the body for immediate action." Emotions are usually fleeting with relatively well-defined commencements and endings. Some authors have classified emotions into primary/basic and complex types of emotions. While there are *six primary emotions namely—happiness, anger, sadness, fear, disgust, and surprise; complex type of emotions include altruism, guilt, shame, and jealousy.* Basic/primary emotions have three major characteristics—(1) they have certain common elements as regard to the context in which they occur even though there can be individual and cultural differences, (2) they are likely to be observable in other primates too, though some are unique only to humans, and (3) they can be aroused rapidly even before one gets aware of them. Various components of each type of emotions are—firstly its subjective experience, secondly the associated physiological changes, and thirdly the associated behavioral changes. For example, for fear, there occur a subjective feeling of fearfulness, physiological changes in the form of sweating and palpitations, and associated behavioral changes in the form of running away or getting frozen. There exist individual variations in experiencing each type of emotion based on the emphasis one attaches to it. It has been postulated that the experience of emotion-arousing stimuli is processed by the thalamus of the brain, which in turn sends impulses to the cortex and hypothalamus. While cortical processing of emotions leads to the conscious awareness of the emotion, impulses sent to the hypothalamus lead to autonomic physiological changes. Some psychologists believe that experience of emotions is derived from physical changes occurring in the periphery, which are considered primary and some others believe that emotions result from mental processes primarily while physical changes are secondary. Studies have proved that the autonomic nervous system and endocrine system of the body are linked with emotion processing and presentation.

The manner of expression of emotions may be either inborn or culturally learned. Some facial stereotypes, like smiling and crying, have been found to be common, even among visually impaired individuals, who have no means of copying them. However, some expressions are unique to some cultures like raising eyebrows in surprise or taking tongue out in surprise, which vary from one culture to another. Cultural forces also impact how individuals describe and classify what they are feeling. Extreme positive or negative emotions can affect the performance of an individual. Assessment of emotional state of an individual is a very basic step of mental state examination in psychiatry. Any intense emotional state can pose risk to self and others and hence needs to be taken care of.

Awareness

Awareness is the primary quality of mind, which allows us to directly know, perceive, feel, or to be conscious of events either within oneself or the surrounding. It is a relative concept and can be focused either on an internal state or on external events. Being aware of oneself is known as self-awareness and it is regulated by both central and peripheral nervous system of the individual. Self-awareness is probably unique to human beings. Impaired awareness is seen in a number of neuropsychiatric disorders like delirium, dementia, traumatic brain injury, acute psychosis, severe depression, acute stress reaction.

Sense of Self, Time, and Reality

Sense of self, time, and reality can be collectively conceptualized as specific facets of consciousness awareness. Consciousness of the self is the ability to experience oneself as distinct and different from all other nonself-entities. Disturbance of sense of self has two aspects—one is awareness of existence and activity of the self and another is awareness of disturbance of being separate from the environment. In normal individuals, disturbance of awareness of self can occur during severe exertion, anxiety, sensory deprivation and during substance intoxication (Cannabis, lysergic acid diethy-lamide—LSD). It has been commonly seen in patients with panic disorder, dissociative disorder, depersonalization–derealization syndrome, and psychosis.

Sense of time is closely linked with the concept of self and its relationship with the external environment. Disorder of time has been divided into two types—disorder of objective time (disorder in orientation to time, time duration, and chronology) and disorder of subjective time (disorder of experience of flow of time, direction of time, uniqueness of time, and quality of time). In general, disorder of objective time occurs in organicity and disorder of subjective time occurs in functional psychosis and affective disorders. Sense of reality also has to be acknowledged as an independent dimension of conscious experience. Our convictions and actions depend on the degree of sense of reality that is experienced with any phenomena. Sense of reality has to be contrasted against the dreamy states and illusory states. This concept of reality is of increasing relevance in modern times when the gates of unlimited virtual world has been opened by the Internet. Disorder of sense of reality is seen in many clinical states.

Intelligence

Intelligence has been defined by Wechsler as the capacity of an individual to act purposefully, to think rationally, and to deal effectively with the environment. Piaget has defined intelligence as an adaptive process, which involves an interplay of biological maturation and interaction with the environment. Intelligence is usually measured by the intelligence quotient (IQ), which is calculated by mental age/actual age × 100.

There are several theories of intelligence, which have suggested different types of intelligence such as:
- Fluid intelligence (ability to solve new problems and use logic in new situations)
- Crystallized intelligence (ability to use learned knowledge and experience)
- Emotional intelligence (ability to recognize own emotions and those of others and label them appropriately).

Many psychological tests have been developed to measure intelligence and estimation of intelligence is an essential component of the mental state examination in psychiatry. Intelligence has now been considered to be a composite of specific abilities rather than a unitary function. Intellectual factors are quite essential in the management of various psychiatric disorders.

Language

Language is the means of verbal communication between human beings. Language is exclusively a human property and to be meaningful, there should be use of proper words and syntax. Language is an important form of expression of one's thoughts and emotions inclusive of one's needs and problems. It can be affected by various neurological and psychiatric disorders. Common neurologic disorders, which affect language, are sensory and motor aphasias. Language disorder in psychiatry is seen in schizophrenia and other psychotic disorders. Disorder of language is not the same as disorder of thinking, even though the disorders of thinking can be accessed only through the medium of language. Every individual is endowed with a neurological substrate for language, upon which different sociocultural influences act upon to allow emergence of different languages in different societies and geographical regions. Language is a very important mental faculty of human beings, as it is the chief bearer of the progress of our culture and civilization.

Motivation

In simpler words, motivation is the drive that produces a goal-directed behavior. Motivation is closely associated with the stimuli that direct the initiation, course, strength, and perseverance of a behavior.

Table 3.2: Theories of motivation.

Theory of motivation	Based upon	Example
Instinct theory of motivation (McDougall, 1960)	Humans are motivated by a variety of their innate instinctual drives, which are automatic, spontaneous, and untrained processes and these control/direct human behavior	A human mother will attempt to provide comfort to her crying baby till he/she calms down. According to instinct theory, it is a mother's instinct to provide comfort to her child
The homeostatic drive theory (Cannon, 1929)	A state of imbalance occurs when the basic biological needs of body are not fulfilled leading to driving oneself to such behaviors for restoration of internal balance or homeostasis	Voluntary nature of eating and drinking when hunger and thirst arise
Drive-reduction theory (Hull, 1943)	Any behavior that reduces the drives will be repeated by animals and humans, as the reduction of the drive serves as a positive reinforcement or acts as a reward for the behavior that caused such drive reduction	Searching for water to drink when one is thirsty or looking for food when hungry
The incentive theory	Stresses on the role of environment in motivating behavior, i.e., it suggests that one is driven into action by outside incentives	Studying for examination to get a good rank/praise, running a race to get a prize/recognition
The cognitive theory (Vroom, 1964)	Proposes that motivation in individuals is influenced by both intrinsic and extrinsic forces that energize them to move	A person would be motivated to work in office, based on his internal desire to improve/seek promotion as well as with an expectation of reward from his superior based on his past experiences

Three basic categories of motives have been recognized by many philosophers and scientists, i.e., biological/primary (hunger and the regulation of food intake), incentive-seeking (core needs for physical, emotional, and cognitive stimulus), and learned (motives learnt through reward and punishment, or by observation of others). There are several theories of motivation. The important theories are the homeostatic drive theory, the instinct theory, the incentive theory, the cognitive theory, and the drive reduction theory. The **Table 3.2** lists down these common theories and their propositions.

Attachment

Attachment is an emotive bond between a newborn and its caregiver leading to the newborn's experience of comfort, security, and safety in presence of its caregiver and suffering when temporarily disconnected. It has been proposed by many behavioral scientists that attachment is a significant building block for development of later healthy relationship and adult personality. It plays a major role in emotional and social development of an individual. There are many schools of thought on attachment. While psychologists view attachment as a secondary drive originating from basic instinct drives like hunger (for example, attachment to mother occurs because she supplies food to the baby), behavioral scientists view attachment as arising from the newborn's physical needs for food and warmth, both of which are provided by the mother and supposed to be occurring as a result of conditioning. Many animal and human experiments have been carried out to establish attachment by prominent scientists like Harry Harlow, John Bowlby, Mary Ainsworth, etc. It has been proved that attachment serves to help children's exploration of the environment. A secure attachment is necessary for the overall development of an individual, i.e., those who are securely attached in the childhood tend to be more confident, friendly, and mature later on. Various forms of anxiety like stranger anxiety and separation anxiety have been based on the principles of attachment and these have been incorporated in the developmental milestones of children. Research has shown that early attachment patterns can have a significant impact on later behavior, for example, children with an insecure attachment often continue to have difficulty with relationships as adults because they are preoccupied by their own emotional uncertainty. Attachment shapes the emotional regulation, cognitive schemas, and stress vulnerability of an individual.

Personality

Personality has been defined as the unique pattern of emotional and behavioral features by which each individual can be distinguished from others. It is one of the fundamental parts of the psychological sciences. Since the time of Sigmund Freud, special importance has been given to personality development. Several hypotheses have been proposed regarding the development of personality. Child psychologists assume that the child's inherited biology, i.e., temperament, is an essential foundation for the child's later personality. But, psychoanalysts view that variation in the sensual and aggressive drives of the Id, which are biological in nature along with differences in parental interactive influences, leads to the variations in personalities. There are many theories of personality and some important ones are mentioned in **Table 3.3**.

Defense Mechanisms

Defense mechanisms are a major component of the psychoanalytic theory. These have been used to understand psychopathology using psychodynamic concepts. Concept of defense mechanisms began with Sigmund Freud. In his theories of the mind, he postulated certain unconscious ego processes that he called defense mechanisms. Freud has suggested that defense mechanisms are the ways and means by which the ego wards off displeasure and anxiety and exercises control over impulsive and instinctual behavior. Later, Vaillant defined defense mechanisms as the habitual, unconscious, and sometimes pathological mental processes, which are employed to resolve conflict between instinctual needs, internalized prohibitions, and external reality. Four types of defense mechanisms have been described by Vaillant. They are narcissistic defenses, immature defenses, neurotic defenses, and mature defenses. Details of these have been summarized in **Box 3.1**.

Defense mechanisms have been postulated to be helpful in order—(1) to keep effects within bearable limits during sudden alienation in one's emotional life, e.g., during sudden awareness of heightened intimacy with or dependence on a taboo person, (2) to restore psychological homeostasis by postponing or deflecting sudden increases in biological drives, e.g., aggression toward parents during adolescence, (3) to obtain a time-out to master changes in self-image that cannot be immediately integrated, e.g., puberty, major surgery, and (4) to handle irresolvable conflicts with persons living or dead of whom one cannot bear to take leave.

Table 3.3: Theories of personality.

Theory of personality	Description

Type theory of personality (Hippocrates, BC 400), (Friedman, 1977)	• *Hippocrates*:
	  – Characterized human behavior in terms of four temperaments—each linked with a specific bodily fluid
	  – The phlegmatic type (sluggish) with phlegm, sanguine type (optimistic) associated with blood, the choleric (angry) type with yellow bile, and the melancholic type (sad and depressed) with black bile
	  – The personality of an individual is determined by the quantity of each of the four bodily fluids
	• *Friedman*: Two types of personality—
	  – *Type A personality*—those who are insecure about status, excessively time conscious, hostile and aggressive, highly competitive, and incapable of being relaxed
	  – *Type B personality*—those typically work steadily, enjoy achievement and focus less on winning or losing in competition

Trait theory of personality (Eysenck, 1970; Cloninger, 1986)	• *Eysenck*: Personality could be described based on three central factors—psychoticism, introversion–extroversion, and neuroticism • *Cloninger*: Three main personality traits—harm avoidance, reward dependence, and novelty seeking

Psychodynamic theory of personality (Freud, 1923)	• *Freud* suggested a three-part personality construct consisting of:
	  – The *id* (concerned with the gratification of elementary instincts)
	  – The *ego* (intervenes between the demands of the id and the restrictions of society, i.e., superego)
	  – The *superego* (through which parental and social values are adopted internally)
	• There is a constant element of conflict between the three and these conflicts are the primary determinants of personality

Box 3.1: Defense mechanisms.

Narcissistic defenses: These defenses permit one to effectively rearrange external experiences to eliminate the need to cope with reality. Also, commonly known as psychotic defense mechanisms. These are:
• *Denial:* Protecting oneself from unpleasant reality by refusing to perceive. E.g., a person with alcoholic liver disease refuses to accept that he has a problematic drinking behavior and can control it.
• *Projection:* Attributing one's own thoughts, feelings, or motives to another. E.g., an angry man might accuse others of being hostile to him.
• *Distortion:* Grossly reshaping external reality to suit inner needs. It includes hallucinations and wish fulfilling delusions.

Immature defenses: These mechanisms lessen distress and anxiety provoked by threatening people or by uncomfortable reality. Usually seen in severe depression and personality disorders. These are:
• *Acting out:* Direct expression of an unconscious wish or impulse in action, without conscious awareness of the emotion that drives that expressive behavior.
• *Blocking:* Temporarily or transiently inhibiting thinking.
• *Hypochondriasis:* An excessive preoccupation or worry about having a serious illness.
• *Introjection:* Identifying with some idea or object so deeply that it becomes a part of that person. It aims to obliterate the awareness of the object being persistently there at the outside. E.g., when a person becomes depressed due to the loss of a loved one, his feelings are directed to the mental image he possesses of the loved one.
• *Passive-aggression:* Expressing aggression toward others indirectly through passivity, masochism, and turning against the self.

Contd...

Contd...

- *Regression:* Temporary reversion of the ego to an earlier stage of development rather than handling unacceptable impulses in a more adult way. E.g., an adult has a temper tantrum or loses his temper when he does not get his way.
- *Somatization:* Converting psychic derivatives into bodily symptoms and tending to react with somatic manifestations, rather than psychic manifestations.
- *Schizoid fantasy:* Tendency to retreat autistically into fantasy to avoid intimacy and to resolve inner conflicts. E.g., a socially inept and inhibited young man imagines himself chosen by a group of women to provide them with sexual satisfaction.

Neurotic defenses: These mechanisms are considered neurotic, but fairly common in adults. Such defenses have short-term advantages in coping, but can often cause long-term problems in relationships, work, and in enjoying life when used as one's primary style of coping with the world.

- *Displacement:* Shifting an emotion or drive from one idea or object to another that resembles the original in some aspect or quality. E.g., a worker, angry at his boss, obviously unable to direct his anger and hostility to his intended target, comes home, and yells at his wife. She, now, also angry and upset, displaces her anger on the child, who then further displaces it on their pet dog.
- *Dissociation:* Temporary drastic modification of one's personal identity or character to avoid emotional distress. E.g., fugue states and conversion reactions after a traumatic event.
- *Externalization:* Tendency to perceive in the external world and in external objects elements of one's own personality, including instinctual impulses, conflicts, moods, attitudes, and styles of thinking.
- *Repression:* Keeping distressing thoughts and feelings buried in the unconscious. E.g., a person is asked—"how do you get along with your mother" and he responds, "just fine" as he turns pale. Negative feelings about the mother are so unacceptable that they block his awareness.
- *Isolation:* Separation of feelings from ideas and events. E.g., describing a murder with graphic details with no emotional response.
- *Rationalization:* The process of constructing a logical justification for a decision that was originally arrived at through a different mental process. E.g., a person after failing to get into a law school may justify himself by saying: "I would have hated being a lawyer anyway."
- *Reaction formation:* Mechanism in which anxiety-producing or unacceptable emotions are replaced by their direct opposites. E.g., one who is strongly attracted to pornography, but has moral or religious obligations to avoid it, might become its staunch critic.
- *Inhibition:* Inhibits ego functions consciously to evade anxiety arising out of conflicts with impulses and superego.
- *Sexualization:* Endows sexual significance to an object or function.
- *Intellectualization:* Avoiding unacceptable emotions by focusing on the intellectual aspects. E.g., focusing on the details of a funeral as opposed to the sadness and grief. Intellectualization helps to protect us against anxiety by separation from the painful or stressful events, hiding the emotions.
- *Undoing:* Trying to reverse or undo a feeling by acting in some opposite or compensatory manner. E.g., a youth with obsessive–compulsive disorder (OCD) reciting the alphabet backwards to undo his sin of sexual thoughts and feelings.
- *Controlling:* Attempting to manage or regulate events or objects in the environment to minimize anxiety and to resolve inner conflicts. E.g., excessive orderliness in office.

Mature defenses: These are commonly found among emotionally healthy adults and are considered mature, even though many have their origins in an immature stage of development. They have been adapted through the years in order to optimize success in life and relationships. The use of these defenses enhances pleasure and feelings of control. These defenses help us to integrate conflicting emotions and thoughts, while still remaining effective.

- *Altruism:* Constructive service to others that brings pleasure and personal satisfaction.
- *Anticipation:* Realistically anticipating or planning for future. The mechanism is goal directed and implies careful planning or worrying and premature but with realistic affective anticipation of dire and potentially dreadful outcomes.

Contd...

Contd...

- *Asceticism:* Eliminating the pleasurable effects of experiences and using moral elements to assign values to specific pleasures. Gratification is derived from renunciation, and asceticism is directed against all base pleasures perceived consciously.
- *Humor:* Overt expression of ideas and feelings (especially those that are unpleasant to focus on or too terrible to talk about) that gives pleasure to others. It is usually done by comedy to overtly express feelings and thoughts without personal discomfort or immobilization and without producing an unpleasant effect on others.
- *Sublimation:* Refocusing of psychic energy away from negative outlets to more positive outlets. Freud considered this defense mechanism the most productive. E.g., a person with high aggression becomes a soldier. It can be understood as aggression is an unwanted impulse and by becoming a soldier, this behavior is socially approved.
- *Suppression:* Consciously or semiconsciously postponing attention to a conscious impulse or conflict. Issues may be deliberately cut off, but they are not avoided.

There has been a waning in the inputs provided by psychodynamic concepts in present day psychiatry since the 1960's. This is reflected in the present as atheoretical trend in the current classificatory systems (DSM and ICD classificatory systems). Possible reasons could be because of the increased explanatory power of alternative models with the growth of science, such as the biological model, cognitive model and behavioral model. However, still defense mechanisms remain important in understanding psychopathology and normal human behavior.

BASIC SOCIOLOGICAL SCIENCES RELATED TO PSYCHIATRY

Sociology is the study of societal behavior or civilization, including its beginning, growth, association, networks, and institutions. The pattern of interaction of society and human behavior has been explained by several sociological theories. The application of some of these sociological theories in mental health has evolved over the years. The relationship between society and individual mental health has been understood in two possible ways by sociologists. They are—(1) the mental health of people is partially or wholly shaped by societal influences otherwise known as social causation and (2) the mental health status of people is determined by the deviant role that they get to adopt inadvertently because of social labeling, which is further maintained by consensually validated expectations of role stereotypes by the society.

Social Causation Theory

It explains that social factors are responsible for the occurrence of mental illness. Social factors like social class, gender, race, living situation, occupational status, and social stressors have been proved to be related with various psychiatric disorders in several studies.

Labeling Theory or Social Reaction Theory

It places emphasis on the socially adopted roles of the individuals. It was proposed by Scheff and states that behavior, which is commonly thought of as symptomatic of mental illness, is seen as a form of deviance from normal and is labeled as mentally ill. The labeled person later on takes on the role of being a mentally ill and this role is maintained by the persisting views of others.

Other sociological determinants of mental health include *migration, impact of culture, role of family, community, social roles, social class, aggression, and spirituality.*

Migration

Migration is a social phenomenon, which has existed since the origin of human beings on earth. People migrate for several reasons and migration has a great impact on one's life. Many factors like lack of preparedness, difficulties in adjusting to the new place, cultural differences, etc. can have a long-standing impact on the mental well-being of an individual. Lee had postulated the "push–pull" theory, which lists out some factors like unemployment, lack of opportunities, famine, political fear, loss of wealth, natural disasters, etc. that push people from their native place and some factors like better living conditions, new job opportunities, improved education, superior health facilities, industrial prospects, etc. attract or pull people to new place. Studies from all over the world have found high rates of psychiatric disorders among migrant populations. Most often, it has been seen that insecurity feelings and nonavailability of their peer groups lead to mental health consequences.

Culture

It has been well defined as "shared learned behavior, which is transmitted from one generation to another for the purposes of individual and societal growth, adjustment, and adaptation; culture is represented externally as artifacts, roles, and institutions, and is represented internally as values, beliefs, attitudes, consciousness, and biological functioning". Every culture seems to have certain conceptualization of good mental health or ideal functioning. There is a significant impact of culture on the causation, presentation, treatment options, outcome, and course of mental illnesses. Culture can influence an individual's understanding and experience of his/her symptoms. Culture also influences notions about causes of symptoms, together with individual attributions regarding personhood, e.g., boundaries of self, self-discipline, and social obligations. This plays an essential role in understanding how an underlying psychiatric disease process is articulated in behavior, how it is handled, how long it lasts, and how it is shunted about in the social systems. Culture can affect in multiple ways— (1) can shape a specific pattern of conduct in individuals of a community (like encourages certain styles of conduct while suppressing others; a phenomenon that also affects the shaping of abnormal states, e.g., trance and possession states, (2) can lead to specific interpretation of one's symptoms, which can influence a positive or negative orientation of the behavior as per interpretation according to traditional concepts/beliefs. This has a bearing on the diagnosis because it influences the decision regarding presence or absence of an "illness", e.g., Dhat syndrome, Koro, etc., and (3) alternatively culture can influence acceptance of certain individual specific peculiarities as normal such as Suchibai syndrome, or (4) can lead to certain culture-specific new interventions.

Cultures also have an impact on the meaning that an individual imparts to his/her illness and one's method of making sense of the subjective experience of illness and suffering. Cultures can also affect one's motivation to seek treatment, one's ability to cope up with his/her symptoms, and the pathways one takes to get help from the society/family.

Family and Relationships

Family is the first and foremost institution for socialization of children, establishing intimate relationship, learning of values, and finding support in all spheres of one's life. Family is an integral part of society and acts as a micro-level society in itself. The members of the family share confidence, advice, trust, and intimacy among themselves and have an emotional, physical, spiritual, and intellectual bonding with one another. All the members have specific roles to play in a family and there exists a power hierarchy within the family system. The basic principles of socialization, i.e., the creation of shared beliefs and ideas, develop initially in one's family. Any deviance in any part of an individual in fulfilling one's role within the family can lead to breakdown of the entire family structure and can cause disharmony among the members of the family. Problems in relationships among family members have been regarded as an ongoing stressor and considered to be an etiological factor in several psychiatric disorders ranging from acute psychosis to depressive illness. Interventions targeting at the family dynamics are as essential as interventions focused on individuals with mental health problems.

Community

Community is the core of social sciences. Community is a group of people staying in a geographically defined area, such as a neighborhood or a city, who interact with one another, for example, as friends, colleagues, or neighbors. The members of the community share many common beliefs and follow certain common behaviors/traditions. Social life is incomplete without community. There exists a wide range of social, political, economical framework within a community,

which is essential for the smooth social functioning of an individual. Community also provides social support to an individual. Social isolation, loneliness, discrimination, inequality, etc. are some of the social factors, which can lead to mental health problems in individuals. Community also can act as a two-way sword—on one hand, it can be supportive enough to facilitate early identification of abnormal behavior and treatment-seeking, while on the other hand, it can be a source of problem due to stigma attached to mental illness and thus be an impediment to help-seeking and recovery from mental illness. So, enhancing community participation by creating proper awareness regarding mental health problems is very essential in overcoming the barriers of stigma and other societal impediments prevalent in the community. Various community mental health clinics have started to grow up in the recent years because of the realization that mental health problems are better treated in the community rather than in the mental hospitals.

Aggression

Aggression has been defined as an overt behavior that involves threat or action that may potentially or actually cause pain, withdrawal, or loss of resources. Violence is aggression that has extreme harm as its goal including possible death. In animals, aggression plays an important role in mate selection, protection of offspring, and for the survival of the group. In humans, aggression is considered as a part of normal repertoire of behavior that generally manifests in response to a threat that is dangerous and imminent. The line between pathological and normal forms of aggression is often blurred. Inappropriate aggressive behavior often represents serious mental and social problems. Two main theories, Frustration Aggression Theory and Social Interaction Theory, have been postulated to explain aggression. As per the Frustration Aggression Theory, frustration occurs when motivated behavior is thwarted or blocked or when the goals are not reached. Frustration always leads to aggression and each aggressive behavior is caused by frustration. The social interaction theory explains that aggressive behavior as a socially influenced behavior and is the result of threats to high self-esteem, especially to unwarranted high self-esteem. People who suffer from mental illness commit violent acts more than twice as often as individuals without a psychiatric diagnosis. Aggressive and violent behaviors place enormous financial burdens on health services and pose danger for patient, caregivers, and treating team. The etiologies of aggressive and violent behavior are numerous, but it is very important to identify them in each individual case, as the management in both acute and long-term setting depends on this information. Acts of aggression have been included in the diagnostic criteria of intermittent explosive disorders, antisocial personality disorder, and conduct disorder.

Social Class

Social class has been defined on the basis of income, education, occupation, and area of residence. One of the most consistent relationships in the psychiatric epidemiology is the inverse relation between social class and mental illness and it has been found so in schizophrenia, depression, and substance use disorders. Two explanations for this observation have been suggested, which are the stress explanation and the selection explanation. As per the stress explanation, the rates of mental illness are higher in low socioeconomic status because of high-environmental adversities, such as unemployment, poverty, social disadvantage, homelessness, etc., generating higher quantum of stress in this class and as per the selection explanation, persons with mental illness drift down into or fail to rise out of their low social class. Recent studies have also found that the risk of psychiatric disorder is inversely related to social class.

Social Roles

Social roles have been defined as a set of expectations for people who occupy a given social position or status. Roles are a significant component of social structure. For example, police are expected to protect us and apprehend criminals. Role conflict occurs when incompatible expectations arise from two or more social positions held by the same person, for example being a coach and a parent to a member in the team. Such conflict can also occur among individuals moving into occupations that are not common among people with their ascribed status. Role expectation is the generally accepted social norms that prescribe how a specific role is ought to be played and role performance is the actual behavior of a person playing a role. Role strain occurs when incompatible demands or excessive demands are generated within a single role held by a person. Analysis of social roles has a significant importance in the overall management issues in persons with mental illness.

Spirituality

Spirituality is a unique dimension of subjective human experience, which also manifests in different forms within every community and society. Spirituality has been conceptualized as relating to matters of meaning and purpose in life, truth, and values.

Spirituality and religion have often been used interchangeably, but they are not the same. A religious person may be spiritual because most religions have a spiritual core, but every spiritual person may not be subscribing to any religion. Being spiritual is an individual pursuit, whereas being religious implies being affiliated to an organized set of beliefs and practices. Religion is concerned with socially and traditionally shared beliefs and experiences but spirituality is concerned with one's own experiences, feelings, and thoughts arising out of his search for the ultimate reality or ultimate truth. Spirituality is increasingly being included as an integral component of comprehensive health and as an effective modality for prevention and treatment of psychiatric conditions. Spirituality can help patients to develop a positive view of self to make sense of difficult situations, provide hope, encourage forgiveness, and enhance social relatedness. Spirituality as a concept has been explored in the self-help groups like alcoholic anonymous and similar other groups. Obtaining information about the spiritual beliefs of an individual is also quite essential while evaluating a person with mental health conditions, as it may have some bearing on management strategies.

INTERFACE BETWEEN PSYCHOLOGY, SOCIOLOGY, AND PSYCHIATRY: THE BIOPSYCHOSOCIAL MODEL

Psychology and sociology are two important disciplines of great relevance to psychiatry. There exist various overlapping theories between the two, and both are inseparable from each other. In almost all psychiatric patients, there are psychological factors and sociological factors, which are responsible for genesis of the illness; similarly, these factors are also required for the understanding the illness as well as also for its treatment. On the whole, in simpler words, a complete psychosocial history, psychosocial under-standing of the illness, and psychosocial interventions are essential for a holistic management of an individual with any mental illness. Also, it has now been well established that almost all psychiatric disorders also have a biological basis, i.e., have definite changes in brain and its neurotransmission systems. Hence, there exist biological determinants, psychological determinants, and sociological determinants for mental illness in an individual. This has been the central premise of the *"biopsychosocial"* model as proposed by Engel.

Continuous feedback loops co-exist between all the three domains of this model to maintain the internal equilibrium. They are equally responsible for the genesis of any psychiatric disorder. For the same reason, all these three dimensions are also judiciously used in the management of such disorders. If we take the example of a common psychiatric disorder, such as depression, we find that there are biological factors, like genetic propensity and neurotransmitter dysfunctions along with psychological factors like faulty coping styles, insecure attachment, poor attention, socially learned behaviors, etc., which combine with existing social factors like adverse life events, poor social support from the society, interpersonal problems in the family, etc., to give rise to symptoms of depression. If treatment is focused only on symptom remission by pharmacological means then it is inadequate as one is not trying to target at the genesis of depression and hence the same illness is likely to recur if appropriate steps to handle the psychological and social issues are not taken care of properly and adequately. Here, lies the importance of the biopsychosocial model of mental illnesses. A biopsychosocial treatment approach considers etiological factors in the domains of all the three dimensions of determinants. Only such management plans, which include relevant determinants from all the dimensions as mentioned above, can be said to be holistic and complete.

CONCLUSION

Undergraduates should imbibe the art of exploring various psychological and social factors behind each psychiatric disorder they come across. *These principles of psychosocial sciences are also applicable to physical illnesses.* Basic psychosocial sciences are the foundation and cornerstone of psychiatry; the understanding of any psychiatric disorder is incomplete without the understanding and application of the psychosocial sciences in that disorder. One should make it a routine habit to use various psychosocial principles in understanding and management of psychiatric disorders.

TAKE-HOME MESSAGES

- Basic psychological sciences include the principles of learning, perception, attention, memory, emotions, motivation, attachment, personality, awareness, language, intelligence, and defense mechanisms.
- Basic sociological sciences include sociological theories of social causation and labeling, migration, role of culture, family and relationships, community, social class, social roles, aggression, and spirituality.
- Learning is a relatively permanent change in behavior that occurs as a result of prior experience and is usually of three basic types—behavioral/conditioning, observational and cognitive learning.
- Perception is an active process, which involves the interpretation of the information gathered from the different sensory organs of the body and is dependent on two processes "bottom-up" processing and "top-down" modulation.
- Attention is the selective focus of conscious awareness on a specific stimulus.
- Memory is the capability to store and later recall previously learnt information and practices. Memory processing occurs in three stages—encoding, storage, and retrieval.
- Emotions are the reactions, which are personally experienced as robust feelings and usually organize the body for instant action. Six primary emotions are happiness, anger, sadness, fear, disgust, and surprise.
- Motivation is the drive that produces a goal-directed behavior and is an important determinant of the beginning, course, strength, and persistence of a behavior.
- Attachment is an emotive bond between a newborn animal and its caregiver, which ensures newborn or animal's experience safety, security, and comfort in the presence of its caregiver and suffering when temporarily disconnected. Early attachment patterns (secure/insecure) can have a significant impact on later behavior and mental health status.
- Personality is the distinctive pattern of emotional and behavioral features by which each individual can be differentiated from others.
- Intelligence is the capacity of an individual to act purposefully, to think rationally, and to deal effectively with the environment.

- Defense mechanisms are the habitual, unconscious, and sometimes pathological mental processes, which are employed to resolve conflict between instinctual needs, internalized prohibitions, and external reality. There are four types of defense mechanisms, i.e., narcissistic defenses, immature defenses, neurotic defenses, and mature defenses.
- In any mental/psychiatric disorder, there are psychological factors and sociological factors, which are responsible for genesis of the illness and are required for understanding the illness and also essential in the treatment of the individual.
- There exist biological determinants, psychological determinants, and socio-logical determinants of mental illness in an individual, which is otherwise known as the "biopsychosocial" model.
- There is a necessity to realize that psychiatric thinking about the mental disorder is not exclusively biological and there are various psychosocial models to explain and help in management of psychiatric disorders.

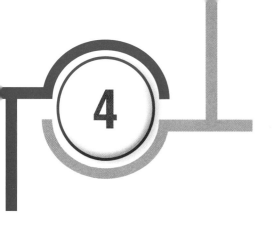

Mental Health and Mental Disorders

Rajesh Sagar, Ananya Mahapatra

INTRODUCTION

The World Health Organization (WHO) defines health as "a state of complete physical, mental, and social well-being, and not merely absence of disease or infirmity." The WHO has included mental health in this overarching definition of health in general, since its inception. Mental health has been considered to be an integral as well as essential part of the overall health of an individual. As suggested in the definition of health, mental health is not simply the absence of mental illness. It encompasses various aspects of mental well-being in life in general. It is also intimately connected to physical health. However, the construct of normal mental health is a difficult concept to define.

CONCEPT OF MENTAL HEALTH

It is important to define mental health in order to delineate its multiple domains and aspects. The WHO has proposed that mental health is "a state of well-being in which the individual realizes his or her own potential, can cope with the normal stresses of life, can work productively and fruitfully, and is able to make a contribution to her or his community".

Mental health forms a part of the basic foundation for general well-being and effective functioning for a person at an individual level as well for a community as a whole. A mentally healthy person would generally have affective warmth, would be at peace with himself and others, would be energetic and have a sense of buoyancy, be flexible, and would generally be responsible, sensible and cooperative. All these attitudes would generally get reflected in his capacity to work, capacity to play, and capacity to love within and outside family relationships. Mental and physical health are interdependent. Neither mental nor physical health can exist on its own, in isolation of the other. As an extension to that, mental, physical, and social functioning of an individual are also interdependent. Mental health and mental illnesses are dependent on various biological, psychological as well as social factors, which vary from individual to individual. How these factors interact is an important factor determining the mental health as well as the risk of developing mental illness.

LINK BETWEEN PHYSICAL AND MENTAL HEALTH

The relationship between mental and physical health has been demonstrated by a large number of research studies in the last few decades. For example, various studies have shown the link between depression and cardiac as well as vascular diseases. It has been demonstrated that patients suffering from medical disorders who have a negative attitude toward their illness, have a poorer outcome in terms of remission and recovery as compared to those who have a more positive attitude toward their illness. Also there is now ample evidence to suggest that the mental state and emotional status of an individual is an important factor that determines the course of recovery from physical illness. They are also important for satisfactory maintenance of physical health. Mental disorders may also act as predisposing or precipitating factors for physical illnesses. There is now strong evidence that depression and certain personality traits may act as risk as well as poor prognostic factors for heart disease. Acute stress as a trigger for myocardial infarction or sudden death has also been reported in individuals with heart disease.

Just as poor mental health may contribute to either causation of or poorer outcomes from a physical illness, the reverse is also true. Medical disorders may also lead to causation of mental disorders. Individuals suffering from chronic medical conditions, often develop mental disorders such as anxiety, depression, etc. Secondly, many medical disorders may sometimes present with symptoms suggestive of a mental disorder. Thyrotoxicosis may present with panic attacks, hypothyroidism may present with symptoms suggestive of depression, etc. Similarly, a WHO study conducted in 15 centers all over the world demonstrated that medical conditions associated with persistent pain are four times more likely to be associated with anxiety or depressive disorders.

Besides the inter-relationship between physical and mental health, there are various psychosocial factors, which interact in complex ways and affect the outcome of both physical as well as mental illnesses.

Poor social support has been shown to exert influence on the state of physical as well as mental health. Traumatic/stressful events in early childhood, nutritional deficiencies, etc. have also been associated with the development of mental disorders. Stigma and depression are commonly experienced by patients living with mental illness, which adds to the loss of quality of life as well as adversely affects the outcome.

There are two main pathways through which a person's mental and physical health mutually influences each other over time, while simultaneously interacting with social and environmental influences. The first pathway is directly through physiological systems, such as the neuroendocrine and immune system of the body. The second pathway is through an array of health-related behaviors, which includes lifestyle factors such as sleeping and eating patterns, levels of physical activity, sexual practices, etc. This pathway also includes reaction pattern of individuals to physical illnesses, treatment seeking behavior, compliance to prescribed treatment, etc. While these two pathways influence health through distinct trajectories, they also interact with each other in concert with factors from an individual's psychosocial environment.

In an integrated and evidence-based model of health, mental health, including emotions and thought patterns, emerges as key determinants of overall health. Anxious and depressed moods, for example, have been shown to adversely affect the endocrine and immune functioning of an individual leading to increased risk of development of various physical illnesses. While the exact mechanisms of these pathways are yet to be fully delineated, it is unequivocally established that poor mental health plays a major role in the altered functioning of various physiological processes which in turn may increase predisposition for development of physical as well as mental illnesses.

VARIOUS DEFINITIONS OF MENTAL ILLNESS

Various attempts have been made to define mental illness; however, there is no universal definition of the same, neither is there a clear consensus among the existing definitions. Some of the accepted definitions of mental illness are:

- Mental illness has been defined in Diagnostic and Statistical Manual-5 (DSM-5) as a syndrome characterized by a clinically significant disturbance in an individual's cognition, emotional regulation, or behavior that reflects a dysfunction in the psychological, biological, or developmental processes underlying mental function.
- The National Institute for Mental Health (NIMH) defines mental illnesses as developmental brain disorders with genetic and environmental factors leading to altered circuits and altered behavior.
- The Mental Healthcare Act 2017 of India has defined mental illness as "substantial disorder of thinking, mood, perception, orientation, or memory that grossly impairs judgment, behavior, capacity to recognize reality or ability to meet the ordinary demands of life, mental conditions associated with the abuse of alcohol and drugs, but does not include mental retardation which is a condition of arrested or incomplete development of mind of a person, specially characterized by subnormality of intelligence."

Majority of mental disorders begin in adolescence or early adulthood. However, it often remains undiagnosed for substantial period of time. This prevents early treatment and often leads to poorer outcomes. Research endeavors are being made to look for ways to diagnose mental disorders early so that treatment can be instituted at the earliest, thereby improving outcomes. In this regard, it is important for clinicians to have a clear concept of the core and cardinal features, applicable to all mental illnesses in order to differentiate it from normal and culturally accepted ways of reacting to life events and psychosocial circumstances. For any clinical condition to be called a mental disorder, it is important to have evidence for change from the baseline state of the individual and also evidence that such changes in the psyche and behavior of the individual are leading to significant distress, dysfunction, or danger to self.

There are various kinds of mental disorders, which present with individual cluster of signs and symptoms. However, all mental disorders possess certain common characteristics:

- It is a recognized, clinically diagnosable condition.
- It is associated with significant cognitive, affective, or psychosocial impairment.
- It results from developmental, biological, and/or psychosocial factors.
- It can be managed using established treatment approaches (i.e. prevention, diagnosis, treatment, and rehabilitation).

MENTAL DISORDERS
Epidemiology

Mental and substance use disorders are one of the leading causes of disability worldwide. About 23% of all years lost because of disability is caused by mental and substance use disorders. About half of the mental disorders have been shown to begin before the age of 14. Overall, neuropsychiatric disorders are among the leading causes of worldwide disability in young and adult population. Paradoxically, developing nations, which have the highest percentage of population under the age of 19, have the poorest level of mental health resources. Because of this, these regions have a significant "treatment gap", meaning thereby that a significant proportion of people with mental illness remain undiagnosed as well as untreated in these countries. This adds to the magnitude of global burden of diseases. It further leads to reduced productivity and suboptimal level of well-being of the society as a whole.

Classification of Mental Disorders

The earliest attempts to classify psychiatric disorders can be traced back to the text of *Ayurveda*. Thereafter a myriad of classifications has been furnished by philosophers such as Plato (4th century BC) and Asclepiades (1st century BC), and ancient systems of medicine. The evolution of psychiatric classificatory systems over centuries has led to the addition of newer illnesses. At present, the two most accepted systems of classification of mental disorders in use are the International Classification of Diseases, (ICD), developed by WHO and DSM, developed by American Psychiatric Association (APA), respectively. These classificatory systems have been systematically updated in order to keep up with the emerging evidences generated through research. The most recent iterations of the two which are currently in use are as follows:

1. *ICD-10 (International Classification of Diseases, 10th Revision, 1992)* is the WHO's classification of all diseases and related health problems inclusive of psychiatric disorders. Chapter 'F' of the ICD-10 deals with the classification of psychiatric disorders as mental and behavioral disorders and codes them on the basis of an alphanumeric system from F00 to F99. ICD-10 is now available in several versions including one for research criteria, primary care, etc. and it is freely available.

2. *Diagnostic and Statistical Manual-5*: It is the fifth edition of the DSM published by the APA in 2013.

As per the ICD-10 classification, major mental disorders are listed as follow:

- *Organic mental disorders*: Delirium, dementia, organic amnestic syndrome, etc.
- *Mental and behavioral disorders due to psychoactive substance use*: Acute intoxication, harmful use, dependence syndrome, etc. due to psychoactive substance use.
- *Schizophrenia, schizotypal and delusional disorders*: Schizophrenia, schizoaffective disorder, persistent delusional disorder, etc.
- *Mood (affective) disorder*: Depressive disorder, bipolar disorder, etc.
- *Neurotic, stress-related and somatoform disorders*: Anxiety disorders, phobic disorders, obsessive-compulsive disorder, dissociative (conversion) disorders, somatoform disorders, adjustment disorders, and other neurotic disorders.
- *Behavioral syndromes associated with physiological disturbances and physical factors*: Eating disorders, nonorganic sleep disorders, sexual dysfunctions (not caused by organic disorder or disease), etc.
- *Disorders of adult personality and behavior*: Specific personality disorders, habit and impulse disorders, gender-identity disorders, disorders of sexual preference, etc.

- *Mental retardation*: Mild, moderate, severe, and profound mental retardation
- *Disorders of psychological development*: Specific developmental disorders of speech and language, specific developmental disorders of scholastic skills, specific developmental disorders of motor function, and pervasive developmental disorders
- *Behavioral and emotional disorders with onset usually occurring in childhood and adolescence*: Hyperkinetic disorders, conduct disorders, mixed disorders of conduct and emotions, tic disorders, etc.

Description of Common Mental Disorders

- *Schizophrenia*: It is a severe mental illness that primarily affects a person's perception of reality, behavior as well as cognition. Schizophrenia causes distortions in the perception of reality; a person may have auditory or visual hallucinations, be fearful and withdrawn, have delusions and exhibit inappropriate or disorganized behavior. The essential features of schizophrenia include the presence of specific psychotic features such as delusions and/or hallucinations, formal thought disorder, and a significant deterioration from a previous level of functioning in such areas as work, interpersonal relations, biological functions, and self-care.
- *Mood disorders*: These are distinguished by disturbances in mood state, which affect the physical, mental, and social functioning of an individual.
  - *Depression*: Depressive episodes are characterized predominantly by sadness of mood which is sustained and invariable, decreased interest in previously pleasurable activities, decreased energy, difficulty with attention, and concentration; slowed thinking and movements; reduced appetite and disturbed sleeping patterns; and feelings of hopelessness, helplessness, worthlessness, and other negative cognitions. A depressive episode if severe in intensity is often associated with thoughts of self-harm or suicide. The onset of depression often occurs during the late 20's, but it can occur at any age. Women are twice as likely to be diagnosed with depression as compared to men. Genetic influences, traumatic life events, and nutritional deficiencies, such as magnesium or vitamin B_{12} deficiency, are established risk factors for depression. Depression can also occur as a natural reaction to loss, especially the death of close family members or friends, heavy financial loss, etc. Depression is also known to be associated with various medical disorders such as hypothyroidism, Parkinson's disease, and terminal illness such as cancers, etc. In many cases, depression may develop without an identifiable cause or precipitating event.
  - *Bipolar disorder*: It is characterized by cyclical changes in the persistent mood of an individual, e.g. high phases (mania) and lows phases (depression) or a combination of both (mixed state) interspersed by periods of mostly near total normality. Alteration in mood states may sometimes occur very frequently or even within hours or days (rapid cycling and ultradian cycling), or may be separated by months to years.

A manic phase is characterized by euphoric or irritable mood, decreased need for sleep, increased activity, over-talkativeness, elevated self-esteem, grandiose ideas, increased libido, etc. Patients may spend huge sums of money or make elaborate plans, which are unrealistic, or indulge in high-risk behaviors during this phase. A manic episode may also be associated with psychotic symptoms such as delusions and hallucinations.

In a depressive phase, the person experiences persistent low mood, and other symptoms as described above.

- *Anxiety disorders*:
  - *Generalized anxiety disorder (GAD)*: It is described as persistent and excessive worry about routine life events and activities which lead to impairment in functioning. GAD is associated with physical symptoms such as tremulousness, muscle tension, headache, nausea, and autonomic symptoms such as palpitation, feeling of dizziness, etc.
  - *Obsessive compulsive disorder (OCD)*: OCD is characterized by intrusive and repetitive thoughts known as obsessions which a person recognizes as his own but considers as unwanted, leading to distress. These are invariably associated with certain ritualized and repetitive pattern of behaviors, which a patient is unable to control. They are known as compulsions.
  - *Panic disorder*: Panic disorder is characterized by abrupt onset of intense but brief anxiety attacks, often associated with a sense of doom, in the absence of a medical cause or a trigger. The patient also experiences "anticipatory anxiety" regarding similar attacks in the future.

- *Substance use disorders*: Substance dependence is a disorder featured by maladaptive patterns of mood, physical as well as cognitive symptoms which are associated with, generally prolonged use of psychoactive substances, such as alcohol, cannabis, tobacco, sedatives, opiates, amphetamines, inhalants, etc. A person with this disorder gives precedence to the substance use over other activities in life, experiences an intense craving for the substance, and neglects other pursuits in life leading to significant impairment in psychosocial functioning.

- *Eating disorders*:
  - *Anorexia nervosa* is a disorder in which a person refuses to maintain minimal body weight with respect to age and height, is intensely afraid of gaining weight, and has significant misperceptions of body image. Severe restriction of dietary intake leads to malnutrition, severe nutritional deficiencies which can culminate in death in extreme cases. It is often associated with comorbid depression or anxiety symptoms.
  - *Bulimia nervosa* is a disorder characterized by a cyclical pattern of rapid spurts of binge eating, followed by guilt and subsequent purging. This is often associated with inappropriate methods of purging such as self-induced vomiting, improper use of laxatives, etc. which can lead to medical complications.

Disorders Diagnosed in Childhood

- *Autism spectrum disorder*: This encompasses a spectrum of neuro-developmental disability, associated with stereotyped patterns of behavior and a restricted repertoire of interests, as well as difficulties in language and communication. The symptoms of this disorder appear at an early age, characterized by poor eye contact, inability to bond with peers and stereotyped movements. It is often associated with intellectual impairment of variable degree.

- *Attention deficit hyperactivity disorder (ADHD)*: Children suffering from ADHD show symptoms of inattention characterized by an inability to pay attention to details; difficulty in sustaining interest in a given task or play or to follow instructions. They get easily distracted and are often forgetful. They also exhibit symptoms of hyperactivity/impulsivity, typically characterized by being fidgety, inability to wait for one's turn, and repeatedly interrupting conversation of others.
- *Mental retardation*: Mental retardation is a condition characterized by arrested or delayed development of mind, because of which a child is unable to develop intellectual and socioadaptive functioning that is expected of his age. There is difficulty in acquiring language, motor as well as socio-cognitive skills. It is often associated with various genetic syndromes and hereditary metabolic conditions.

Consequences of Mental Disorders

Mental disorders lead to reduction or loss of functioning in various domains of life, which include educational, socio-occupational, familial, financial, and other areas. It also prevents an individual from fully realizing his potentials and contributes positively to society as per his abilities. The adverse consequences of mental disorders can be categorized as per certain terms outlined by the WHO.

- *Impairment*: It refers to a pathological defect, which can be physical or mental.
- *Disability*: Limitation of physical or psychological function that arises from the impairment, e.g., poor self-care in a patient with chronic schizophrenia.
- *Handicap*: It refers to the social dysfunction caused by the impairment and disability, e.g., loss of job due to mental illness.

Besides the dysfunction caused in multiple domains of life, mental disorders also lead to stigma and discrimination in society because of the prevalent misconceptions and myths about mental illnesses.

- *Stigma*: Stigma is defined as a sign of disgrace or discredits, which sets a person apart from others. The stigma of mental illness remains a powerful negative attribute in almost all societies, though of variable degree. Stigma also gets attached to the caregivers as well as to the mental health professionals. The impact of stigma is a kind of double punishment to the mentally sick. It leads to distress, to discrimination, and to deterioration in the quality of life of people with mental illness. It works as an impediment to health-seeking and also adversely affects the treatment-outcome.

Treatment of Mental Disorders

Treatment can be broadly divided into pharmacological and nonpharmacological. Within pharmacological domain, there are many medications that offer relief for various symptoms of mental disorders. In most cases, these drugs influence the action of brain neurotransmitters, such as serotonin, norepinephrine, and dopamine. Nonpharmacological methods like psychotherapy and behavior therapy have also been proved to be effective. Various forms of psychotherapy are available geared toward specific disorders. In addition, various other biological treatments are also available such as electroconvulsive treatment, repetitive transcranial magnetic stimulation, deep brain stimulation, psychosurgery, etc.

CONCLUSION

Mental health is an integral component of general health. Mental disorders are real but, currently, are mostly diagnosed on the basis of cluster of signs and symptoms, because their etiologies are not fully understood. For the same reason, they get associated with a plethora of myths and misconceptions in the minds of general public. Also, mental disorders are often linked with negative and stigmatizing attitudes which lead to isolation, discrimination, and significant distress to the patients. The role of positive mental health in contributing to our overall well-being, quality of life as well as to social capital, needs to be recognized. In between mental health and mental disorder, there exists a substantial size of subsyndromal conditions, which also cause significant suffering to the individual and are a source of additional burden to the society.

TAKE-HOME MESSAGES

- Mental health is an integral part of general health and well-being of individuals, which is a very important determinant of optimal functioning of society.
- Mental health is also intricately linked with physical health in terms of causation as well as course of illnesses. They are mutually interdependent.
- Mental disorders lead to significant morbidity as well as psychosocial impairment for the patients. Stress to their caregivers for chronic conditions is an important consideration.
- Mental disorders are diagnosed on the basis of cluster of specific signs and symptoms. They are of several types. Their etiologies are not fully understood.
- Treatment of mental disorders is possible, generally by drugs and psychotherapeutic interventions. It is important for full rehabilitation of the individual.
- Mental health resources in developing countries are very limited, even though the size of their need is very large.

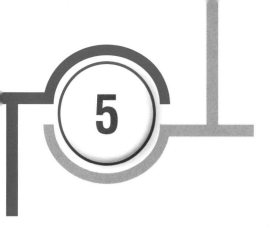

Classification and Clinical Evaluation

Samir Kumar Praharaj, PSVN Sharma

INTRODUCTION

Classification of clinical entities has to be preceded by their identification. Such entities are generally referred to as either a disease, a disorder or a syndrome. A *disease* refers to those abnormal health conditions, which result from injury to tissues because of internal or external factors. The underlying etiology and pathogenesis for most of the diseases is known. A structural pathology is also implied in a disease. A *disorder* refers to clinically recognized set of symptoms or behaviors, which is associated with distress and impairment in functioning. A *syndrome* is a collection of signs and symptoms that occur together more frequently than by chance. For both "disorder" and "syndrome", the underlying etiopathogenesis is quite often unknown and there may be no gross structural pathology. Diabetes mellitus is an example of a disease; as it is mostly associated with structural and/or functional pathology of pancreas. The pathological consequences of long-standing hyperglycemia leading to end organ damages, along with its pathophysiology, are mostly known. In contrast, most of the mental conditions are described as "disorders" or "syndromes" and not as "diseases", as the pathophysiology for them is still not known. For example, we know the signs and symptoms of depressive disorder and the associated neurochemical abnormalities. However, the long-term pathological consequences of these conditions are far from clear. Similarly, the pathophysiology of how these changes occur is poorly understood. However, as we understand more about these conditions by using sophisticated investigative technologies, subtle brain abnormalities are becoming apparent. However, Alzheimer's disease, which is the most common type of dementia, is an exception to the above-mentioned general observation, because here the pathology is known.

CLASSIFICATION OF MENTAL DISORDERS

Mental disorders are classified into various categories and subcategories as in other branches of medicine. Classification of illnesses is generally based on either etiology or clinical features or treatment response. Among them, the most useful one is that based on etiology.

Purpose of Classification

Classification of disorders subserves many purposes. Firstly, it is intended to facilitate uniform clinical practice so that specific treatment can be advised for specific conditions. Classification also enhances better communication among professionals about the disorders, as everyone uses a common, agreed upon, language. Classification, with its well-defined diagnostic criteria, is essential also for research on mental disorders, because it allows for formation of homogeneous research samples to begin with. Classification also aids in planning and evaluation of mental health service delivery.

Organic versus Functional Disorders

A distinction is commonly made between organic and functional psychiatric disorders. Organic disorders refer to conditions where there is an identifiable brain pathology, whereas, functional disorders refer to those without a demonstrable pathology. For example, a brain tumor causing psychiatric symptoms is an organic psychiatric disorder. When psychiatric symptoms appear without any other neurological or medical disorder, it is a functional psychiatric disorder, such as schizophrenia or depression. However, such distinction between organic and functional disorders is *fallacious* as all disorders ultimately either arise from brain or have a neurophysiological substrate, which reflect disruptions in brain circuitry. The organic conditions may cause structural and irreversible disruptions of neural circuits, whereas functional disorders may cause reversible disruptions. In organic conditions, pathology may be seen in structural neuroimaging, whereas functional neuroimaging techniques are required to image *functional changes* in nonorganic conditions. Even though organic psychosyndromes can often be independently identified based on their distinguishing features, sometimes organic conditions may present with features indistinguishable from functional psychosyndromes.

Systems of Classification

International Classification of Diseases, tenth edition (ICD-10), is the most widely used system worldwide, whereas some countries have their own local systems such as Diagnostic and Statistical Manual (DSM) in USA or Chinese Classification of Mental Disorders (CCMD) in China. There is a clinical version (blue book) and a research version (green book) of ICD-10. Current classification of mental disorders is based on symptom descriptions and not on the etiology, i.e., it has an *atheoretical approach*. Thus, there are operational criteria for specific disorders, which increase the *reliability* of psychiatric diagnoses. It implies that two different persons examining the index patient will reach at the same diagnosis. The mental disorders currently listed in ICD-10 have considerable empirical evidence and are based on extensive field trials, thus improving the *validity* of diagnosis. Also, there is *clinical utility* of making clinical diagnosis, as it helps in treatment planning.

The *F chapter* in ICD-10 refers to mental disorders. The major group of disorders includes organic disorders, substance use disorders, psychotic disorders, mood disorders, neurotic and stress-related disorders, personality disorders, eating and sleep disorders, and child psychiatric disorders. The disorders are organized according to a *hierarchical model (of Fould)*, which means that the preceding disorders in ICD-10 subsumes the ones following them (e.g., organic disorders have precedence over psychotic or mood disorders). However, currently there is more emphasis on diagnosing all disorders that are present as it has been noted that most disorders have high rates of comorbidity. All the disorders in ICD-10 are assigned an *alphanumeric code* (e.g., F20.0 refers to paranoid schizophrenia). The major categories in ICD-10 are summarized in **Table 5.1**.

Table 5.1: Major categories in ICD-10 Chapter V.

Code	Disorders
F0	Organic and symptomatic mental disorders
F1	Mental and behavioral disorders due to psychoactive and other substance use
F2	Schizophrenia, schizotypal, and delusional disorders
F3	Mood (affective) disorders
F4	Neurotic, stress-related, and somatoform disorders
F5	Behavioral syndromes and mental disorders associated with physiological dysfunction
F6	Disorders of adult personality and behavior
F7	Mental retardation
F8	Disorders of psychological development
F9	Behavioral and emotional disorders with onset usually occurring in childhood or adolescence

Multiaxial System

Multiple axes of diagnoses are used to describe the other associated disturbances on other dimensions in addition to the primary psychiatric disorders, inclusive of disturbance at medical and psychosocial levels along with the disabilities caused by them. This system is in tune with the biopsychosocial understanding of the illnesses. This facilitates the coordination of interventions executed by different health professionals (e.g., psychiatrists, clinical psychologists, and social workers). ICD-10 has formulated three axes to fully describe the clinical condition of any individual—axis I includes clinical syndromes, axis II has disabilities, and axis III describes contextual factors. Clinical syndromes include both physical and mental disorders; disabilities include occupational, social, and other disabilities. Contextual factors include the environmental/circumstantial and personal lifestyle/life management factors that influence the disorder.

ICD-10 Primary Healthcare Version

The primary care setting is the most likely place where the need for identification and service delivery for most of mental disorders is likely to be felt, because only a small proportion of patients will have the opportunity to be able to consult a specialist psychiatrist. To cater to these needs, there is a primary healthcare version (ICD-10 PHC) for use by general practitioners and nonpsychiatrists. It is similar to the blue book, but the organization is less complex and it lists the diagnostic features of common disorders that are encountered in general practice. The primary care classification consists of 24 categories, which includes common presentations in general medical care settings (**Table 5.2**). ICD-10 PHC consists of diagnostic and management guidelines for each category, flowcharts, symptom index, patient leaflets, and medication cards.

LIMITATIONS OF CLASSIFICATION

The current classificatory systems are far from perfect. There are concerns about the diagnostic validity of psychiatric disorders. The boundaries between disorders are not absolute and conditions falling between diagnostic categories have been described. For example, schizoaffective disorder has features of both schizophrenia as well as affective disorder. Substantial number of patients fall in the NOS or the "not otherwise specified" category, thereby undermining the validity of diagnostic criteria of mainstream diagnostic categories. Although atheoretical in principle, some disorders do imply specific etiology, such as stress-related disorders, organic mental disorders, and substance use disorders. It has been found that most people with a mental health problem, often also fulfill diagnostic criteria for two or more other mental disorders. They are at present

Table 5.2: ICD-10 primary healthcare categories.

Code	Disorders
F00*	Dementia
F05	Delirium
F10	Alcohol use disorder
F11*	Drug use disorders
F17.1	Tobacco use
F20	Chronic psychotic disorders
F23*	Acute psychotic disorders
F31	Bipolar disorder
F32*	Depression
F40*	Phobic disorders
F41.0	Panic disorder
F41.1	Generalized anxiety disorder
F41.2	Mixed anxiety and depression
F43*	Adjustment disorders
F44*	Dissociative disorder
F45	Unexplained somatic complaints
F48.0	Neurasthenia
F50*	Eating disorders
F51*	Sleep problems
F52	Sexual disorders
F70	Mental retardation
F90	Hyperkinetic disorder
F91	Conduct disorder
F98.0	Enuresis

*More than one ICD code is included

updated. The next version (ICD-11), which is based on extensive field studies and practitioner surveys, and is harmonized with DSM-5 is expected to come into effect from 1st January 2022. There is, at present, more emphasis on the *clinical utility* of the classification system. Utility includes value in communication among practicing professionals, researchers, and policy makers; implementation in clinical practice in terms of accuracy, ease of use and feasibility; and finally usefulness in clinical management decisions and record keeping.

Beyond the Classification System

Psychiatric disorders (e.g., depression and schizophrenia) are most likely not a single entity, but a heterogeneous group of conditions that are clubbed together based on a predefined and identifiable syndrome. Hence, classification of disorders beyond ICD-10 may have some heuristic value. For example, subtyping of depression into melancholic (endogenous) or nonmelancholic (reactive) depression may have different therapeutic implications. The former, which is more biological may preferentially respond to tricyclic antidepressants or electroconvulsive therapy, whereas, the latter may have psychosocial etiology and require psychotherapeutic interventions.

generally conceptualized as comorbid conditions; however, it may not be reflective of true comorbidity, instead it may just be an artifact of the current system of classification. Nevertheless, in the absence of any alternative etiology-based classification, we have to use the currently available system, which is the best at present and is also clinically useful.

As the classification evolves with advancement of knowledge about the disorders, these manuals are periodically

Advances in Nosology

Developments in neuroscience and genetic research may unravel newer diagnostic entities or newer ways of classifying in future and a more etiologically-based classification may evolve. Studies have found specific gene alterations leading to schizophrenia-like psychosis. However, in majority of schizophrenia patients, multiple genes are involved, each having a very small effect.

Thus, higher the number of such genes one has, higher would be the risk for developing schizophrenia.

As the clinical phenotypes that we know today may limit research in the field of neurobiology, several other approaches have been suggested. One of them is based on the Research Domain Criteria (RDoC), which is a research framework for new approaches to investigating mental disorders along various dimensions. There are five major domains that are being studied—negative valence system, positive valence system, cognitive system, systems for social processes, and arousal/regulatory systems.

CLINICAL EVALUATION

The diagnosis of psychiatric disorders is mostly clinical, based on *interviews* with the patient and their relatives as well as observations made during such interviews as regards general behavior and speech. The description of signs and symptoms in psychiatry, i.e., *descriptive psychopathology*, forms the basis of all diagnosis. The interview is summarized into two components— history and mental status examination (MSE). Medical and psychological investigations may be required occasionally to aid the diagnosis. As in all other branches of medicine, *clinical reasoning* is required to arrive at the final diagnosis after ruling out all other possible alternatives, known as differential diagnosis. However, it is important to remember that there is a whole person behind all the symptoms and signs, and they appear in the context of the unique characteristics of the individual. Hence, they are always colored by the *personality*. Symptoms are also colored by the cultural milieu, therefore cultural sensitivity is important to understand some of the mental phenomena. Some symptoms that are observed could simply be expressions of *cultural practices*. Some general principles of diagnostic interviews are outlined here.

Confidentiality

It should be ensured that confidentiality is maintained for the interview and this has to be explicitly stated to the patients. This helps in building good doctor-patient relationship. The exceptions include emergency situations when the life of patient or others are in danger. Also, wherever possible, privacy is ensured while conducting the interviews. This may not be always possible in wards or busy clinics. However, discussing sensitive matters should always be done in private.

Rapport

This is a bidirectional empathetic relationship between the psychiatrist and patient. Rapport is essential for all diagnostic interviews. *Empathy* means being able to understand what the other person experiences in a particular situation. Proverbially speaking, it is like putting oneself in the other person's shoes. Verbally one may respond by "yes, I understand", or nonverbally by head nodding or leaning forward, which makes the patient feel understood. Throughout the interview, the psychiatrist should maintain objectivity. Empathy is different from *sympathy*, which refers to feeling pity on someone who is suffering, without a deeper understanding. Also, it is different from *identification* when one gets emotionally involved with the patient's experiences and loses objectivity, which is detrimental to the diagnostic interviews.

Safety

Although most psychiatric patients are not violent, there may be occasional instances of unprovoked anger. Therefore, safety is of paramount importance during interviews. There should be an easy way out of the room in case of any eventuality, i.e., the interviewer should have access to the door. Also, while interviewing a violent patient, it is better to have another person in the room. If there is any suspected weapon with the patient, security personnel need to be informed before starting the interview.

HISTORY

As in other fields of medicine, history is the most important aspect of clinical evaluation of patients with mental disorders. Because of the nature of illness not everyone will be able to narrate their story of illness adequately and reliably. Hence, collateral information from family members or other informants is of paramount importance to improve the *reliability and also adequacy.* Sometimes, it may be necessary to interview multiple informants to get a coherent picture about the illness as well as the individual characteristics of the person. Information is deemed to be *adequate* when enough information is available to arrive at a diagnosis. In the beginning, it is essential to know the reason for current consultation, as to whether they have come on their own, referred by someone or there is some clinical or social urgency.

It is advisable to start the interview with *open-ended* questions, which allows for more than one possible answers such as, "tell me about your problem or what brings you here today?" and allow the patient to speak about their problems. This can be followed later by *closed-ended* questions, which allow for limited options. These latter questions are built upon the leads obtained by the open-ended questions. For example, if a patient reports of sleeping difficulty during open-ended initial questioning, it can be followed up later with specific questions

such as whether there was difficulty falling asleep, midnight awakenings, or waking up early in the morning, which refer to initial, middle, and terminal insomnia, respectively. However, it is important to conduct an interview in a *conversational style*, where the flow is maintained along with covering all pertinent questions in a flexible sequence. This makes the patient feel understood in contrast to more interrogational style of interviews, which use a checklist approach to elicit symptoms.

All the information required may not be elicited with a single interaction, and sometimes multiple interviews may be required. The style of the interview also needs to be modified depending on the clinical situation. For a hostile and uncooperative patient, detailed evaluation may need to be deferred. Similarly, a patient with depression may require prompting several times to elicit information.

History of Presenting Illness

Patients and their relatives should be asked about the *chief complaints separately as* their concerns and perception of the problem may be different. It should be documented separately in a chronological order. The *history of presenting illness* is an elaboration of the chief complaints and other related symptoms, which are being considered, based on the diagnostic possibilities. The subjective complaints are typically reported by the patient, whereas, the behavioral observations need to be obtained from the informants. Eliciting *negative history* is important as it narrows down the differential diagnosis for the presenting symptoms. Also, the effect of the symptoms on the socio-occupational functioning and interpersonal relationships is evaluated. There may be *precipitating factors* for the current symptoms, which can be medical (e.g., head injury) or psychosocial (e.g., life events such as job loss or death of loved one). Sometimes the *mode of onset* provides a clue. For example, acute onset of illness (less than 2 weeks) is common in mood disorders, whereas, insidious onset (longer than 2 weeks) is seen in schizophrenia. The *course* and *progression* of illness should also be obtained. Episodic course is common in mood disorders, whereas, continuous course with periodic exacerbations is observed in schizophrenia. If treatment was received, the details of medications (dose and duration), compliance, response, and adverse effects help guide treatment planning. It is important to enquire whether any traditional healing methods have been tried. Elucidation of predisposing and perpetuating factors may also help in long-term management.

Past and Family History

The *past history* of medical and psychiatric disorders may sometimes provide clues to the diagnosis of present episode. For example, past history of episodes of mania and depression suggests a diagnosis of bipolar disorder. Medical conditions are often comorbid with several psychiatric disorders. For example, cardiovascular disorders and metabolic syndrome are more prevalent among people with schizophrenia or bipolar disorder. Also, several atypical antipsychotics are associated with increased rate of metabolic syndrome. Any history of past surgeries is also recorded.

Family history of psychiatric disorders or medical disorders provides information on possible genetic contribution. Thus, a family history of schizophrenia in a patient presenting with psychosis strengthens the possibility of diagnosis of schizophrenia. Similarly, history of suicide in a family member increases the suicide risk of the patient. Also, family history of good response to a mediation may help in making a choice of drug. In those with family history of diabetes or hyperlipidemia, atypical antipsychotics should be used with caution as it increases the risk for metabolic syndrome. It is also important to enquire about any adverse events in the family such as parental death, separation, divorce, disharmony, etc., which increase the risk of several mental disorders. Similarly, history of abuse or neglect during childhood makes the person vulnerable to developing mental disorders at later age. Family traditions and beliefs may be useful in understanding symptoms and their presentations. An understanding of available social support is necessary in most cases for planning treatment. Also, it is known that negative expressed emotions such as critical comments and hostility increase the risk of relapse.

Personal History

Birth and developmental history is important for several psychiatric disorders. Influenza infection during second trimester of pregnancy has been implicated in schizophrenia. Obstetric complications leading to fetal anoxia is documented in those later developing schizophrenia and bipolar disorders. Delay or deviation in developmental milestones is characteristic of intellectual disability (previously known as mental retardation) or autism spectrum disorders. Presence of childhood disorders such as attention deficit hyperactivity disorder or conduct disorder increases the risk of substance use during adulthood. Several of anxiety disorders in adults have their first manifestation during childhood, which can present with features such as school refusal or selective mutism. Those with specific learning disorders have history of poor academic performance during school years. Other conditions such as nocturnal enuresis or bedwetting, which is seen more often during childhood, is considered as an example of delayed maturation.

Occupational history including the type of jobs, performance at job, and changes in job may provide clues to the degree of impairment because of illness. Chronic absenteeism and other job related problems are common in those with mental disorders. Enquiring about current sources and amount of income helps in identifying any possible financial distress and also helps in treatment planning. *Legal history* is relevant to many conditions and may provide clues to diagnosis as well. It is imperative to document all legal cases, both past as well as current ones.

Sexual history is also important for many psychiatric conditions. Eliciting sexual history requires sensitivity and privacy, and sometimes need to be deferred for subsequent interviews. In those with mania, an increased libido is reported, whereas, in depression it is reduced. Many psychotropic medications result in sexual adverse effects. *Menstrual history* provides information about some aspect of reproductive and endocrine status of the person, which may have a bearing on management.

Premorbid personality is an important component of psychiatric evaluation. It refers to the major traits a person has prior to the onset of mental disorder. The information regarding the personality can be obtained from the patient himself, but often it needs to be corroborated with the informant's version. It is evaluated by asking questions about the strengths and weaknesses a person has, the ease with which a person forms and maintains relationships, changes in mood states and ability to tolerate criticisms, their attitudes toward work and other responsibilities, their

fantasy life, and other habits. There are three main clusters of personality disorders—those with odd and eccentric behavior, those who are overly dramatic and manipulative, and the third group is characterized by anxious and avoidant types. In children and adolescents, instead of personality, temperamental characteristics are assessed.

MENTAL STATUS EXAMINATION

The goal of MSE is to elicit current psychopathology, extending up to past 1 week. This includes the patients' subjective experiences as well as the observable behavior. The method of *empathy* is the key to understanding subjective experiences, which are otherwise inaccessible for observation. The major areas that are examined include general appearance and behavior, cognitive functions, thought, mood, perceptions, and insight **(Table 5.3)**.

General Appearance and Behavior

General appearance refers to the patient's overall appearance including personal

Table 5.3: Mental status examination.

S. No	Components
1	*General appearance and behavior*: Appearance, cleanliness, dressing, eye contact, rapport, attitude, motor behavior, and involuntary movements
2	*Cognitive functions*: Consciousness, attention and concentration, orientation, language, memory, abstraction, judgment, calculation, and intelligence
3	*Speech and thought*: Spontaneity, speed, productivity, form, possession, and content
4	*Mood and affect*: Quality, depth, range, reactivity, and communicability
5	*Perception*: Distortions and deceptions
6	*Insight*: Awareness, attribution, and acceptance

hygiene, grooming, etc. which gives a clue to the level of self-care that may be deteriorated because of psychosis, depression, or dementia. They may be shabbily dressed, have offensive body odor, untrimmed beard, and nails. In contrast, those with anankastic personality may be neatly dressed. Also, the attitude toward the examiner during the interview gives clue to the diagnosis. A paranoid patient may be hypervigilant and secretive, avoids direct eye contact with the examiner, whereas, a manic patient may be overfamiliar, playful, and distractible. Those with histrionic traits are usually colorfully dressed and could be overtly seductive during the interview.

Motor behavior may be reduced (hypoactivity) or increased (hyperactivity) in patients with depression or mania, respectively. The hyperactivity seen in mania is usually goal-directed and not aimless as in schizophrenia. Furthermore, patients with schizophrenia may have awkward motor behaviors. *Catatonic symptoms* are primarily motor symptoms such as posturing, mutism, stupor, or excitement. These signs may be apparent in those with schizophrenia or mood disorders. *Abnormal involuntary movements* may be clues toward diagnosis of organic conditions (e.g., movement disorders) or adverse effect of psychotropic medications (e.g., tardive dyskinesia). They include tremor, chorea, athetosis, tics, dyskinesia, and myoclonus.

Cognitive Functions

Cognitive functions are tested initially, as rest of mental state evaluation would become meaningless in persons with cognitive impairments. The domains tested are attention and concentration, orientation, language, memory, abstraction, judgment, and calculation. Initially, the *level of*

consciousness is ascertained. Sometimes, when patients have altered level of consciousness such as stupor and coma, rest of MSE is deferred till the clinical condition improves. Also, if the patient is heavily sedated because of medications or otherwise, it may not be possible to conduct a meaningful MSE.

Attention refers to the ability to focus on the subject at hand. It is inferred from the way patients react when conversation is initiated. In some patients attention can be aroused easily with minimal stimulus, whereas, some may require repeated efforts. Also, whether attention is maintained for some time to allow meaningful conversation to occur is also recorded. This sustained attention is known as *concentration*. Attentional impairment is the hallmark of delirium. Some patients with schizophrenia or mania can have poor attention. These patients are distracted easily during conversation. A simple bedside test for attention can be naming the days of week backward.

Orientation refers to the patient's awareness of himself in the context of his environment. It is tested for time (day, date, and month), place (building, floor, and city), or person (people around him). The most sensitive for clinical testing among these is orientation to time, which is lost early, followed by loss of orientation to place and still later to person. On behavioral observation, disorientation may be suspected when they appear confused and scan the environment repeatedly. Disorientation is seen in cognitive disorders such as delirium or dementia. It is unusual to have loss of orientation to person with preserved orientation to time and place. In such situations, either dissociative disorder or malingering is suspected.

Language function testing includes testing for fluency, comprehension, repetition, naming, reading, and writing.

Among these, naming is the most sensitive and is lost early in certain organic mental disorders such as Alzheimer's dementia. It is tested by asking to name objects, colors, or body parts. Most of the language function is apparent during normal conversation with the patient. Spontaneity in conversation gives clues to the fluency. To test comprehension, simple yes/no questions (e.g., is it raining outside?) or pointing commands (e.g., point to the fan) are used. Reading and writing may be less useful in those with no formal education. In persons with motor or Broca's aphasia, fluency, repetition, and naming are lost, whereas, comprehension is preserved. In those with sensory or Wernicke's aphasia, comprehension, repetition, and naming are lost, whereas, fluency is preserved.

Assessment of *memory* is done for immediate, recent, and remote events. Immediate memory is tested with repeating a telephone number. In delirium, immediate memory may be impaired. Recent memory for *verbal* material is tested with unrelated words recall, whereas, *visual* memory is tested with the hidden object test. Typically, words are given or objects are hidden in front of the patient, following which they are asked to recall them after 5 minutes. Remote memory for personal and impersonal events is tested separately. The organic disorders of memory, i.e., *organic amnesias*, follow Ribot's law, i.e., memory of recent events are lost first than remote memories. In contrast, *functional amnesias* will have patchy loss of memory or loss of remote memories when recent memory is preserved. It is commonly associated with anxiety, depression, and occasionally with dissociative disorder.

Abstraction refers to the ability to deal with concepts, be able to think in terms of attributes, aspects, and classes of a particular object or situation. Concrete or literal thinking is the opposite of abstraction. Clinically, proverb interpretation is a sensitive test for abstraction. Normally, the patient should be able to provide the implied meaning of the proverbs. In those with schizophrenia, the responses can be concrete, i.e., they give the literal and surface level meanings.

Judgment refers to the ability to make sensible decisions, to choose rationally from alternative options, both at personal and social levels. *Personal judgment* is assessed by asking about their future plans. Similarly, *social judgment* is evaluated by observing how they interact with others. Test judgment is evaluated by providing a problem situation and getting his response. *Fund of information* is examined by using simple general knowledge questions. The choice of questions should be based on the background and education level of the patient.

Calculation is evaluated by testing additions, subtractions, multiplications, or divisions, which are presented either verbally or in written form. Simple arithmetic problems can also be given, e.g., if cost of a pen is 6 rupees, how much would a dozen cost? Clinical assessment of *intelligence* is based on the results of cognitive function testing, specifically, abstraction, comprehension, judgment, fund of knowledge, and calculation.

Speech and Thought

Speech is described under amount or productivity, rate or speed, loudness or volume, and tonal fluctuations. Increased productivity of speech or volubility is characteristic of mania, whereas, reduced productivity may be a feature of depression, anxiety, or psychosis. Fast or pressured speech as well as loud speech is typical of mania. Reduced tonal fluctuations or monotonous speech is characteristic of depression or psychosis. Also, the reaction time may be increased in those with depression, i.e., take more time to respond to questions. Just the opposite is seen in patients of Mania who have increased spontaneity.

Thought disorders may be described under disorders of stream, form, possession, and content. The normal *form of thought* is linear, organized, and goal directed, which makes them coherent. In those with flight of ideas, typically seen in mania, patient moves from one idea to another in rapid succession, which is connected superficially through similarities of sound, such as punning and rhyming. Those with circumstantiality give unnecessary details to answer of questions, which may not be relevant or necessary; however, they do not lose the goal. Tangentiality refers to answers to questions which are off the mark, i.e., there is loss of goal direction. Loosening of association refers to thoughts that are poorly connected and are quite difficult to understand. This is seen in those with schizophrenia and other psychotic disorders. Occasionally, patients with psychosis coin new words or use conventional words in an idiosyncratic way, known as neologisms.

Disorders of thought possession include obsessions and thought alienation phenomena. Obsessions are recurrent, intrusive thoughts, which are considered by the patient as irrational and generally absurd. Obsessions can also be an image or an impulse. Even though these thoughts, images, and impulse are considered as one's own, but they enter into mind against resistance, thereby signifying inadequate control of the individual. Obsessions are usually accompanied with or followed by compulsions which are mostly motor and sometimes mental acts that are aimed at reducing the distress associated with obsessions. Obsessions and compulsions are characteristic of obsessive-compulsive disorder. In thought insertion and withdrawal, which are true thought alienation phenomena, patient experiences thoughts being inserted or withdrawn from their mind by some external agency. Similarly, thought broadcasting is experienced as thoughts being known to others. These thought alienation phenomena are characteristic of schizophrenia, and need to be distinguished from depersonalization, a nonpsychotic symptom, where patient reports these to be "as if" experiences.

Thought content includes dominant preoccupations, anxious and depressive cognitions, and delusions. Delusions are false, unshakeable beliefs, which are not shared by others from same sociocultural background and held with conviction despite evidences to contrary. These are hallmark of psychosis. Several types may be seen based on content including delusions of persecution, reference, grandeur, jealousy or infidelity, somatic, etc. Delusions may be bizarre which are completely implausible, or nonbizarre which, though plausible, are completely untrue. Bizarre delusions are more common in schizophrenia, whereas, nonbizarre delusions are seen in delusional disorders. Those having delusions usually have high preoccupation and conviction about the belief, and consequently may sometimes act on their delusions. This is in contrast to delusion-like ideas, which may be held with less conviction, and can be challenged easily. In psychotic depression, delusions of guilt, sin, poverty, illness, or nihilism may be observed. Depressive cognitions include ideas of hopelessness, helplessness, and worthlessness. Sometimes, passive death wishes or active suicidal ideas are present in those with depression.

Anxious cognitions include worries about future or about impending catastrophe as in panic attacks.

Mood and Affect

Mood is the subjective feeling state over the past week as reported by the patient, whereas, *affect* mostly refers to the cross-sectional observed emotional state as seen objectively. The quality of affect can be euphoric or irritable in mania, depressed or irritable in depression. Similarly, anxious affect is characteristic of anxiety disorders. In those with acute psychosis, affect may be irritability, fearfulness, or perplexity. Affect may be labile in mania, where there is rapid shift from one extreme to another, such as from sadness to euphoria. Affect may be blunted or flat in those with schizophrenia, in which there is minimal or nearly absent expression of emotions. Occasionally, in schizophrenia, affect may be inappropriate to the situation or incongruous to the content of thought.

Perceptual Disorders

The disorders of perception include illusions and hallucinations. *Hallucinations* are false perceptions in absence of sensory stimuli. They have all the qualities of true perceptions and occur along with them. They can occur in any sensory modality, such as auditory, visual, tactile, olfactory, or gustatory. Auditory hallucinations of certain types, such as voices commenting on one's action or voices discussing about the patient in third person are characteristics of schizophrenia. Patients recognize them as true perceptions and may act on them. Hallucinations are said to be prominent, if they occur frequently, throughout the day as in schizophrenia, or fleeting as in other psychotic disorders. True hallucinations need to be distinguished from *pseudohallucinations*, which occur in

mind's subjective space, are not as vivid as hallucinations and patients retain insight to the phenomena. Presence of prominent visual hallucinations, specifically in absence of auditory hallucinations, should prompt a search for organic causes of the disorder. *Illusions* are misinterpretations of stimuli, and are not diagnostic of any specific illness. They may be seen in normal persons, in delirium or in psychoses. Other forms of sensory distortions are also possible, such as micropsia or macropsia, where the objects appear smaller or larger than they actually are.

Insight

Insight is the degree of understanding about the mental disorder held by the patient. It includes *awareness* of the symptoms, *attribution* of the symptoms to mental disorder, and *acceptance* of treatment (the 3As of insight). If the patient is aware of the symptoms, attributes to mental condition, and accepts treatment, then he/she has *full insight*. If the patient is aware of symptoms but attributes to medical condition or do not accept treatment, it is *partial insight*. If the patient does not acknowledge the symptoms then there is *nil insight*.

Physical and Neurological Examination

A general physical examination would reveal signs of medical conditions, which may be contributory, a consequence or simply incidental to the psychiatric disorders. In patients with depression, presence of pallor or goiter may point toward anemia or hypothyroidism, which may be the underlying cause. Minor physical anomalies such as high-arched palate or low-set ears point toward possible developmental origins of psychiatric disorder. A thorough systemic examination is needed for most of the psychiatric patients and will be guided by the presenting symptoms. For example, those with panic symptoms with prominent dyspnea, a careful assessment of respiratory and cardiovascular system is needed. Similarly, those with history of alcohol abuse, medical complications such as hepatomegaly, signs of cirrhosis and portal hypertension, polyneuropathy, etc., are important. Sometimes, persistent horizontal nystagmus may be the only clue to the possibility of a prior episode of Wernicke syndrome.

Neurological Examination

A thorough neurological examination is necessary in all patients, to identify possible organic (medical or neurological) etiology for psychiatric syndromes. Examination of cranial nerves, motor, sensory, autonomic, gait, and stance are essential components of this segment. Also, primitive reflexes such as grasp reflex or palmomental reflex provide clues to frontal lobe dysfunction. Examination for extrapyramidal symptoms is necessary to document adverse effects of antipsychotics. Antipsychotics may cause Parkinsonism or akathisia during the initial period, or can lead to tardive dyskinesia with long-term use.

Lobar function tests are done to localize the lesions of cerebral cortex. Many psychiatric syndromes are seen with frontal and temporal lobe lesions. Specifically, prefrontal cortex lesions lead to either a pseudodepressive syndrome (dorsolateral lesions) or pseudopsychopathic lesions (orbitofrontal). Signs of frontal lobe dysfunction include perseveration, presence of release reflexes such as grasp reflex, gaze impersistence (inability to maintain extremes of gaze), and alternating motor tasks (e.g., pronation-supination movements). Temporal lobe lesions can result in memory deficits (visual or verbal).

FORMULATION

Making a case-formulation is a process in which the unique positive and negative features from the history and examination of each individual case are brought out in a coherent and chronological manner, so as to reach a diagnosis or suggest differential diagnosis. This is different from case-summary, wherein all relevant information is covered in a summarized fashion. A well-formulated case makes it easy to develop a comprehensive management plan.

Differential Diagnosis and Diagnosis

In many situations, if a specific diagnosis is not forthcoming, it is acceptable to have differential diagnosis starting from the most probable to least probable. Discussing the points in favor of a diagnosis as well as the points against it helps to narrow down the differential diagnosis and finally arrives at the correct diagnosis. The diagnosis may be *definite,* if the patient fulfills the criteria for a particular disorder. However, in absence of sufficient information or evidence, a *provisional* or working diagnosis is acceptable so as to facilitate treatment.

Management Plan

Next step is to outline a management plan. This includes investigations and treatment which is based on the diagnosis. The decision to treat is followed by the evaluation of locus (i.e., inpatient or outpatient), focus (i.e., target symptoms), and modus (i.e., pharmacological or nonpharmacological) of treatment. Investigations can be either psychological or medical (laboratory, imaging, etc.). Psychological investigations may include projective tests that use semistructured or unstructured stimuli (e.g., Rorschach test), or objective tests which are well-structured paper and pencil tests (e.g., Minnesota Multiphasic Personality Inventory). Basic laboratory investigations may include complete blood count, liver and renal function tests, blood sugars, and lipids. Other investigations may be indicated based on the clinical presentation. Urine drug screen may be indicated in young patients presenting with behavioral abnormalities. Structural neuroimaging such as computed tomography (CT) and magnetic resonance imaging (MRI) scan are indicated if the presentations are atypical (e.g. late onset psychosis) or if symptoms are consistent with a space occupying lesions or other neurological disorder. Electroencephalogram (EEG) may be ordered, if seizures are suspected. Treatment modalities include pharmacological (medications), psychosocial (psychotherapies or counseling), or somatic (electroconvulsive therapy).

CONCLUSION

Classification of mental disorders is essential for diagnosis, management as well as research and professional communication. Current classification is based on symptoms and signs and is purely descriptive. Therefore, the diagnosis of mental disorders is purely clinical. The clinical evaluation consists of careful history taking and systematic MSE to delineate the subjective experiences as well as the objective phenomena, which constitutes descriptive psychopathology. A proper physical and neurological examination will help in identifying most of associated medical conditions. Investigations may be necessary to find medical or neurological cause for the psychiatric syndrome.

TAKE-HOME MESSAGES

- Health conditions requiring medical attention may be either a disease, a disorder or a syndrome.
- Classification of clinical entities has to be preceded by their identification, which requires a set of consensually agreed upon criteria. ICD prepared by WHO and DSM prepared by APA (American Psychiatric Association) are two such internationally recognized system which provide the diagnostic criteria for individual clinical categories and their classification.
- All system of classification serves the purpose of ensuring uniformity of diagnosis, enhancing better communication and also facilitates better record keeping and verifiable and comparable research.
- Psychiatric disorders are also labeled as organic or functional. Organic disorders refer to conditions where there is an identifiable brain pathology, whereas, functional disorders refer to those without a demonstrable pathology.
- Two major system of classification used internationally are ICD, authored by WHO and DSM authored by American Psychiatric Association (APA).
- The diagnosis of psychiatric disorders is mostly clinical, based on *interviews* with the patient and their relatives to obtain the history and MSE based on observations made during clinical evaluation. General physical and neurological examinations are also very important for total management of the case.

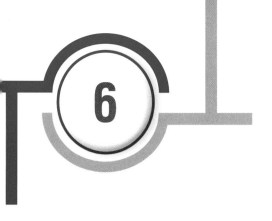

Communication Skills for Effective Medicare

Baxi Neeraj Prasad Sinha

INTRODUCTION

Communication is defined by the Oxford dictionary as "the imparting or exchange of information by speaking, writing, or using some other medium," while communication skills have been defined as "the ability to convey or share ideas and feelings effectively."

In the medical field, experts have regarded "communication" as a psychobehavioral phenomenon where the emphasis is placed not only on the verbal but also on the nonverbal aspects of behavior and written transfer of information during the process of communication.

Good communication is the cornerstone of good medical care and can lead to positive clinical outcomes, while poor communication skills can be associated with difficulties for all parties including poor patient satisfaction, adverse clinical outcomes, and legal challenges to the doctor and the clinical team.

"Communication" can be discussed across several levels and in different ways. One such way is to explore the various interfaces where a doctor needs to communicate in medical settings.

- Communication of the doctor with patient and caregivers, is used to:
  - Establish an effective therapeutic relationship and rapport.
  - Elicit accurate and pertinent clinical information promptly.
  - Discuss various aspects of treatment like options, pros, and cons including side effects, expenses, and making sure patient expectations from the treatment are realistic.
  - The roles and responsibilities of doctor and treating team including the boundaries and limitations
  - Achieve a shared understanding of all aspects of the treatment.
  - Communicate hope, positive emotions, and instill trust which is important for holistic care.
- The doctor also needs to communicate simultaneously with other members of the medical team, which includes:
  - Direct communication with immediate team (like nurses and ward staff)
  - Indirect communication, e.g., written requisitions for investigations, writing laboratory reports, prescriptions, and discharge summary
  - Keeping accurate clinical records to facilitate future care and fulfill medicolegal requirements
  - Teaching and training members of the medical team.
- Communicating with third parties and the public:
  - Communicating with patient's insurers, employers, and other authorities lawfully and appropriately

- Raising public awareness, use of social media, and so on.

It is most important to realize that communication is a multiway process, so the doctor must make active efforts to understand what others are trying to convey back to the doctor. Active listening is vital; it helps to take notes while listening and summarize what has been discussed so that all parties have a shared understanding. A nonjudgmental approach should be used, and assumptions should not be made based on the way a person looks. If in any doubt, clarifications should be sought early, help from others should be requested when needed (e.g., help from interpreters when confronted with an unfamiliar language, dialect, or phrases).

Illness is often associated with stress, not only for the patient but also for caregivers, which can adversely affect communication. A person under stress can become less attentive, not being able to recall details immediately, have emotional changes like irritability and anger. In such situations, the patient or their caregivers might appear to lack objectivity and rationality and appear inconsiderate. However, the clinician must maintain a cool, neutral, and sympathetic disposition. The doctor needs to be aware of and be equipped to deal with such situations, asking for help when needed.

Medical and surgical conditions may be associated with comorbid mental health conditions, such as anxiety states, depressive illness, dementia, etc., whether formally diagnosed or not. Hence a focus on communication skills training especially targeting communication skills that can be beneficial in the presence of some common mental health disorders can be rewarding for medical students irrespective of the medical specialty they choose to specialize in the later stages of their career.

IDENTIFYING AND ADDRESSING COMMON ERRORS IN COMMUNICATION

Errors in Communication can arise from:

- *Individual factors:* Language difficulties, unfamiliarity with subtleties and nuances of local culture and customs, speaking too fast or loudly, not being sensitive to and aware of patient's privacy (so patients may not share pertinent information), continuing to speak without checking degree of shared understanding, using excessive medical jargon, lack of training for communication in complex situations (like breaking bad news), poor reading or writing skills or poor handwriting, closed body posture, being perceived as having less interest, severe tiredness, high-stress levels, either party getting distracted by phones or other persons, etc.

- *Environmental factors:* Busy clinic environment, less than optimal lighting, lack of privacy, noisy surroundings, and poor general systems (e.g., letters or requests for investigations not reaching in time, severe staff shortage, high workloads, etc.).

Addressing Common Errors in Communication

Doctors need to identify areas of improvement in terms of communication skills and seek help/work to improve those. It may be difficult to identify one's own "blind spots" in communication skills, therefore obtaining regular structured and anonymous multisource feedback from colleagues, patients, and caregivers can be a helpful strategy for reflection and self-improvement. Specific training targeted for more complex topics like communicating bad news is usually helpful.

Communicating Bad News

A doctor is often faced with conveying bad news to the patient or caregiver. This could include communicating:

- A catastrophic diagnosis (like severe extensively metastasized cancer)
- A poor prognosis or outcome (e.g., need to amputate a limb or poor response to life-saving treatment)
- To caregivers about the death of their loved one.

For such situations, there is evidence to suggest that dedicated training can be helpful. Focusing on the needs and expectations of patients and caregivers is important. Breaking bad news can be a stressful task for the doctor but it must be done in a caring and sensitive manner. Training can take the form of didactic lectures, small group discussions, and practicing role-playing case scenarios during teaching sessions under the supervision of experienced teachers or dedicated specialized training.

COMMUNICATION SKILLS FOR UNDERGRADUATES

The importance of learning and improving communication skills in undergraduate years cannot be overemphasized. Something as fundamental as successfully passing the undergraduate medical training hinges on being able to (1) accurately write answers for question papers in examinations on time, (2) articulate verbal responses to complex questions during the viva voce, and (3) demonstrate skills in practical examinations where the trainee needs to interact with patients/subjects as well as examiners.

It is only natural to expect doctors to be able to easily extrapolate this ability to the clinical field in later years; however, it is often not so straightforward.

Communication with Other Colleagues, Teaching, and Training

An important aspect of communication in medicare involves interacting with other team members who have different education and training levels. Doctors are often called upon to provide teaching and training to colleagues in the multidisciplinary team (MDT) which can comprise of nurses, technicians, administrators, and other members of staff who may or may not have clinical training. To communicate effectively with MDT, one of the first steps is an awareness of the ability level of our colleagues, be it nurses or other staff members, medical students, or doctors.

For a successful teaching session, it is important to have clear aims and objectives and a structured plan for the lesson. The topic should be introduced, discussed, and concluded within the allotted time, while retaining the interest of the audience and handling questions confidently. Audience participation techniques, like posing questions to the audience to gauge their level of understanding, can be helpful. These skills can be learned and improved upon with practice and training during undergraduate years and beyond.

Having a good command of language and confidence in the use of modern technologies and teaching aids, like computerized slides and audiovisual equipment, is an important skill which can be improved by practice.

Written Communication to Other Parties

Medical communication often requires the ability to communicate complex information succinctly to other parties, for example, writing reports for medicolegal purposes. It is important to keep the intended audience in mind while writing a clinical report.

Sometimes doctors will be called upon to provide medicolegal reports to police or write reports to patient's employers. While writing reports especially for nonmedical colleagues, it is good practice to explain the medical technical term briefly in the beginning and to write the full-expanded terminology at first use of any acronym.

We must remember that the information we gain from patients during our work as doctors is confidential and should be disclosed only if there is consent from the patient or there are other legally valid reasons to release the confidential information. Further, we must also be mindful as to how our patients or their caregivers might feel when they read our written report at a later date, once they happen to find or receive a copy of the report.

EFFECTIVE COMMUNICATION SKILLS WHEN HELPING PATIENTS WITH MENTAL HEALTH CONDITIONS

Many common mental disorders are diagnosed primarily on patient history and mental state examination, both demand good communication skills.

Mental health settings may at times present unique challenges for the doctor as regards communication. The patient can be in a state of significant distress, highly anxious, depressed, or suffering from acute psychosis (i.e., may be harboring delusions and/or experiencing hallucinations); or may have limited cognitive abilities associated with reduced ability to understand and interpret complex language (e.g., dementia). Quite often the accompanying person, who may be a family member, a friend, or a concerned caregiver, may himself be in a state of great stress as mentioned earlier. It might lead to narrowing of his attention span

that is dominated by preoccupations for the wellbeing of his patient.

Some simple tips for effective communication include opening the conversation with appropriate pleasantries (something as simple as saying "Hello" or greeting the patient in their local language), using simple language, checking if the patient is understanding what is being discussed, for example, by requesting them to summarize what we have discussed so far in their own words. It is also important not to be patronizing and we must give due respect to everyone we engage in communication.

Different mental health conditions can be uniquely challenging in terms of communication in their distinct ways; some tips and strategies which can be rewarding in improving effective communication in those settings are outlined below.

Severe Anxiety States

Heightened states of anxiety can commonly occur in healthcare settings both in mental health as well as in general medical settings. A person having severe anxiety may not be able to sufficiently focus attention and concentrate on what is being asked or said by the doctor, can also struggle to immediately recall details of what has been asked, making effective communication a challenge. However, different strategies can allow meaningful communication even in challenging situations. For example, giving the patient extra time during early stages of the interview can often help by allowing acute anxiety levels to settle down, that extra time can be utilized for supporting the patient and rapport building while also observing the patient's behavior and responses (which can be rewarding for mental state examination). It helps if the doctor remains calm and speaks using simple words, short sentences with brief pauses if necessary. Sometimes questions can be repeated giving time to the patient to understand and respond properly. It is good practice to encourage patients to ask any questions they may have from the doctor and to provide answers and explanations in clear and simple language, avoiding medical jargon as far as practicable.

Severe Depressive Illness

Patients suffering from severe depression can have low mood, poor motivation, and psychomotor retardation, among other features. Thinking processes may be slowed down, compared to the nondepressed states, making it difficult for the patient to process complex information or to accurately answer multistep questions. For example, it can be difficult for a severely depressed person to quickly respond to long questions like, "how do your feelings and emotions change when you are faced with time pressures for completing tasks in your office from your boss who, as you had earlier told me, reminds you of the boy who used to bully you in your school days?" Instead, the same question can be broken down in smaller parts and information can be elicited in smaller chunks. An empathic approach which means trying to understand and share the feeling of others and validating a person's emotions, can be helpful.

Schizophrenia and Related Illnesses

When suffering from acute exacerbation of paranoid schizophrenia, a person may be experiencing auditory hallucinations, wherein the patient could be hearing several voices at the same time while the doctor is trying to ask questions for gathering information and eliciting symptoms. This can make it harder for the patient to concentrate on the doctor's questions. In these situations, if a patient

is struggling to answer basic questions, it is worthwhile to gently ask what is making things difficult; give more time for the patient to respond and use simple language. At times giving written questions can be rewarding. While remaining mindful of patient's educational and literacy levels, written responses can often help evaluate patient's thoughts patterns in terms of grammar and syntax which can reveal some clinical features of schizophrenia like "formal thought disorder," where sentence structure, syntax, or flow of ideas in sentences can be disjointed at times. In long-term chronic or residual schizophrenia, a person may communicate very little or use a limited number of words often in an odd way to express their thoughts and feelings. In such circumstances, asking gently for clarifications, while being watchful for features of frustration and irritability, and using nonverbal techniques like pictures or hand gestures to supplement the spoken and written words can be helpful.

Dementia and Cognitive Impairments

A person with severe dementia may have limited cognitive ability to understand and retain complex information for longer periods. Commonly a person with severe dementia may also have sensory impairments like hearing loss or poor vision; at times, the person can present with behavioral difficulties like aggression which can be challenging. Often these can be understood as their way of communicating their needs and distress in a backdrop of declining cognitive functions.

Several techniques can be used in these situations to improve the effectiveness of communication. Remaining calm but vigilant is the key. In persons suffering from dementia, assessment of sensory impairments, especially the visual and auditory functions, are very important.

Sometimes simple practical strategies can improve communication and be rewarding, for example, checking if their hearing aid is working properly, are they wearing their correct prescription glasses, have they had anything to eat, how their bowel and bladder functions are, and so on. Having patience, avoiding distractions, talking about one thing at a time, looking for signs of frustration, and being ready to revisit the interview at a different time of the day can be useful.

Apart from using simple verbal communication, the use of written material, or pictorial diagrams can be helpful, such printed information or leaflets can be given to the patient for future reference to aid their memory.

Autistic Spectrum Disorder

Persons having autistic spectrum disorder can have different language patterns and/or some differences in reciprocal social interaction, which could be associated with challenges in communication.

It usually helps to speak in very clear language using simple, nonambiguous words and short sentences. It is worthwhile starting by taking the person's name so the person knows that the doctor is addressing him. Direct eye-to-eye contact may at times be poor, so it is important to ensure that he is paying attention before starting to ask questions. Talking about their interests is often helpful. The possibility that statements may be interpreted differently by different people must always be kept in mind. Some people can take the literal meaning of words and struggle with alternate meanings and be confused. Care should be taken to ensure that the context is understood correctly by the patient in all situations.

Communicating with Children

Children of different age groups can present with special challenges especially when they are also having various mental health difficulties. It can at times be difficult to gain their rapport and elicit the right information within a short period. Strategies like taking more time for the appointment, offering repeat reviews, use of nonjudgmental attitude, and interviewing in calm surroundings with children friendly furnitures, like desks and chairs suited to their age, availability of common toys, coloring pens, and papers can be helpful.

Encouraging the child to draw some pictures, then sensitively discussing the situation around that can be helpful as a communication technique when it is difficult to elicit relevant clinical information by direct verbal questioning. Starting the conversation with a topic of child's interest like their hobbies can be rewarding. It is important to be aware of the child's language and literacy levels and how it matches with their stage of development.

Communication in the Presence of Different Disabilities

It is very important to be sensitive to the needs and preferred methods of communication of persons with various disabilities, for example, intellectual disability, learning difficulty, or mental retardation. It is important to use clear simple phrases and give people the time they need and not rush them for answers otherwise it can be counter-productive and cause more distress to the person we are trying to help. Sometimes it becomes necessary to continue the assessment in more than one setting if needed.

We can come across many other situations where special communication skills can be helpful. For instance, where a patient has language or speech difficulty or other sensory impairments, visual, or auditory, along with mental health issues, can be difficult situations. Different and often multiple strategies to overcome such challenges need to be employed on a case to case basis. The general principles of prioritizing our patients and keeping their individual needs at the center of what we are doing, usually paves the way for effective communication. Taking help of suitable tools and their adaptations, such as use of braille or sign language interpreters and so on as needed on a case to case basis, can be helpful.

Violent/Mute or Uncooperative Patients

A discussion about communication skills in the field of mental health will be incomplete without a discussion of how to attempt to perform and record a meaningful mental state examination for patients who may be mute or uncooperative. This could take the form of severe agitation or violent behavior or when a person hardly speaks or remains mute.

In such situations, Kirby's method for mental state examination can be invaluable, which can be briefly summarized under the headings of (1) general reaction and posture, (2) facial movements and expression, (3) eyes and pupils, (4) reaction to what is said or done, (5) muscular reactions, (6) emotional responsiveness, (7) speech, and (8) writing.

Kirby's method is a structured way of observing the mental state of uncooperative patients and recording the same in clinical records which can be helpful for risk assessment and treatment planning as well as for communicating the same with other clinicians and for comparison at a later

date as to whether there is improvement or deterioration in the person's presentation.

Communication with the Public

A doctor may need to communicate complex information to the public, for instance, to raise mass awareness via newspapers, television, radio, or social media. While each communication medium can have its strategies, in general terms, it is important to maintain a professional stance and ensure accurate information is conveyed in simple language, with minimal use of medical jargon, done confidently in a manner that retains the interest of the public. It is good practice to mention sources of further information like accredited websites from where interested people can get more detailed information.

Globalization of Healthcare and Use of Interpreters

The doctor's ability to understand, speak, and read the patient's local language/mother-tongue and awareness of subtle nuances of local culture and practices can be extremely valuable.

However, many doctors get trained or work in different regions, where the predominant language may be different from their mother tongue. Often people migrate and need to access healthcare in a different country where the team does not speak their language. This globalization of healthcare brings its challenges in terms of establishing effective communication. The use of trained language interpreters for communicating in different languages is showing an increasing trend. Telephone/web-based language interpretation services are also available in some places.

Doctors need to realize the limitations in the use of interpreters who primarily help with language translation and to resist the temptation of requesting the interpreters to also analyze what the patient is saying, especially in mental health settings. Such boundaries of practice and expectations from different professionals should be made clear at the outset to all parties to reduce the chances of misunderstanding and miscommunication.

Sometimes a patient's caregiver turns out to be bilingual and offers to act as an interpreter. Ideally, if facilities of formally trained interpreters are available then it is not advisable to use a caregiver as an interpreter as there could be a conflict of interest, for example in cases of suspected domestic violence if the perpetrator is also the interpreter then the issue is obvious.

Use of Social Media for Communication

Social media has gained significant prominence in the modern age. Professionals and members of the public use social media for voicing opinions and to follow trends as well as to communicate with others. Doctors need to be aware of codes of conduct for responsible use of social media and follow similar principles of professionalism while communicating via social media as they would be doing while communicating in person in any other public forum, maintaining the standards of good medical practice as doctors. The General Medical Council of the UK has published a very useful guide for doctors for the use of social media.

CONCLUSION

Communication skills include our verbal, nonverbal, and written abilities to interact not only with patients but also their families, other caregivers, other professionals, public authorities, and general public at large.

Communication in medicare is a skill that needs to be developed during the undergraduate training years. Effective communication can improve patient engagement; earn their trust and adherence with the treatment, thereby improving clinical outcomes. The converse is also true, i.e. poor communication skills can lead to misunderstandings and mistrust toward the doctor and further to poorer clinical outcomes. This may further lead to legal claims of negligence or malpractice toward the doctor and clinical team.

Mental health settings can present challenging situations that demand more adept use of advanced communication skills. However, beginning from the days of undergraduate medical training to the professional journey as a specialist, we are constantly dependent on our communication skills for our clinical work of providing effective and optimal medicare to our patients and also for the advancement of our career in general. We should constantly try to examine and improve our communication style and skills based on personal experience and feedback from our colleagues and consumers of our services.

TAKE-HOME MESSAGES

- Good communication skills are the cornerstone of effective medicare.
- Communication skills training is important in undergraduate years and continued improvement throughout professional life is highly desirable.
- Effective communication in medicare involves multiple parties like the patient, caregivers, other members of the medical team, and other competent authorities and includes verbal, nonverbal, and written communications.

- Complex situations such as breaking bad news can benefit from dedicated training for advanced communication skills.
- Illness can often be associated with high-stress levels which demand high-quality communication skills.
- Mental health settings can present with challenging situations that demand especially good communication skills because of the altered mental states of recipients of these services such as those with severe anxiety states, schizophrenia, dementia, autistic spectrum disorders, and those who are violent, mute, or uncooperative.

- With the globalization of medical care doctors needs to adapt to changing demands generated by advancing technologies, expanding use of social media, and need of interpreters because of multilingual and multicultural settings.
- There is a need to maintain professional behavior, patient confidentiality, and sensitivity to legal and ethical issues while communicating in medical settings.
- Effective communication can lead to improved clinical outcomes while poor communication skills may be associated with a breakdown in therapeutic relationships and claims of medical negligence against the doctor and clinical team.

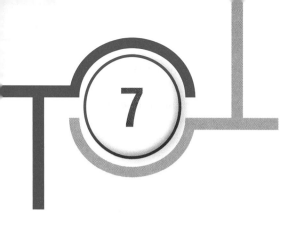

7

Organic Brain Syndromes

Malay Kumar Ghosal

INTRODUCTION

One of the most dreadful mistakes that a psychiatrist can make is missing a medical/neurological diagnosis and continuing to treat the case as a primary psychiatric disorder. A psychiatrist must always keep in mind that a medical diagnosis has a precedence over a psychiatric diagnosis in the hierarchy. This attitude also has a bearing on the emphasis in the management plan. Delirium appearing in old age will have an entirely different management protocol from delirium appearing after alcohol withdrawal, though they might appear similar superficially. A liaison with the specialists from other respective disciplines is often called for as the psychiatric disorder may sometimes be caused by the underlying biological factors. The current chapter deals with the psychiatric disorders predominantly caused by and/or temporally associated with various medical/neurological conditions and their management plans.

DISTINGUISHING FEATURES

When a patient comes to a doctor with behavioral abnormalities or irrelevant speech, the first question the doctor should ask himself is whether he is dealing with a case of organic brain syndrome. That means whether the symptoms are manifestations of any underlying brain disorder. Though at present almost all psychiatric disorders are known to have underlying neurobiological correlates, and therefore organic versus functional distinction is blurred, but still for practical purposes we can classify the mental disorders into organic (where we can find some underlying systemic or brain disorder as a cause of the mental disorder) and functional (where no such cause can be found).

So how to differentiate organic from functional at the outset? There are some symptoms, which are telltale signs of organic brain syndrome. These include:

- Impairment of memory, language, etc. However, at times, schizophrenia mimics language impairment and is difficult to differentiate.
- Altered sensorium and impairment of consciousness.
- Incontinence of stool and urine.
- Any neurological deficit or difficulty with gait; impairment of recognition of people.

But there are some subtle signs for differentiation also:

- Underplaying the symptoms. That means objective signs and symptoms are more than the subjective complaints.
- Hallucinations in visual, gustatory, or olfactory modalities. Though they are found in functional psychosis, yet they are more common in organic brain syndromes.

- 'La belle indifference' that means the patient is least concerned about his deficits. This is a common feature of dissociative disorder, but there are some caveats.
- Ability to provide the history of present illness systematically and in chronologically correct sequence usually goes against organic brain disorders.
- Sudden change in personality in adult life is a clue to some organic brain syndrome.
- Sudden appearance of neurotic symptoms in adult life without any significant psychosocial stress is a pointer to organic brain syndrome.

The dictum is better to err on the organic side. That means it is always better to misdiagnose a functional disorder as organic disorder than vice versa.

After deciding that the patient is suffering from some organic brain disorder, we have to answer some more questions:

- Is the disorder acute, subacute, or insidious in onset?
- Whether the impairment is focal or diffuse? In focal syndromes, usually one cognitive function is differentially more damaged, e.g., speech is impaired but memory is relatively intact.

If we can decide on these issues, it will help us to diagnose the underlying disorder. For example, acute and focal disorder is usually due to vascular events like stroke, whereas acute and diffuse disorders are usually delirium from different encephalopathies. In subacute and diffuse causes, one has to think of autoimmune encephalitis, or other causes of rapidly progressive dementias. In subacute and focal causes, one has to think of some quickly expanding brain tumors. In insidious and focal cases, one has to think about other space occupying lesions (SOL) and if it is insidious and diffuse, degenerative dementias should be considered.

The other important clue for diagnosis is the temporal profile of development of symptoms. There are several ways by which the symptoms can develop.

- Gradually progressive in nature, means there is gradual deterioration of symptoms—degenerative disorders, expanding SOLs
- Stepwise—repeated vascular events
- Relapsing and remitting—demyelinating, inflammatory
- Remitting—transient vascular events, metabolic.

History should be taken from the patient as well as informants. The sequence of events should be elicited thoroughly. Then one should perform thorough clinical examination. All the systems should be examined but particular emphasis should be given on the neurological examination. Mental state examination with examination of the cognitive functions should be done properly. There are many good screening instruments available. Mini-mental state examination (MMSE) and Addenbrooke's Cognitive Examination (ACE) are two commonly used instruments for assessment of cognitive functions.

GLOSSARY OF SOME TERMS

Cognition

Cognition is a term which has its origin from gnosis, meaning to know. To know the environment, and everything that is around oneself. So it basically refers to an information processing mechanism. Very simplistically we can compare it with a computer. A computer has an input, a processor, a storage system, and an output. Here the input is perception, the processor is thought process, the storage system is memory and the output is language. So cognition is sum total of all these functions and many more things.

Amnesia

Amnesia is impairment of memory. Memory is very important for our day-to-day work or existence. If you think of a state where you have lost your memory, you can imagine how difficult it would be to perform our daily activities. The memory is not a unitary concept. One type is called declarative memory; the other type is called non-declarative memory. The declarative memory is what you are conscious about, e.g., you can remember, "Yesterday evening, I had a dinner with my friend". Nondeclarative memory is the memory, which you are not conscious of. The example is how you have learnt to ride a bicycle.

The cerebral localization of declarative memory is medial temporal lobe, more specifically hippocampus. Nondeclarative memory has its localization in basal ganglia, cerebellum, amygdala, etc.

Amnesia can be anterograde, where the impairment of memory is after the brain insult or retrograde when the impairment is before the brain insult. For example, after a head injury a patient cannot remember anything about the next two days. This is anterograde amnesia. Again head injury patients often cannot remember what has happened several minutes before the head injury. This is retrograde amnesia.

Usually the patient or the informants complain about amnesia in the following manner:

- They misplace things, usually in some unusual places, and sometimes they forget that they have misplaced the things altogether.
- They forget to pass information to others.
- They make mistakes in shopping list, when they go to market.
- Sometimes they even forget that they have taken meals.

- As they forget things, they repeatedly ask the same question.
- As they forget, where they have misplaced documents, money, etc., they come with the explanation that people are stealing their things.
- They forget the topography and geography of a place and many a times they lose their way when coming back home or going to some very familiar place.

Apraxia

It is failure to execute coordinated move-ments, in the absence of motor weakness, sensory impairments, coordination problem, and comprehension problem. A person is unable to comb his hair, faces problem in brushing his teeth, cannot open lock using keys, etc. There are different types of apraxia such as ideomotor apraxia, ideational apraxia, dressing apraxia, constructional apraxia, etc. Elaborating on each type is beyond the scope of this chapter. Many areas of the brain are responsible for praxis but the most important area is dominant parietal lobe. This knowledge is needed for ultimately understanding as to which part of the brain is damaged and that will help in understanding the pathology and diagnosis.

Agnosia

It is failure to recognize an object, despite having no impairment in primary sensory apparatus or comprehension ability. That means a person has no impairment in visual system but cannot recognize an object if placed in his visual field.

Most common agnosia is visual agnosia, though it can occur in any sensory modality. The person cannot recognize the object, if it is being presented in his visual mode, but can recognize if presented in other sensory modalities. The person cannot tell that it is a pen if shown to him, but can name it if he is allowed to grasp it. This is usually due to a disconnection between the primary visual cortex (occipital lobe) and the visual association cortex (temporal lobe). There are two pathways from visual cortex, one dorsal pathway going to parietal lobe is "where pathway". This denotes the location of the object. The other is ventral pathway, going to the temporal lobe, "what pathway". This denotes the nature of the object. This pathway is damaged in case of visual agnosia. If there is a visual agnosia, the person has difficulty in identifying the objects, which are used in day-to-day activities. So there is impairment in activities of daily living.

A special type of agnosia is prosopagnosia, where a person cannot identify the face of a person. The person cannot identify his close relatives and many a times tells his wife to be his mother or his son to be his brother. He is also unable to identify the photos of different personalities from different fields, and also unable to match the face photographed from different angle. The area involved is inferior occipitotemporal region, commonly known as fusiform gyrus.

Aphasia

This is a higher order language dysfunction; damage at the level of cortex. There are mainly two language areas. One posterior, meant for comprehension of language. Other is anterior for expression of language. The posterior language area is the posterosuperior part of the temporal lobe (Wernicke's area) and also Heschl's gyrus. The main output area, anterior language area is situated in the posterior and inferior frontal convolution; commonly known as Broca's area. These two areas are connected by a network, arcuate fasciculus. If there is a damage to the Broca's area, the speech becomes hesitant, omission of words leading to a telegraphic speech, word finding problem, leading to repetition of the same word, known as verbal stereotypy. If there is damage to the Wernicke's area, the person will have comprehension problem. He will also speak incoherent. He will sometimes replace one word with another, called paraphasia. Instead of telling mango he may tell orange. These patients are many a time mistaken for schizophrenia. The acute onset, paraphasic errors and other localizing signs of brain damage may help to differentiate the two conditions.

Executive Function

When we do any work, there are two parts. What is to be done (1), and (2) how it is to be done? The how part is executive function. Like an executive officer who does not do any work by himself, but commands and organizes the whole work, there is an area in brain which does the same thing. It commands lower brain areas to do things. Its function is organization, sequencing, planning, etc. For example, I am planning a tour to Shimla. I have to plan my holiday, decide over the route (railway/flight), selection of the spots to be visited, etc. These are executive functions, and the brain area subserving this function is the dorsolateral prefrontal cortex. In executive dysfunctions, there are myriad of symptoms. The person cannot manage his day-to-day functions, keeps things haphazardly, takes extra time in cooking (as his organizational capacity is poor), unable to continue conversations efficiently, unable to give opinion in important household affairs and many other things.

DEMENTIA

Dementia is a syndrome and it is characterized by three groups of symptoms:
1. *Neuropsychological:* Amnesia, aphasia, apraxia, agnosia, and executive dysfunctions

2. *Neuropsychiatric:* Also known as behavioral and psychological symptoms of dementia (BPSD). This includes agitation, psychotic symptoms, depression, sleep disturbance, etc.
3. *Impairment of activities of daily living:* If there is no impairment of activities of daily living, then the syndrome will not qualify for dementia. Dementia is one of the most common problems of the elderly, and with the increase in number of aged population, the number of people suffering from dementia is also increasing. This is a huge burden to the society at large. With the breakdown of joint families and urbanization of people, the caring of people with dementia is also a great problem. Many a time the caregiver is the spouse, who himself is pretty old, which imposes a severe burden, both physical and psychological, for the person concerned.

There is a rapid growth of dementia population worldwide, but India is going to bear the brunt of highest rate of growth of dementia people. The prevalence of dementia varies widely in India from as low as 0.62% to as high as 3.54%. There are many reasons for this discrepancy. However, before further discussion on the topic, a few words on "mild cognitive impairment (MCI)" are very much needed.

Mild cognitive impairment—MCI falls between normal cognitive aging and dementia. There is some possibility of a disease-modifying agent for Alzheimer's disease (AD) being developed in near future. In that case the diagnosis should be done as early as possible. So the concept of MCI has gained popularity. There are three outcomes of MCI. It may remain static, may progress to dementia, or may revert to normalcy. So the concept is still fluid to some extent. However, there is some consensus on the diagnostic criteria of MCI.

- Subjective memory complaints corroborated by an informant
- Objective memory impairment
- Intact activities of daily living
- Normal general cognitive function
- Not demented.

However, it has been found that about 10–15% of MCI subjects progress to dementia every year. But the total conversion to dementia falls slightly below 50%. Among the many predictors of conversion to dementia, the most important predictor is the ApoE4 status. That means those who have homozygous ApoE4 status, they are most likely candidates for progression to dementia. No definite treatment is available. Treatment of vascular risk factors, physical exercise, and cognitive intervention may be helpful.

Causes of Dementia

The most common cause of dementia is Alzheimer's disease (AD). Other common causes of dementia are diffuse Lewy body dementia (DLBD), vascular dementia (VaD), frontotemporal dementia (FTD), etc. These are all primary neurodegenerative dementias.

There are other types of dementias, which are secondary to other causes, and sometimes they are treatable also. Though the percentage of treatable dementias is about 10% only, yet due to their reversibility, it is very important to diagnose potentially reversible causes.

Common Causes of Dementia

- Alzheimer's disease
- Vascular dementia
- Diffuse Lewy body dementia
- Frontotemporal dementia
- Dementia due to Huntington's disease (HD) and Parkinson's disease (PD)

- Nutritional deficiency, e.g., vitamin B_{12} deficiency, Wernicke–Korsakoff syndrome, etc.
- *Infectious disease:*
  - Meningoencephalitis
  - Herpes simplex encephalitis (HSE)
  - Human immunodeficiency virus (HIV)
  - Neurosyphilis
  - Prion disease, e.g., Creutzfeldt–Jakob disease (CJD)
- *Endocrine disorder:*
  - Hypothyroidism
  - Addison's disease.
- Traumatic brain injury
- Space occupying lesion in the brain.

Dementia can also be classified as cortical and subcortical varieties. In cortical dementias, as the name suggests, it involves mainly the cortical areas like frontal, temporal, or parietal areas. The prototypes are AD, FTD, etc. In subcortical dementias, the main areas involved are basal ganglia, thalamus, and brain stem. The common types are PD, HD, PSP (progressive supranuclear palsy), etc. There is a triad of symptoms in subcortical dementia. They are dementia, depression, and movement disorder.

ALZHEIMER'S DISEASE

The most common type of dementia is AD. sixty percent of all dementias are AD. It affects mainly older people. With the increasing number of old age population in the community, the number of AD patients in the community is also increasing. Urbanization and breaking down of the joint families are causing a huge burden on the care givers, most of whom are also old.

Epidemiology

The prevalence and incidence of AD increase with increasing age and over 65 there is more rapid increase. There is wide variation in the prevalence of dementia from 0.34 to 1.31% over 60 years at different parts of India. In USA, dementia is the third most common cause of death and carries an enormous burden to the healthcare system. As per WHO and World Bank studies, dementia constitutes 4.1% of the global burden of disease. The healthcare cost amounts to several billion dollars in UK and USA and supersedes the cost for heart disease, stroke, or cancer. The developing countries will have to bear the brunt of increasing growth of dementia population in near future.

Risk Factors

The common risk factors are advancing age, female sex, poor socioeconomic condition, and poor education level. Curiously turmeric, which contains curcumin may have a protective role in development of dementia.

Course and Outcome

Alzheimer's disease being a neurodegenerative disorder runs a chronic downhill course. Average life expectancy after the onset of the disease is 7–10 years. Early- onset AD has a poorer prognosis.

Neurobiology

The hallmarks of AD are amyloid or neuritic plaque, which is extracellular and neurofibrillary tangle, which is intracellular. It has long been debated which one is the primary pathology, but now the consensus is in favor of amyloid plaque.

The amyloid plaques are aggregation of protein which are folded into a specific shape known as beta-sheet secondary structure. Initially, it was thought that these were made up of starch and so the name because of their staining properties. Amyloid plaque contains 41–43, commonly 42-amino acid polypeptide, which is found in abundance in

AD and is known as beta-amyloid protein. It has been found in normal ageing brains also, but usually there is quantitative difference. They are found in different cortical regions of brain.

Neurofibrillary tangles are hyper-phosphorylated tau proteins and are found intracellularly. The tau proteins are normally associated with microtubules present within neurons, and responsible for signal transmission. When they are deranged, they are associated with destruction of neurons.

The AD patients show cerebral atrophy. The main areas affected are the medial temporal lobe and hippocampus. The hippocampus is the area responsible for human memory. Other cortical areas, mainly the association cortex, e.g., parieto-temporo-occipital region, are atrophied also.

Formation of Beta-amyloid

Beta-amyloid, which is a 42-amino acid polypeptide, is the main underlying factor for pathogenesis of AD. The mechanism has been unraveled to some extent recently. Amyloid precursor protein (APP) which is a much larger polypeptide and is found in brain is processed by three enzymes. They are alpha-secretase, beta-secretase, and gamma-secretase. If APP is primarily acted upon by alpha-secretase and then gamma-secretase then it forms nontoxic soluble metabolite. But if APP is acted upon initially by beta-secretase and then gamma-secretase then toxic beta-amyloid is formed. This beta-amyloid then through a cascade mechanism leads to the formation of neurofibrillary tangle and ultimately death of the neurons.

The neurotransmitter, which is mostly found to be deficient in AD, is acetylcholine. The nucleus basalis of Meynert is the nucleus involved. Hence, one of the main therapeutic targets is to increase the level of acetylcholine by giving acetylcholine esterase inhibitors.

Clinical Features and Diagnosis

The diagnosis of AD is mainly through exclusion. First of all, it should qualify for the diagnosis of dementia. That means apart from memory impairment, there should be impairment in at least another domain manifested as apraxia, agnosia, aphasia, or executive dysfunction. Then the onset should be insidious, if a person can pinpoint the exact onset, in all probabilities the diagnosis is not AD. Next there should not be any pointer that the condition may be secondary to any other condition from clinical features as well as investigations. It should also not be temporally associated with any vascular insult to the brain, or associated with any focal neurological deficit.

Assessment of Cognitive Functions

The two commonly used instruments for screening of cognitive functions are:
1. Mini-Mental State Examination
2. Montreal cognitive assessment test

Treatment

There are three approaches to treatment:
1. *Pharmacological treatment for cognitive dysfunction:*
   - Cholinesterase inhibitors—donepezil, rivastigmine, and galantamine
   - N-methyl-D-aspartate (NMDA) receptor antagonist—memantine
2. *Nonpharmacological management:* Different sorts of behavioral modification therapy based on A (antecedent)—B (behavior)—C (consequence) model
3. Pharmacological management of behavioral and psychological symptoms.

Antidepressants and antipsychotics, mainly atypical antipsychotics, are used to manage the psychiatric problems and behavioral symptoms associated with AD.

But one has to keep in mind that food and drug administration (FDA) has issued a black box warning for the use of antipsychotics in dementia, because there are chances of increased cerebrovascular accidents and mortality associated with antipsychotics in dementia. So, minimum dose should be used for a minimum duration.

FRONTOTEMPORAL DEMENTIA

Frontotemporal dementia is very important from psychiatric point of view, as many of the cases present with psychiatric features at the onset. At one time, it was thought to be a rare disorder. It was known as Pick's dementia. Recent epidemiological studies, however, have shown that FTD is quite common among non-AD dementias and more so among the patients of young onset dementia. FTD is subdivided into three types as per the clinical features and cerebral localization of pathology:

1. *Behavioral variant of FTD (bvFTD):* In such cases, the patient presents with change of personality and disinhibited behavior, such as passing some obscene comments unbecoming of him, taking away food from the plates of guests, etc. He himself is unaware of the change, which means his insight is lost. Memory problem is not very prominent at the onset, though with passage of time memory is also impaired gradually. So it is very important to find out the chronological history, which faculty is getting impaired after which. Many a time the patient shows repetitive and stereotyped behavior similar to compulsive behavior of obsessive compulsive disorder. Other symptoms are hyperorality, and food cramming and forced eating. The patient puts a bolus of food into the mouth before finishing the first. Lack of sympathy and empathy for the near and dear ones is also commonly present. The prefrontal cortex and anterior cingulate cortex are the main brain areas involved.

2. *Semantic dementia:* Here the patient gradually loses the concept and meaning of the objects, also known as semantics. He has impaired knowledge of the particular objects, its name, its use, etc. So many a times, the patient uses "this" or "that" instead of an object. This is the history given by the informants, but one has to ask the specific question to get the information. The person cannot name an object presented to him either visually or through any other modalities and also unable to tell the use of the object, or cannot point to the object on naming the object. The left anterior temporal lobe is the brain area involved.

3. *Progressive nonfluent aphasia (PNFA):* Here the patient initially presents with articulatory problem. He also has word finding problem and phonemic paraphasia. Here words are replaced with similar sounding words, like pen with hen or grass with bus, etc. The patient also has agrammatism, so when he speaks or writes the grammatical rules are not followed. The brain area involved is left posteroinferior frontal lobe.

Many neurodegenerative disorders are proteinopathies. It means there are intracellular accumulations of abnormal proteins in the neurons. AD is a tauopathy, where hyperphosphorylated tau is accumulated within brain cells. Similarly DLBD and PD are synucleinopathy, it means there is abnormal accumulation of alpha-synuclein protein in the neurons. But, FTD is heterogeneous regarding proteinopathy. There are groups where tauopathy is present but in other patients another protein transactive response DNA binding protein of 43 kDa (TDP-43) is involved. There are other proteinopathies also, but it is beyond the scope of this book. There is no known treatment for FTD, only sometimes the symptomatic management of behavioral problems can be done.

VASCULAR DEMENTIA

Vascular dementia is the second most common dementia after AD. It is more common in the developing countries such as India. The reasons for this are that the risk factors for VaD such as diabetes and hypertension are not adequately treated. There are three types of presentations of VaD:

1. *Single strategic stroke:* Here there is a stroke in a strategic area of brain, causing cognitive decline. One of the common areas is thalamus.
2. *Multi-infarct dementia*: Here multiple small infarcts, many of them lacunar in nature lead to dementia. The onset is more acute than AD and the course is usually of a step-ladder pattern of deterioration. There may be associated neurological signs and symptoms. The patients may show emotional incontinence in the form of pathological laughter or pathological crying, due to associated pseudobulbar palsy. The MRI shows multiple small lacunar infarcts, many of which are not visible in computed tomography (CT) scan.
3. *Subcortical VaD:* This is also known as Binswanger disease. In this case, there are ischemic changes in the deep white matter of the cerebral hemisphere. They are visualized in the T2-weighted image of the MRI as white matter hyperintensity. Many a times, they present with depressive features and progresses to dementia.

As the frontal subcortical circuit gets damaged, executive dysfunctions are more prominent than episodic memory impairment. There may be associated apathy, gait disturbance, pyramidal signs, and urinary incontinence. So sometimes they are mistakenly diagnosed as normal pressure hydrocephalus (NPH).

There is no specific treatment for VaD. However, control of vascular risk factors reduces the risk of development of VaD to some extent. Acetyl salicylic acid and/or clopidogrel are used to prevent further stroke.

DELIRIUM

Delirium is one of the most common clinical condition for which a psychiatrist gets a referral in the general hospital setting. Many a time, delirious patients are considered to be suffering from psychotic condition. It is basically an acute confusional state. If treated properly, many of the delirious patients recover, but otherwise it carries a high-mortality rate.

The most common risk factor of delirium is advanced age. A person over 85 years has several fold increased chance of developing delirium than a person less than 65 years. Delirium is commonly found in postoperative patients and also in patients getting treatment in ICU. Persons with cognitive dysfunction are also highly vulnerable to develop delirium.

The etiologies of delirium are myriad. Dementia is one of the most common predisposing conditions for delirium. Delirium superimposed on dementia is a clinical challenge for diagnosis. Delirium is differentiated from dementia on three main points:

1. Acute onset
2. Fluctuating nature of symptoms
3. Altered sensorium.

The common causes of delirium are:

- Infection (encephalitis of various etiologies, systemic infection)
- Trauma (head injury)
- Vascular (stroke, vasculitis)
- Autoimmune (encephalitis, collagen vascular disorder)
- Metabolic (dyselectrolytemia, hepatic encephalopathy, and uremia)
- Drugs (withdrawal of sedative, hypnotic drugs, alcohol withdrawal, and overdose)
- Neoplasm (SOL of brain, paraneoplastic syndrome).

It is very important that one should diagnose the exact cause of delirium, because that is the key to successful treatment.

Clinical Features

There is impairment of attention. This results in lack of concentration (from impairment of sustained attention), distractibility (impairment of focusing attention), and perseveration (impairment of shifting attention). There is altered consciousness. Patient is often disoriented to time, place, and person. Usually, the disorientation to time is the most common. Patient cannot tell the time of the day, or month, or year properly. There is fluctuation of symptoms, with worsening toward night. This is known as sundowning. The delirious patients often pick up the bed clothes involuntarily and aimlessly. This is known as *floccillation* which is very characteristic of delirium. Sometimes they are afraid and seem to suffer from persecutory delusions. They think that people around them are enemies and behave in an aggressive manner. They are often restless, try to get down from bed, and take away catheter, intravenous drip, Ryle's tube, etc. These are the main reasons of referring a delirious patient to a psychiatrist. There is also reversal of the sleep wake cycle.

The patient sleeps in the daytime, and remains awake at night. Sometimes the patient is very anxious, at other times apathetic. There are three subtypes of delirium:

1. Hyperactive—restless, agitated having delusions, and hallucinations.
2. Hypoactive—listless, apathetic. Often misdiagnosed as depression or dementia.
3. Mixed

Management

The proper management of delirium can save life, so it is very important. Before proper treatment, one should do some investigations to clinch the proper diagnosis. These are:

- Complete blood count—to rule out infection
- Fasting blood glucose/urea/creatinine/ LFT/glycemic, renal, and hepatic status
- Serum electrolytes—dyselectrolytemia, particularly hyponatremia
- Urinary ketones—ketoacidosis
- Urinary drug screening
- Electroencephalogram (EEG)
- Neuroimaging.

Apart from finding and treating, the cause of delirium, there is often dire need for controlling the behavioral part. Here both pharmacological as well as nonpharmacological methods are used.

Nonpharmacological methods include finding out any sensory impairment, if present and to take care of that. While speaking to a delirious patient, one should talk clearly, slowly, and slightly loudly, as many of the times their attention is impaired. It is prudent to keep the bed near the glass window of the ICU, so that one can be aware of the outside environment, which helps one to remain oriented with time to some extent. Restraint should be minimum and only if the need is extreme. The environment should be noise free and there should be a low level of lighting at night.

Whenever any drug is used one should keep in mind that the drug may cause further impairment in his sensorium and so it will be difficult for the clinician to asses. Also, many a time, the patient has disease of other organs such as heart, liver, lungs, or kidney. So, one has to be careful while choosing the drug. Haloperidol has the highest evidence behind it in treating delirium, though now second-generation antipsychotics such as olanzapine, risperidone, or quetiapine are also used. Benzodiazepines should be avoided as there is no evidence of improvement in delirium, on the contrary it can cause deterioration. They are useful only in cases of delirium caused by alcohol withdrawal or seizure.

Outcome of delirium is varied. It may be complete recovery, persistent cognitive impairment, long-term hospitalization, or death.

AMNESTIC SYNDROME

In this case, there is differential impairment of memory, both recent and remote, though other cognitive functions are relatively intact. If other cognitive functions such as speech, praxis, gnosis, or executive functions are also impaired, then the syndrome will be either dementia or delirium. The brain area which is damaged is either hippocampus or hypothalamic diencephalic region.

The two most common causes of amnestic syndrome are Wernicke–Korsakoff syndrome and HSE. In the former, the diencephalic system is damaged and in the latter the hippocampal system is damaged.

Sometimes it is difficult to distinguish this type of amnesias from psychogenic amnesia. Here are the differentiating points:

- In psychogenic amnesia, usually the memory impairment is selective for some emotional events.
- The psychogenic amnesia does not obey Ribot's law, a law which states that recent memory is more impaired than remote memory.
- Sometimes, in psychogenic amnesia, the person is unaware of his personal identity. In organic amnesia personal identity is the last to get impaired.

Wernicke–Korsakoff Syndrome

This is a syndrome found in patients of alcohol dependence syndrome. Wernicke's syndrome and Korsakoff's syndrome are actually on a continuum. Wernicke's syndrome occurs in the acute phase and Korsakoff's syndrome occurs if the Wernicke's syndrome is not treated properly and adequately. The Wernicke's syndrome is characterized by a triad of symptoms given below:

- Ataxic gait
- Global confusion
- Extraocular ophthalmoplegia.

If the syndrome is not adequately taken care of, then it progresses to Korsakoff's syndrome, which is characterized by following features:

- Amnesia—recent memory is more impaired than remote memory. Both anterograde and retrograde amnesia occur.
- Confabulation—the patient tells lies to fill in the gaps in the memory but he himself is not consciously aware of this.
- Peripheral neuropathy.

The Wernicke–Korsakoff syndrome may occur in nonalcohol-dependent people sometimes, such as chronic malnutrition, patients undergoing bariatric surgery, or undergoing dialysis. The underlying cause is vitamin B_1 (thiamine) deficiency, and the treatment is also thiamine supplementation.

HERPES SIMPLEX ENCEPHALITIS

This encephalitis is caused by herpes simplex virus. It usually damages the frontal and temporal lobes of the brain. Sometimes HSE is mistakenly diagnosed as a case of functional psychiatric disorder, as initially it may present with psychiatric symptoms. There is usually necrosis, hemorrhage, and gliosis of the affected brain areas.

The clinical feature is usually characteristic of acute encephalitis, with fever, seizure and altered sensorium. But in a good number of cases, psychological features are the initial presentation. Sometimes, it is some behavioral oddities, at other times frank psychotic features. They are due to the involvement of frontal and temporal lobes.

Persons who recover from the acute phase sometimes develop amnestic syndrome. This is due to the fact that medial temporal lobe is often affected in HSE. Sometimes they develop Kluver–Bucy like syndrome. Kluver–Bucy syndrome is typically seen after damage to bilateral anterior temporal lobes of the brain. The symptoms are hypersexuality, hyperorality, hyperphagia, visual agnosia, and docility.

Diagnosis of HSE is done by polymerase chain reaction (PCR) to detect the HSE virus in the cerebrospinal fluid (CSF). The EEG shows periodic lateralized epileptiform discharge (PLED). MRI brain shows hyperintensity in T2 images in the temporal and frontal region.

Herpes simplex encephalitis is treated with the antiviral drug acyclovir. Many a time, the treatment is started empirically, because the diagnostic confirmation by PCR of CSF HSE virus is time consuming and prognosis of patients if they remain untreated is poor. However, many patients who recover from the acute phase are left with post-HSE sequelae, e.g., cognitive impairment, seizure, etc.

NEUROPSYCHIATRIC ASPECTS OF EPILEPSY

Epilepsy means recurrent (more than one) unprovoked seizure. A seizure is the excessive, hypersynchronous, disorderly discharge of neurons in the brain, which is self-limited and which is associated with some behavioral manifestation. Seizure type is classified as generalized and focal or partial. A generalized seizure is a seizure where the discharge is simultaneously recorded from both the cerebral hemispheres and a focal seizure is where the discharge is recorded to arise from one part of one cerebral hemisphere. A focal/partial seizure can be simple or complex, depending upon whether the sensorium is altered or not. In case of complex partial seizure, the sensorium is altered but in simple partial seizure it is not. Altered sensorium is manifested by either unawareness of the surrounding and unresponsiveness to external command or with subsequent amnesia. In case of generalized seizure, there is always loss of consciousness. The partial seizure, particularly the complex partial seizure, is more important from the perspective of psychiatry as many psychiatric manifestations are commonly associated with complex partial seizure. Though the complex partial seizure may originate from any of the four lobes of brain, yet the seizures that arise from the temporal lobe and frontal lobe are more important from the psychiatric point of view.

The common interfaces of psychiatry and epilepsy are many:
- Neuropsychiatric problems associated with epilepsy
- Seizure phenomenon which can present as psychiatric problems
- Pseudoseizures—they present like seizures but are not true seizures.

Neuropsychiatric Comorbidities of Epilepsy

Cognitive Impairment and Epilepsy

Some epileptic patients become cognitively impaired. Likewise, persons suffering from intellectual disability have higher prevalence of epilepsy. The reasons for cognitive impairment in epilepsy are myriad. The underlying brain pathology may be the common etiology of both cognitive impairment and seizure. Recurrent seizures itself can cause cognitive impairment. Some antiepileptic drugs such as topiramate, phenobarbitone may cause cognitive dulling.

Patients having cognitive impairment in epilepsy are said to be suffering from epileptic encephalopathy. The epileptic encephalopathy may be static, where the cognitive impairment remains stable over years or progressive when there is gradual deterioration of the cognitive functions with passage of time. Some of the progressive epileptic encephalopathies are:

- West syndrome
- Lennox–Gastaut syndrome
- Dravet syndrome
- Landau–Kleffner syndrome.

The details of these syndromes may be had from any standard neurology textbook.

Psychosis

It may be postictal, where the psychosis occurs after an attack of seizure or it may be interictal, where psychosis occurs in between fits, without any preceding seizure. The psychotic symptoms may be like schizophrenia. The treatment of interictal psychosis is antipsychotic agent with low seizure precipitating potential like risperidone or haloperidol. In case of postictal psychosis, usually the treatment is controlling the seizure only.

Depression

Another common psychiatric comorbidity of epilepsy is depression. Recently, it has been postulated that there is a bidirectional relationship of depression with epilepsy. That means those with epilepsy have increased chance of developing depression and also patients suffering from depression are more prone to develop epilepsy. Depression in epilepsy is associated with increased suicidal risk. The treatment is mainly selective serotonin reuptake inhibitors (SSRI). They are effective as well as carry a low seizurogenic potential.

Seizure Manifestations as Psychiatric Symptoms

Some psychic symptoms may present as aura in simple or complex partial seizure. They are:

- *Dysmnesic symptoms:* Patients present with déjà vu (feeling of familiarity in unfamiliar setting) or jamais vu (feeling of unfamiliarity in familiar setting).
- *Cognitive symptoms*: Presenting with feeling of unreality of the environment (derealization) or self (depersonalization).
- *Hallucinations:* Visual, auditory, gustatory, olfactory, or tactile all types of hallucinations can occur.
- *Affective*: Fear and joy are the emotions the patients may feel; sometimes one feels orgasmic pleasure also.

Seizure and Pseudoseizure

Another common problem one has to face in clinical practice is dissociative fits (previously known as hysterical fits). It is very important to differentiate true fits from this type of pseudoseizures. The points, which are helpful clinically, are:

- In dissociative fits, the semiology or the presentation is nonstereotyped, that means in different episodes they present with different types of fit.

- Dissociative fits usually last much longer than true seizures. True seizures rarely exceed 3–5 minutes whereas dissociative fits can last up to several hours.
- The loss of consciousness and amnesia are usually not total in dissociative fits. Many a time, the patient says that he can hear what other people are talking but cannot himself speak.
- Dissociative fit is usually not associated with self-injury or incontinence, and commonly does not occur in sleep.
- Sometimes, the dissociative fit can be precipitated by suggestion.

But sometimes, it is very difficult to distinguish between true seizure and dissociative fit, and then one has to take the help of video EEG, which is the gold standard for differentiating the two.

The mainstay of treatment of dissociative fit is psychotherapy, but sometimes, psychopharmacological help is needed for associated depression or anxiety.

HUMAN IMMUNODEFICIENCY VIRUS AND NEUROPSYCHIATRIC DISORDERS

Human immunodeficiency virus/acquired immunodeficiency syndrome (HIV/AIDS) is a disease, which was discovered for the first time in 1980 in USA and in 1986 in India. It has proved to be a real menace for human race. As per the 2016 WHO report, there are 36.7 million cases suffering from HIV infection, of which majority are in the sub-Saharan Africa. In India, about 21 lakh people are living with HIV/AIDS, but the good news is that HIV epidemic in India is showing a downward trend recently. Among those people living with HIV/AIDS (PLWHA) in India, 88% of patients contacted the disease through heterosexual route of infection. Only north east states of India have more transmission through using of infected needles in intravenous drug users (IDU). Other routes of contacting infection are vertical transmission from mother to child and contaminated blood transfusion.

Recently HIV/AIDs have changed from being a fatal disorder to a chronic treatable condition. As a result PLWHA are living longer with the highly active antiretroviral therapy (HAART). Many of such persons are having neuropsychiatric sequelae. Psychiatry is very important for both prevention and treatment of HIV/AIDS patients. As the transmission of infection is very much related with the most pleasurable human act and also related to high-risk behavior patterns among people, so the prevention can only be done through psychological maneuvers.

The three most common neuropsychiatric problems associated with HIV/AIDS are:

1. Depression
2. Delirium
3. Dementia

Depression

Depression is a very common psychiatric problem associated with HIV/AIDS. The prevalence varies from 25 to 40% in different studies. If depression is not properly treated, it contributes to the problem of non-adherence to treatment. In HIV/AIDS treatment, adherence is a very important issue as 95% adherence is the minimum level needed for successful suppression of viremia. Depression also leads to other maladaptive and destructive behavior like substance use and suicide.

The psychosocial issues such as bereavement, stigma, fear of death, feeling of guilt along with disease, and drug-related factors, all contribute to the development of depression. The two common drugs, which are used in HIV/AIDS and can commonly produce depression, are efavirenz and interferon.

The suicide risk among PLWHA is also higher and disclosure of the positivity and initiation of HAART are the two trigger points that can lead to suicide. Stigmatization, bereavement, occupational, and financial problems are other important causes for triggering suicide. And of course depression is very important as we know that about 15% of depressed patients commit suicide.

The treatment of depression in HIV/AIDS is with drugs that have better tolerability and low drug-drug interactions. SSRIs like sertraline or escitalopram and other drugs like mirtazapine are commonly used. The drug treatment should be properly supported with psychosocial therapies.

Delirium

Delirium is also another common problem associated with HIV/AIDS. About 40–50% of AIDS patients have one episode of delirium. Delirium is associated with increased mortality among HIV/AIDS patients.

The common causes of delirium in HIV/AIDS are:

- Opportunistic infections
- Toxoplasmosis
- *Cytomegalovirus* infection
- *Cryptococcus* infection
- Progressive multifocal leukoencephalopathy (PML)
- Tuberculosis
- Malnutrition
- Electrolyte imbalance
- Substance intoxication/withdrawal.

Management should include treatment of specific causes, supportive treatment, and control of psychiatric problems.

Dementia

Neurocognitive disorder in HIV/AIDS has been classified in three groups:

1. *Asymptomatic neurocognitive impairment (ANI):* Here there is very subtle change in cognitive function without any interference with self-care or occupational functioning.
2. *Mild neurocognitive disorder (MND):* It is like MCI.
3. *HIV-associated dementia (HAD):* Here the person fulfills the criteria for dementia.

Dementia is a late manifestation of HIV/AIDS. Higher viral load, female sex, lower educational level, and older age are a few risk factors for development of HAD. The CD4 count is usually below 200/cmm.

The dementia is typically of subcortical variety with the typical triad.

- Movement disorder
- Memory impairment and psychomotor speed impairment
- Depressive symptoms

HIV-associated dementia is a poor prognostic predictor in HIV/AIDS and a good number of patients die within 6 months of diagnosis of HAD. The treatment of HAD is HAART with symptomatic management of other problems.

MOVEMENT DISORDER AND PSYCHIATRY

Basal ganglia and cerebellum were once thought to be the organs responsible for movement and coordination only. Now it has been proved beyond doubt, they are very important organs for cognitive and affective functions also. Psychiatric problems are now recognized as one of the major manifestations of movement disorders. Moreover, on the reverse side, antipsychotic drugs used to treat psychotic disorders can give rise to different movement disorders as their side effects.

Drug-induced Movement Disorders

There are several types of drug-induced movement disorders. They are acute dystonia, Parkinsonism, akathisia, and tardive dyskinesia. There is some temporal relationship between their onset and initiation of the antipsychotic drug. Acute dystonia occurs within hours to days, Parkinsonian symptoms occur within days to weeks, akathisia occurs within weeks to months, and tardive dyskinesia occurs within months to years. As these will be discussed in detail in the chapter of psychopharmacology, it will not be discussed further in this section.

Wilson's Disease

Wilson's disease or hepatolenticular degeneration is an autosomal recessive disorder. Though rare, it is important from the point of psychiatry, as many a times the disease presents with behavioral manifestations. The gene that encodes for Wilson's disease is ATP7B, and is located on chromosome 13. Mutation in the gene results in impaired elimination of copper, leading to deposition of copper in liver, basal ganglia, cornea, and other organs. Depending upon which organ is more affected the manifestation varies. The importance of the disorder is that if diagnosed early, it can be treated successfully to prevent the deterioration.

The clinical features of Wilson's disease are movement disorders like dystonia, tics, rigidity, choreoathetoid movements, tremor, ataxia, etc. The psychiatric manifestations are personality changes, cognitive impairment, depression, and psychotic features. Any child who shows some movement disorder associated with some psychiatric manifestation should be screened for Wilson's disease without fail to prevent a catastrophic outcome.

Liver involvement in Wilson's disease may lead to cirrhosis and hepatic encephalopathy.

Diagnosis is done through slit lamp examination of eye, to detect Kayser–Fleischer (K-F) ring. K-F ring is almost invariably found in the neurological variant of Wilson's disease, so K-F ring is an easy screening test for Wilson's disease. Other tests for Wilson's disease are estimation of serum ceruloplasmin which is low in case of Wilson's disease and estimation of 24-hour urinary copper excretion which is high.

The treatment of Wilson's disease is zinc, and copper chelating agents like penicillamine and trientine.

Parkinson's Disease and Psychiatry

Parkinson's disease is a very common neuro-degenerative disorder leading to involuntary movements. Though it is primarily a movement disorder, recently there is growing body of evidence showing that nonmotor symptoms are common and responsible for the disability associated with PD.

There are four cardinal features of PD:
1. Bradykinesia
2. Rigidity
3. 4–6 Hz resting tremor
4. Postural instability

Among all these features, bradykinesia has been given more importance than other features for the diagnosis of PD. Diagnosis of PD is made if bradykinesia is associated with at least one more cardinal feature. Parkinsonian symptoms are present in other disorders apart from PD. If there are early autonomic features, early cognitive impairment, supranuclear gaze palsy, or repeated history of stroke with stepwise progression, PD is unlikely to be a diagnosis. The tremor is most manifest when the body part is in resting state; it starts from one side of the body and gradually becomes bilateral within an average of 18 months. The other tremor which is also found in PD is postural tremor, but action tremor is not a feature of PD. The rigidity is typically of cogwheel variety, because of associated tremor. There is associated gait abnormality; typically the gait is festinant, the person walks with a stooped posture, with gradually increasing speed, as if he is going to catch his center of gravity. The gait abnormality and associated postural instability may result in repeated fall with resultant injury.

The psychiatric disorders associated with PD are:

- Depression
- Psychosis
- Cognitive impairment.

Depression in Parkinson's Disease

Depression occurs in 30–40% of PD patients. As psychomotor retardation is a common feature of depressive disorder, and PD is also associated with bradyphrenia (slowness of mentation) and bradykinesia, there are some overlaps of clinical symptoms. So many a times, one disorder may be mistakenly diagnosed for other one.

There is no linear relationship with the clinical stage of PD and depression. Female sex, right hemi-Parkinsonism, and past history of depression have been found to be the risk factors for depression.

Antidepressants like SSRIs or tricyclic antidepressants (TCAs) are effective in treating depression in PD. One should be cautious of the associated anticholinergic side effects and orthostatic hypotension when treating with TCA.

Psychosis in Parkinson's Disease

Psychosis in PD is a tricky situation as treating psychosis with antipsychotics may increase the Parkinsonian symptoms, and some anti-Parkinsonian drugs may precipitate psychotic symptoms.

Visual hallucinations are common, they are usually well-formed and complex. Auditory hallucinations are also not uncommon. Delusion of theft, infidelity, and one's house is not his own are the common types of delusions. Increasing cognitive impairment is a common accompaniment of psychotic symptoms. Dopamine agonist drugs like pramipexole and bromocriptine are notorious for giving rise to psychotic symptoms.

The treatment is with antipsychotic drugs having low extrapyramidal symptoms (EPS) potentials like quetiapine and clozapine. The dose is usually very small. Pimavanserin is a new drug which holds promise for treating psychosis in PD.

Cognitive Impairment in Parkinson's Disease

Parkinson disease dementia is another problem in PD. This is usually a late presentation in PD. If cognitive impairment occurs early in PD then one would have to question the diagnosis of PD. The dementia is typically of subcortical nature.

CONCLUSION

Organic brain syndromes are a group of disorders of great significance to psychiatry. They originate in the pathology of brain but manifest with mental and behavioral symptoms. They are placed higher in the hierarchy of psychiatric diagnosis. They have to be ruled out first before making a psychiatric diagnosis. Dementia, delirium, and amnestic syndromes are the three major diagnostic categories included in this group. Epilepsy and movement disorders are two entities which fall in the borderland between neurology and psychiatry, which require insights from both disciplines for proper understanding and management.

TAKE-HOME MESSAGES

- Medical and neurological disorders as a cause of psychiatric syndromes are very important and therefore must be ruled out first.
- Impairment of consciousness, orientation, memory, and control over sphincters are important distinguishing features of organic brain syndromes.
- Aphasia, agnosia, apraxia, and disorders of executive functions are other important indicative features.
- Alzheimer's disease, FTD, and VaD are three important types of dementia. Dementia is akin to chronic brain failure leading to gradual downhill course.

- Mild cognitive impairment is in between dementia and normal aging. Certain percentage of MCI cases do progress to dementia. Others, either remain static or revert back to normalcy.
- Delirium is the acute variant of brain failure manifesting primarily with impairment of attention, lowered sensorium, and fluctuating course. It is almost always secondary to a medical or surgical illness.
- Epilepsy may be associated with a psychiatric syndrome as ictal, postictal, or interictal phenomena. Epilepsy has to be distinguished from pseudoseizure based on detailed description of semiology.
- The major neuropsychiatric syndromes associated with HIV/AIDS are depression, delirium, and dementia.
- Parkinson's disease, Wilson's disease, and drug-induced movement disorders are three important conditions where a psychiatric syndrome and movement disorder are found to coexist.

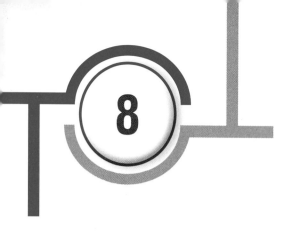

Substance-related Disorders

Atul Ambekar, Piyali Mandal

INTRODUCTION

Alcohol and other psychoactive substances induce change primarily in mental functioning. These substances are used voluntarily by people to experience a change in their mood, cognitive functions, and perception or for achieving pleasure. Repeated consumption of these substances or drugs can cause "addiction" or dependence. At a later stage, the primary purpose of substance use is to avoid or reduce the bodily discomfort resulting from the absence of the psychoactive substance (i.e. "withdrawal") rather than seeking pleasure. As per International conventions, certain psychoactive substances have been listed under the category of the "narcotic drugs" and "psychotropic substances".

Some psychoactive substances are legally allowed for trade and consumption within a country and hence are called licit substances. Alcoholic beverages and nicotine (tobacco) are considered licit in most of the countries. In certain parts of India, consumption of alcohol is illegal. On the other hand, the substances for which trade and consumption are strictly prohibited (for nonmedical and nonscientific purpose) are called illicit (or illegal) substances. Many narcotic drugs (such as heroin, ganja, charas, cocaine, etc.) fall in this category.

The World Health Organization (WHO) lists substance use disorders for the following classes of substances:

- Alcohol
- Opioids (opium, heroin, morphine, pethidine, buprenorphine, codeine, etc.)
- Cannabis ("ganja", "bhang", and "charas")
- Sedative—hypnotics ("tranquilizers")
- Cocaine
- Other stimulants, including amphetamines and caffeine
- Hallucinogens [e.g., lysergic acid diethylamide (LSD), "acid"]
- Tobacco
- Volatile solvents (typewriter correction and dilution fluids, kerosene, gasoline, petrol, paint thinners, nail-polish removers, etc.) and other organic hydrocarbons (e.g., those in shoe polish, iodex, etc.)

Of these, the common and major substances used in India are alcohol, tobacco, opioids, cannabis, tranquilizers, and recently, volatile solvents.

Common substances of use are briefly described below:

Alcohol: Among all the psychoactive substances known to humankind, alcohol is the oldest and most popular one. The active ingredient is ethyl alcohol (ethanol). Absolute concentration of alcohol varies depending upon the type of drink (**Table 8.1**). Because

Table 8.1: Types and concentration of alcohol.

Types of alcohol	Concentration (%)
Beers (standard)	4–8
Beers (strong)	8–11
Wines	5–13
Distilled spirit (whisky, vodka, gin, etc.)	40
Arrack/country/*desi*	33

Table 8.2: Blood alcohol concentration (BAC) levels and the corresponding acute effects of alcohol.

BAC (in mg/dL)	Acute effects
40–80	Elevation of mood, feeling relaxed, able to talk freely, hand and leg movements may be clumsy, while alertness is reduced, and the users believe themselves to be alert
>80	Users becomes noisy and moody, judgment may be impaired, and driving ability is impaired (with risk of accidents)
100–200	The vision gets blurred, gait becomes unsteady, and users talks loudly though the speech is slurred. Behavior changes like quarrelsomeness, aggression are observed. Motor coordination affected grossly
200–300	*The Blackout phenomena:* Person is unable to remember the experiences when they were drunk
>300	May result in coma, and with further increase in levels, even death may occur

of these variations, therefore, the standard practice is to measure amount of alcohol in "standard units", where 10 mL of absolute alcohol constitutes one standard unit. For comparing different beverages, the common "rule of thumb" is, one standard drink = ½ bottle of standard beer = ¼ bottle of strong beer = 1 glass (125 mL) of table wine = 1 drink (30 mL) of spirits.

The level of alcohol in the blood (i.e., blood alcohol concentration or BAC) determines the physical and mental effects on the person drinking alcohol. These are given in **Table 8.2**.

Opioids: The poppy plant (*Papaver somniferum*) is one of the well-known plant in many parts of the world, which provides opium the prototype opioid. Substances which act like opium in the human body are called "opioids". They have been classified into three broad categories—(1) Those occurring naturally (morphine and codeine); (2) Those produced by modification of natural opioids—"semi-synthetics" (heroin, oxycodone); and (3) Those that are not produced from natural substances but produced synthetically, though they mimics the pharmacological action—"pure synthetics" (fentanyl and methadone). Opium is legally cultivated in some states of India, for its medicinal value.

Upon consumption, opioids initially produce an unpleasant feeling to a naïve user. However, if people continue to use the opioid, they experience a short-duration intense state of pleasure and euphoria called "rush" immediately after they take opioids. Opioids are excellent analgesics (the reason why they are used as pain killers). They also produce decreased responsiveness to the environment—a dream-like state. At very high doses, severe intoxication may occur leading to decreased breathing and even death ("overdose").

Heroin is a common opioid, used by smoking, chasing (inhaled), or injecting (intramuscular or intravenous routes). Opioid medications (analgesic or cough suppressants) are also sometimes used for intoxication or pleasure. These include morphine, pentazocine, cough syrups (with codeine), and buprenorphine. Injecting of opioids along with potential risk of spread of blood-borne infections including human immunodeficiency virus (HIV) is a serious public health risk in many parts of India.

Cannabis: Many parts of the world, including many North and Northeast Indian states, are home to the plant *Cannabis sativa*, which produces various preparations of cannabis. "Cannabinoids" are the active chemical compounds in the cannabis. Among cannabinoids, tetrahydrocannabinol (THC) is the most potent. Different types of cannabis products contain different concentration of THC **(Table 8.3)**.

The effect of cannabis varies with blood level of THC. At low dose, cannabis consumption results in euphoria or a state of well-being, experienced as a dreamy state of enjoyment which is usually followed by a phase of drowsiness. Cannabis can impair coordination and thus tasks like driving or operating heavy machinery can be risky even if cannabis is used at a modest dose. Dexterity and hand steadiness are both adversely affected. With an increase in dose, perceptual and sensory distortions may be experienced. Perception of depth is adversely affected. Auditory and visual stimulus appears more intense along with derealization (an unreal feeling about what is seen or heard) and depersonalization (unreal feeling about one's own body). The sense of passage of time gets affected; time appears to pass much slower than it actually does. Some users may experience "bad trip" (restlessness, fear, and panic). Higher doses may result in delirium (confusion), psychosis, and paranoid ideations (unwarranted suspicion) which may be self-limited.

Nicotine: Among active chemical in tobacco, nicotine is the most important one, which is a very common legally and socially sanctioned substance of use. Tobacco is consumed in various forms: Smoking (cigarette, bidi, hookah, etc.) and smokeless (chewable tobacco, snuff, etc.). Nicotine improves alertness and results in better functioning in continuous repetitive tasks. Other reported effects are relaxation and decrease in fatigue with nicotine use. While trying to quit, smokers report irritability, restlessness, anger and frustration, and difficulty in concentration.

Sedatives/hypnotics: These are often prescribed by medical practitioner for anxiety and sleep disorders. Certain medications like alprazolam, nitrazepam, and pheniramine are widely used at a higher dose than prescribed and also for recreational purpose (without prescription) because of their easier availability and cheap price. These may be used either through oral or parenteral route.

Cocaine: Cocaine comes from the leaves of plant *Erythroxylum coca*, which grows wildly in Latin American region. Its use is largely restricted to the Western countries till date and generally very low in India. It is generally snorted, but can also be chewed and smoked.

Table 8.3: Types of cannabis products.

Cannabis products	Origin	Route of consumption	Concentration of tetrahydrocannabinol (mg %)
Bhang	Dried leaves of the plant	Oral, smoking	1–3
Ganja	Dried flowering top	Smoking	6–20
Hashish	Resinous extract of the plant	Smoking	10–20
Hashish oil	Syrup extracted from resin	Smoking	15–30

Cocaine use is characterized by "rush" (7–10 minutes of intense pleasure). Therefore, people use cocaine in "binges" or "runs" where they take it every few minutes to hours, continuously for 3–7 days.

Stimulants: Like cocaine, stimulants also activate the brain to increase alertness, produce euphoria, improve performance, and decrease fatigue. The prototype drug of this group is amphetamine. Collectively, they are also called as "amphetamine-type stimulants (ATS)".

Hallucinogens: Hallucinogens or psychedelics change how a person sees or hears things (i.e., produce hallucinations). The classic example is LSD, consumption of which has been described to make one "see music" and "hear light". Other substances of this group include phencyclidine (PCP) and ecstasy.

Inhalants: Inhalants produce vapor without heating. Majority of them are easily available everywhere like petroleum products glues, thinners, cleaners, solvents, etc. People use them by "huffing", sniffing, or "bagging" (rebreathing from a bag). Upon inhaling them, people experience a rush and sense of well-being. Within 5–6 minutes, there is an urge to reuse. Chronic use of inhalants is associated with brain damage and multiple liver and lung problems. In India, among children (particularly the street children), the use of inhalants as intoxicant is growing rapidly.

As per the medical model of diseases, substance-related disorders are recognized as biobehavioral conditions which manifest as chronic relapsing noncommunicable disease. Hence, treatment for these conditions, like many other chronic non-communicable diseases (viz., diabetes mellitus, hypertension), only modifies and alters the course of the disease. The concept of "cure" in traditional sense does not apply to these.

This chapter of this textbook is intended to address substance-related disorders for each of the major classes of substances of use described in the International Classification of Diseases-10 (ICD-10) mentioned earlier.

EPIDEMIOLOGY

While psychoactive substances are used in most countries of the world, the extent, patterns, and consequences of use differ from country to country and from time to time. In India, traditionally, the legal substances (such as tobacco and alcohol) are widely prevalent while a sizable minority of people also use illegal drugs (like heroin and ganja).

In India, a nationwide epidemiological survey titled "National Survey on Extent, Pattern and Trends of Drug Abuse in India" was conducted in 2004. The National Household Survey (as a part of the National Survey) reported prevalence of current drug use (past 1 month use) of various drugs as: alcohol 21%, cannabis 3%, opiates 0.7%, any illicit drug use 3.6%, injection drug use (ever) 0.1%, and polydrug use 22.3% among males of 12–60 years age. Among them, 16.8%, 25.7%, and 22.3% were estimated to be dependent on alcohol, cannabis, and opiates, respectively. Among people seeking treatment for drug dependence, prevalence of various substance found was: alcohol 44%, cannabis 12%, and opiates 26%. The National Family Health Survey (NFHS) reports increasing trend of alcohol use among men and tobacco use among women (NFHS-2, NFHS-3). As per NFHS-3 (2005–2006), 40% of males (youth) and 5% of women use tobacco in any form. Nineteen percent of the males smoke tobacco and 30% report smokeless tobacco use. Use of tobacco (in any form) and alcohol increase sharply from age 15 to 24 years.

The first nationwide survey "Global Adult Tobacco Survey" India (2009–2010) reported current tobacco use in any form among 34.6% adults (47.9% males and 20.3% females). Among them, 14% and 25.9% adults are current tobacco smokers and smokeless tobacco users, respectively.

Gender and Age

In contrast to most of the other mental-health conditions, substance use primarily affects men but women are also vulnerable. The critical age-group for the onset of substance use is 15–24 years; majority of users initiate substance use in this period. The young people usually start experimenting with substances which are legal, easily available, and have social approval to some extent (such as tobacco, alcohol, and cannabis). Onset of tobacco use may occur at an even earlier age (12–13 years). Usually, boys initiate drug use, earlier than the girls. After using substances like tobacco and alcohol, some of the people using these substances start taking other drugs like cannabis and opioids as well.

Socioeconomic and Cultural Factors

Socioeconomic and cultural factors influence pattern of substance use at an individual level and also at a population level. Religious and cultural practices influence the risk and pattern of substance use. In some cultures in India, home-brewed alcohol use (Northeastern states) or opium (Rajasthan) use is acceptable.

Comorbidity

Among people using substances, a high prevalence of comorbid psychiatric disorders is found, a phenomenon also known as "dual diagnosis". Some studies have even shown that up to 50% of the substance users have a psychiatric comorbidity. These comorbid disorders include other substance use disorders, antisocial personality, mania, schizophrenia, depression, and anxiety disorders.

ETIOLOGY

Substance use disorders are best understood as biopsychosocial disorders. It is a brain disease wherein the voluntary drug using behavior transforms into a compulsive behavior due to change in the structure and neurochemistry of the user. Multiple etiological factors have been implicated for the development of substance use disorders. They can be broadly divided into internal (biological) and external factors (environmental).

Biological Factors

Genetics

Most of the information available on genetics of substance-related disorders relates to alcohol. Family studies show history of parental drinking poses higher risk of drinking in offspring. Twin studies show that the concordance rate of alcohol use disorders in monozygotic twins is almost two times higher than that of dizygotic twins (58% vs. 28%). Adoption studies, assessing the rates of developing substance use disorders among children of alcohol using parents, have reported that the rate of development of this disorder was four times higher among children with alcohol using biological parents than nonalcohol using biological parents, thus establishing the contribution of genetic factors.

Neurobiology

Some of the neurobiological mechanisms of developing dependence on substances are common across different class of substances and some are specific to each category. The "brain reward system", which is implicated in the etiopathogenesis of substance use disorders, is discussed below.

Animal experiments and neuroimaging studies done on human subjects suggest that primary brain reward pathway responsible for drug seeking behavior appears to be a subset of the mesolimbic projections originating from the ventral tegmental area (VTA) and terminating in the nucleus accumbens (NA). Disturbances of the dopaminergic reward system lead to the increased vulnerability to drug-taking behavior.

Reinforcing effect of psychoactive substances is largely mediated by dopamine. Animal experiments suggest that the reinforcing is largely mediated by dopamine release in the subcortical regions, particularly at NA. The axonal terminal projections are considered the major site where the substances produce their rewarding effect. These terminals are heavily innervated and modulated by synaptic inputs from gamma-aminobutyric acid (GABA)ergic, gluta-minergic, serotonergic, opioid peptidergic, and other neural systems.

Craving is found to be linked to the concentration of dopamine and endorphins in NA and hippocampus. Craving for cocaine and stimulant has been linked to change in level of dopamine concentration and craving for alcohol has been linked to change in levels of endorphin and serotonin.

Psychological Factors

Concept of Self-medication

A model of "self-medication" as an etiological factor in substance use has been proposed. As per this model, many people take drugs to actually try to counteract their "painful feelings". In this light, drug acts as a kind of medication, helping the users to alleviate their emotional problems. By this principle, chronic cannabis users may be seen as self-medicating for anxiety problems. Alcohol may be used to alleviate panic and anxiety. Opioids may be used to control anger and amphetamines to alleviate depression. Cocaine is thought to help overcome fatigue and alleviates depression in some individuals. While such use may provide immediate relief of some symptoms, but in long-term drug use may itself produce other psychiatric illnesses.

Behavioral and Conditioning Factors

Psychologists also see substance use as a "learned behavior" picked up from parents and peers and describe continued use as forms of classical and/or operant conditioning. External and internal cues may play a major role in eliciting drug-related responses. The external cues for drug-seeking behavior come from the environment (e.g., watching an advertisement citing drug use, meeting a drug using friend) and internal cues may be depressed or elevated mood state. These cues get conditioned with substance-related events. Behavioral cues play a significant role in development of dependence to smoking.

Personality-related Variables

Several common personality traits (i.e., patterns of feeling and behaving in particular situations) have been observed in people who take up and continue using drugs. "Low frustration tolerance" and "sensation seeking" are by far the most studied of them. People with low frustration tolerance seek to avoid immediate pain at the cost of long-term stress and defeatism. They take drugs to escape to the simple and inevitable problems of daily life. Sensation seeking, on other hand, focuses on the need for new and varied experiences through risky behavior. Doing things at the spur of the moment without consideration of outcome (impulsivity) and nonconformity to social, rules and norms are integral part of their lives. Many substance users also suffer from inability to experience pleasure from usually pleasurable activities (anhedonia) or understand their own emotions (alexithymia) and therefore require a stronger "high" to feel pleasure. Such personality traits have been postulated to maintain substance use in affected persons.

Environmental Factors

Social/Cultural/Legal Factors

Initial experimentation with substances (irrespective of the type of substance) is influenced by cultural factors, social attitudes, peer behavior, laws, drug cost, and availability. After onset, continued use is influenced by social and environmental factors. However, for the development of dependence, individual vulnerability and psychopathology are probably more important determinants. A substance user is often in conflict with family and authority resulting in pushing him further to the accepting drug using peer group. Legal and policy issues not only govern the availability of drugs, but also often result in more stigmatization of drug users.

Drug-related Factors

All psychoactive substances are not equally addictive. Substances which give more intense pleasure and act quickly are likely to be used repeatedly. Similarly, drugs which give more distressing withdrawal symptoms are more addictive. Thus, it is possible to remain an occasional user of alcohol throughout the life for most alcohol users. Heroin on the other hand provides so much of euphoria upon use and so much distress upon nonuse in a dependent person, that a person has to use it repeatedly.

Additionally using substance through inhalation or parenteral route increases its addictive potential, as compared to using it orally. With parenteral routes, drugs reach the brain within seconds, producing intense pleasure. Within a few minutes, this intense "high" fades, taking the user down to lower, more normal levels. It is believed that this low feeling drives the substance user to repeated drug use to repeatedly attain the pleasurable state.

A major role in initiation and continuation of use is played by availability and social sanction of a particular drug. The very fact that socially sanctioned drugs like alcohol and tobacco are the drugs which are used first indicates that availability plays major role in initiation. Studies have shown that for alcohol and tobacco, to certain extent, consumption has gone down whenever their price has increased.

These factors are not mutually exclusive and development of dependence is usually a result of complex interplay of these factors. Someone may have a genetic vulnerability, due to which he is predisposed to substance use disorders. This individual finds himself in an environment where a substance (say alcohol) is easily available and he also has many alcohol using friends. He may initiate taking alcohol due to pressure by his friends, and after finding that it is pleasurable and reduces his anxiety, may continue to drink. Then, after long periods of continuous use, his body may become physically dependent on alcohol (i.e., in absence of alcohol, he would experience distressing withdrawal symptoms). Now in order to relieve these symptoms as well as to continue experiencing pleasure, he will continue to drink and would ultimately suffer from alcohol dependence.

CLINICAL FEATURES OF SUBSTANCE USE DISORDERS

Individuals with substance use disorders have a variety of combinations of the clinical features described below. However, the clinical picture of the substance use disorder is best understood alongside the consequences produced by its use. Various stages of substance use are described below.

- *Initiation*: People start using substances for a variety of reasons. The common reasons for initiation are experimentation, peer pressure, to experience pleasure, to allay anxiety symptoms, relieving pain, etc.
- *Progression*: From initial infrequent pattern of use, people progress to regular use. The rate and pattern of progression depend upon individual vulnerability, the abuse potential of the substance being used, its availability, and various other such factors. Time taken to become dependent user varies with individual and across substances. Various physical and psychosocial complications start appearing with continued use.
- *Abstinence*: This is a stage when an individual quits substance use. A period of 1 month abstinence is considered clinically significant. Abstinence may be attempted by self (without any assistance) or it may be assisted by medical treatment.
- *Relapse*: Relapse is the process of resumption of previous pattern of substance use after a period of abstinence.

However, all the stages may not necessarily occur in an individual using substances.

The clinical features of substance-related disorders are described below. However, all the features may not be present in an individual at given point of time. To qualify for a categorical diagnosis, one should have a certain number and set of symptoms present within a certain period of time (described later).

- *Craving*: *Craving* is an irresistible urge to use substances, leading to drug-seeking behavior and relapse. It may be spontaneous or induced by the presence of particular stimuli ("cue-induced" craving).
- *Withdrawal*: A cluster of signs and symptoms appear due to cessation of use or after reduction in the amount of consumption of drug. They are often accompanied by a maladaptive behavior change and cause some clinically significant impairment in important areas of functioning. Withdrawal signs and symptoms vary across different class of substances **(Table 8.4)**. Severity of withdrawal is usually related to the amount, duration, and pattern of the substance.
- *Intoxication*: Intoxication produced by a substance is defined as unwanted physiological or psychological effects causing maladaptive behavior (e.g., acute drunkenness in alcoholism, bad trip due to hallucinogens). It is a transient phenomenon which gradually disappears with time and appears only on further use. It is closely related to the dose of the substance. Many psychoactive substances produce various effects at various blood levels (e.g., alcohol).
- *Tolerance*: Almost all of the psychoactive substances that are associated with the development of dependence induce variable degree of tolerance. Tolerance may be physical and behavioral. Physical tolerance is a process in which there is gradual diminution of the effects of a substance consumed at a particular dose, thus creating a need for increasing the dose to get the desired pleasurable

Table 8.4: List of withdrawal symptoms of some common category of substances.

Alcohol withdrawal: Mild
• Anxiety
• Restlessness
• Sleeplessness and tremulousness (peripheral)
• Craving
• Palpitation
• Sweating
• Breathlessness
	Alcohol withdrawal: Severe
	• Known as: "Delirium tremens"
	  – All features of mild withdrawal
	  – Disorientation (unawareness of self and
	    surroundings—time, place, and person)
	  – Hallucinations
	• Seizures (fits—"rum fits")

Opioid withdrawal: • Dilatation of pupils of eyes • Watering from eyes, nose • Vomiting • Loose stools • Generalized body ache • Anxiety, restlessness, and insomnia • Premature ejaculation	*Cannabis withdrawal*: • Nonspecific • General discomfort • Intense craving • Anxiety, restlessness • Sleeplessness
Stimulant withdrawal: • Lethargy • Hypersomnia/sleepiness • Fatigue/sad mood • Craving • Anhedonia	

effect/intoxication, e.g., a person having started with two drinks of whisky to obtain pleasure, has to consume four drinks of the same to obtain the same amount of high with continued use over a period of time. The phenomenon of cross-tolerance also needs to be understood; after developing tolerance for a brain depressant (such as alcohol), people are likely to experience a similar reaction to another brain depressant (such as benzodiazepines). Thus, a person who is tolerant for alcohol and has been drinking heavily needs a higher dose of benzodiazepines for inducing sleep.

For certain substances, users develop more pronounced tolerance to the toxic and aversive effects than the tolerance to the pleasurable and enjoyable effects. For instance, many users develop tolerance to nausea and vomiting associated by opioids, but continue to experience euphoria.

While experiencing the effects of substance, people may learn to perform tasks effectively. This is behavioral tolerance (e.g., ability to walk in normal gait despite higher level of BACs). Phenomena like pharmacokinetic tolerance have been described with reference to long-term alcohol use. This involves adaptations of the alcohol metabolizing enzymes (e.g., alcohol dehydrogenase). The pharmacodynamics or cellular tolerance is the phenomenon where despite high blood concentrations, the nervous system gets adapted for maintaining its function.

HEALTH HAZARDS AND ADVERSE CONSEQUENCES

Substance use is associated with array of adverse health consequences. These may occur even after single use (e.g., road traffic accidents in intoxicated state, accidental arterial injection while injecting drug

Table 8.5: Physical complications of long-term substance use.

Psychoactive substances	Physical complications of long-term use
Alcohol	• *Gastrointestinal*: Fatty liver, alcoholic hepatitis, cirrhosis, esophagitis, acute gastritis, pancreatitis, and malabsorption • *Nutritional deficiencies*: Thiamine, pyridoxine, vitamin A, folic acid, and ascorbic acid • *Hematological disorders*: Anemia, leukopenia, and thrombocytopenia • *Cardiovascular system*: Cardiomyopathy, hypertension • *Central nervous system*: Wernicke–Korsakoff syndrome, dementia, and cerebellar degeneration, peripheral neuropathy, and myopathy • *Metabolic disorders*: Ketoacidosis, hypoglycemia, hypocalcemia, and hypomagnesemia • *Miscellaneous*: Fetal alcohol syndrome, osteoporosis, tuberculosis, psoriasis, and domestic and traffic accidents • *Malignancies*: Oral, esophagus, colon, hepatocellular, and breast (women)

Opiates	• *Related to parenteral drug use*: Cellulitis, thrombophlebitis, endocarditis, septicemia, hepatitis B and C, acquired immunodeficiency syndrome (AIDS), and pulmonary hypertension
	• *Related to inhalation (chasing)*:
	  – Recurrent chest infection
	  – Chronic bronchitis
	  – Pulmonary tuberculosis
	• Poor immune status
	• Nutritional deficiencies
	• Overdose (accidental, deliberate)
	• Accidental injury during intoxicated state

Cannabis	Not associated with any significant medical complications per se. There is a greater likelihood that individuals who use cannabis regularly, might come into contact with drugs with far greater health consequences with regular use of cannabis
Tobacco • Smokeless tobacco • Smoking tobacco	• Oral ulcers • Submucous fibrosis • Oropharyngeal malignancies • Chronic bronchitis • Recurrent chest infection • Lung malignancy

use). The long-term hazards depend upon individual vulnerability and pattern of substance use. The long-term health hazards are listed in **Table 8.5**.

Substance-induced Psychiatric Features

Certain psychoactive drugs can induce psychiatric syndromes (e.g., cannabis-induced mania, alcohol-induced depressive symptoms, alcoholic hallucinosis, and alcoholic jealousy) apart from producing dependence, harmful use, intoxication, or withdrawal. These induced psychiatric disorders often remit within a short period of abstinence from the substance.

They also produce various other psycho-social complications **(Table 8.6)**.

DEFINITIONS AND DIAGNOSES

The WHO (ICD-10) has provided guidelines to make uniform diagnosis for substance-related

Table 8.6: Psychosocial complications of substance use.

Familial	Social	Occupational	Financial	Legal

Conflicts
Inability to
perform
responsibilities
	Social isolation
	decreased
	social
	reputation
		• Absenteeism
		• Loss of skill
		• Loss of job
			• Financial
			  obligations not
			  fulfilled
			• Exhausting
			  savings
			• Selling properties
				• Involvement in illegal activity
				  to procure money for drug use
				• Breaking laws (drunken driving)
				• Drug-related crime (procuring
				  and storing, selling illegal
				  substances)
				• Imprisonment

disorders. Professionals are expected to make a diagnosis by demonstrating the presence of a certain number of diagnostic criteria out of the larger group. Diagnostic categories which could result from use of substances listed earlier are provided below.

Intoxication

As per the ICD-10, intoxication is diagnosed when there are disturbances in the level of consciousness, thought, affect and perception, or behavior. There is scope to further specify which of several common complications of intoxication (e.g., trauma, delirium) are also present. There are also specific sets of diagnostic criteria for intoxication for each of the drug categories. Diagnosis of intoxication with multiple drugs can be made if the generic criteria for intoxication have been met. Intoxication may be indicated as uncomplicated or having associated with the following conditions like—medical complication, trauma, delirium, perceptual disturbances, coma, and convulsion.

Harmful Use

The ICD-10 uses the category of harmful use as a state that constitutes a pattern of substance use that is causing damage to physical or mental health. The diagnosis requires an actual evidence of damage and absence of concurrent diagnosis of the

substance dependence syndrome for the same class of the substance.

Dependence Syndrome

The criteria for substance dependence syndrome have been developed based upon the criteria provided by Edwards and Gross (1976) for the diagnosis of alcohol dependence, which have been applied to diagnose all classes of substance dependence.

Dependence syndrome has been defined as "a cluster of physiological, behavioral, and cognitive phenomena in which use of a substance or a class of substances takes on a much higher priority for a given individual than other behaviors that once had greater value". Dependence is diagnosed when three or more of the following are exhibited at some time during the previous 1-year period:

▪ Tolerance
▪ Physiological withdrawal state
▪ The capacity to control substance use is impaired in terms of its onset, termination, or level of use as evidenced by the substance being often taken in larger amounts or over a longer period than intended, or by a persistent desire or unsuccessful efforts to reduce or control substance use. Thus, an individual may find it difficult to avoid using substances at particular place or time or also to limit oneself to a particular predetermined amount

- Preoccupation with substance use, as manifested by important alternative pleasures or interests being given up or reduced because of substance use, or a great deal of time spent in activities necessary to obtain, take or recover from the effects of the substance
- Continued use in spite of clear evidence of harmful consequences, as evidenced by continued use when the individual is actually aware, or may be expected to be aware of the nature and extent of harm
- Strong desire to use substance (craving).

While, the criteria (1) and (2) are physiological, while criteria (3), (4), and (5) are psychological. Thus, the diagnosis of dependence requires presence of symptoms in both physiological and psychological domains. It should be noted that the criteria for dependence syndrome exist in degrees of severity and are not an all-or-none state.

Once the diagnosis of dependence is made, it may be further specified as below:

- Currently abstinent
- Currently abstinent, but in a protected environment
- Currently on a clinically supervised maintenance or replacement regimen (controlled dependence)
- Currently abstinent, but receiving treatment with aversive or blocking drugs
- Currently using the substance (active dependence)
- Continuous use

Withdrawal State

Withdrawal is usually associated with the dependence syndrome, but not necessarily so. When the general criteria for diagnosing withdrawal have been fulfilled, specific criteria from each category of drugs are to be used. The withdrawal state may be complicated by convulsion or delirium [e.g., delirium tremens (DT)].

Substance-induced Disorders

Many substances may induce psychiatric syndromes and memory disturbances apart from producing dependence, intoxication, or withdrawal. It may be classified into seven subtypes depending upon the symptom profile (e.g., schizophrenia like, predominantly hallucinatory, predominantly depressive symptom, etc.). Amnestic syndrome characterized by chronic and prominent memory impairment of recent memory with preserved immediate recall and occasional loss of remote memory is found among long-term heavy alcohol users.

MANAGEMENT

The guiding principles for management of all psychoactive substance use disorders are similar. However, treatments for different class of substances may vary as the therapeutic agents and complications associated vary across different class of substances. Management also depends upon the pattern and severity of addiction, physical and psychiatric comorbidity, and physical and psychosocial complications in a given individual.

There are several approaches to treat substance use-related disorders. These include pharmacotherapy, psychosocial therapy (behavior therapy, counseling, cognitive therapy, and psychotherapy) or a varying combination of these depending upon an individual's need. The most effective treatment programs involve several types of professionals which include doctors (general physicians and psychiatrists) and often psychologists, counselors, and social workers and combine several array of therapies and other services for comprehensive management. Apart from the professionals community leaders, spiritual leaders and even lay volunteers and ex-patients may play an important role in the treatment process. However, most patients of the substance use disorders can be managed by the general physicians.

Goals of Treatment

Treatment goals are set depending upon the patient profile and may need to be reformulated as the treatment progresses. The most important goal of treatment is quitting substance use (achieving abstinence) along with improvement of physical, psychosocial, and occupational functioning and quality of life.

However, in many cases, the goal may be "harm reduction" wherein the aim of the intervention is the reduction of harmful health, social and economic consequences of continued substance use. Here, the most damaging consequences pertaining to an individual or society is the immediate priority rather than achieving abstinence. Here are few examples of "harm reduction" intervention:

- Providing knowledge and education regarding adverse health consequences
- Reducing the risk of transmission of communicable diseases related to drug use (avoidance of sharing during injection drug use, avoiding injectable route for drug use)
- Avoiding hazardous situations of substance use (such as drunken driving).

Stages of Management

Comprehensive management of substance use problem is done in a phased manner **(Table 8.7)**. Progression to subsequent stages depends upon the individual case profiles.

Table 8.7: Stages of management.				
Stages of management	Duration (average)	Goals	Modalities	Professional involved
Initial	2–4 weeks	• Management of acute intoxication, overdose, and withdrawal • Management of imminent psychosocial crisis (e.g., in-patient admission for homeless patient) • Decline of craving • Initiate restoration of health • Damage	• Pharmacological • Psychological intervention (e.g., motivational interviewing)	• General medical practitioner • Psychiatrists • Psychologists
Middle	3–6 months	• Management of medical and psychiatric comorbidity and reintegration with family	• Pharmacological agents • Psychological intervention	• Psychiatrists • Psychologists
Late	>6 months	• Relapse, prevention, and reintegration into the society • Rehabilitation and improvement in quality of life	• Pharmacological agents • Psychological intervention • Occupational rehabilitation	• Psychiatrists • Psychologists • Psychiatric social worker • Community leaders

Treatment Setting

The treatment for substance use can be provided at various settings such as:

- Specialized treatment setting
- General hospital setting
- Community clinic setting.

Treatment can be rendered both in outpatient and inpatient settings. However, majority of patients can be treated in outpatient settings only. Inpatient treatment is indicated in cases with higher severity of addiction, acute psychosocial crisis (homelessness, abandoned by family), severe physical complications related to substance use, and medical or psychiatric comorbidity. However, basic guiding principles remain same across settings.

Assessment

In general, substance use behaviors form a part of the "personal history", when physicians obtain history of any patient presenting to them. However, in case of substance use disorders, it is the symptoms related to substance use which bring a patient to the physician. The purpose of assessment is to formulate a diagnosis and management plan. A detailed assessment needs to be done at the initial stage. The components of assessment are listed in **Box 8.1**.

Identification/Screening

In treatment settings other than specialized centers, it is a challenge to identify individuals who do not actively seek treatment for substance use problem per se and the

---

Box 8.1: Components of assessment.

- Identification/screening
- Clinical history taking
- Physical examination
- Mental state examination
- Investigations

---

individuals who may seek treatment for problems which are apparently unrelated to substance use, but may have problems with substance use. Brief screening for all attendees in such settings, like a general medical setup, emergency rooms, trauma centers, psychiatric setting, and antenatal checkup or in a legal setup (e.g., prison wards) may improve identification of cases with substance use problem. Screening for various complications associated with problem of drug use is also an essential part of assessment.

Brief questionnaires and interviews with high degree of sensitivity have been developed to identify substance use problem in a relatively short period of time. Such questionnaires have simple questions with a "yes/no" or a "mostly true/not true" type answers. The brevity and simple format of these instruments make them suitable for use in busy settings like primary care or emergency room. Some common screening tests are:

- *CAGE*: For assessing alcohol problems; an acronym of four questions
- *ASSIST*: Alcohol, Smoking and Substance Involvement Screening Test
- *AUDIT*: Alcohol Use Disorders Identification Test
- *MAST*: Michigan Alcohol Screening Test
- *DAST*: Drug Abuse Screening Test.

Choosing one of these instruments depends on the type of population and the setting and where these are to be used. However, even without using these structured instruments, clinicians can ask some simple and basic questions to all patients to explore the history of problems with substance use. While interviewing a patient with such problems, it is important to avoid a judgmental attitude and instead to adopt an empathic approach.

Clinical History Taking

Components of clinical history taking are listed below in **Box 8.2**.

Physical Examination

To look for:

- Evidence of intoxication, withdrawals, and route of drug use (e.g., injection marks in case of injection drug use (IDU)]
- Evidence of physical damage due to drug use or medical comorbidity.

Mental State Examination

To rule out presence of any induced psychiatric syndromes or comorbidity, a full Mental State Examination would require to be done, which has been dealt in a separate chapter.

Investigations

Investigations serve two purposes in drug use treatment.

- Confirmation of presence/absence of substance within body or validation of self-report (e.g., alcohol breath test, thin layer chromatography for other substances)
- Identify and measure physical damage caused by substances (complete blood count, liver function test, etc.)
- Monitoring of blood parameters as prerequisite for pharmacotherapy (liver function test in patients on disulfiram, naltrexone).

The investigations provide an objective measure of the substance used and the extent of health damage. The findings of the investigations are utilized in formulation of management plan and also to enhance motivation of individuals who does not accept their drug use as a problem.

Treatment Modalities

Irrespective of the nature of substance being used, there are two treatment modalities:

1. *Pharmacological treatment*
2. *Psychosocial interventions.*

Pharmacological Treatment

The pharmacotherapy is aimed at:

- Reversing the acute effects (such as intoxication, overdose, and toxicity)
- Relief of withdrawal symptoms
- Reduction of craving
- Relapse prevention
- Restoring the physiological functions.

Pharmacotherapy can be broadly divided into two phases:

1. Short-term treatment (also known as detoxification)
2. Long-term treatment (maintenance).

Detoxification: Pharmacotherapy plays the major role in this phase of treatment. This phase is aimed at reversing the acute effects and providing relief from withdrawal symptoms. Additional health consequences arising out of substance use, medical, and

---

Box 8.2: Components of clinical history taking.

- Patient's sociodemographic profile
- Details of drug use
- Complications associated with drug use
- *High-risk behaviors*: Such as injecting drug use with needle sharing and risky sexual practices
- Details of past abstinence attempts
- *Nature of treatment in the past*: Pharmacological, psychological, or combined
- Reason for previous relapse/s
- Reason for treatment seeking and level of motivation
- Psychiatric illnesses such as mood disorder, psychotic disorder, and personality disorder/traits
- Presence of family history of substance use disorder (SUD), psychiatric illness, and the current living arrangements
- Extent of available social support

psychiatric comorbidity are also managed at this phase.

The ideal way to achieve detoxification is through abrupt discontinuation of drug use and providing specific medications to reduce withdrawal symptoms. Another (less preferred) approach is by gradually tapering off the drug being used. The purpose is to minimize subjective and objective discomfort as this is an important reason for relapse.

Choice of medications for detoxification: Following kind of medications are useful for detoxification **(Table 8.8)**:

▪ Those with cross-tolerance to the substance of use, e.g., benzodiazepine for alcohol and buprenorphine for opioid withdrawal
▪ Those with specific pharmacological properties to suppress withdrawal, e.g., carbamazepine for alcohol withdrawal, clonidine for opiate withdrawal
▪ Those which provide symptomatic relief, e.g., hypnotics (benzodiazepine as well as nonbenzodiazepines, antiemetics, antidiarrheals, etc.).

In general, antipsychotic or antiepileptic medications are not recommended for treating drug withdrawal.

Dose of medications for detoxification: The doses of medicines for detoxification depend upon the expected severity of withdrawal symptoms. This, in turn, depends upon the substance used (potency, half-life), duration since the last intake, severity of dependence (duration, usual amount, route of use, etc.) use of other drugs concomitantly, comorbid general medical or mental disorder, and individual biological and psychological factors.

Long-term pharmacotherapy: This stage intends to facilitate maintenance of the stage of abstinence after the initial phase of detoxification, with the use of prescribed pharmacological agents. The medications used for maintenance can be classified into

Table 8.8: Agents for detoxification.

Substances	Mechanism of action/purpose			
	Cross-tolerance	Suppression of few withdrawal symptoms (no cross-tolerance)	Symptomatic treatment	For complicated withdrawal
Alcohol	• Oral long-acting benzodiazepines (diazepam, chlordiazepoxide) • Lorazepam is preferred for patients with alcoholic liver disease	β-blocker	–	Parenteral benzodiazepines
Opioids	Buprenorphine (sublingual)	A-2 adrenergic agonist (clonidine)	Antidiarrheals, hypnotics	–
Benzodiazepine	Oral long-acting benzodiazepines	–	–	–
Nicotine	Nicotine gum, lozenges, and transdermal patches	–	–	–

Table 8.9: Pharmacological agents for long-term maintenance treatment.

Types of agent	Types of substance	Examples
Deterrent	Alcohol	Disulfiram
Anticraving		Acamprosate, fluoxetine, and naltrexone
Agonist	Opioids	Methadone, buprenorphine
Antagonist		Naltrexone

Box 8.3: Steps for management of delirium tremens (DT).

- Immediate hospitalization
- *Treatment of choice*: Intravenous benzodiazepines
- *Doses*: Diazepam 10 mg every 20 minutes, till sedation achieved or withdrawal symptoms subside. Further doses of diazepam (oral or intravenous) depend upon the reemergence of withdrawal symptoms
- *Supportive treatment*: Injectable thiamine; correcting dehydration and electrolyte imbalances
- *Environment*: Calm and quite, protective
- Attempts for reorienting the delirious patients (DT usually responds to treatment within 2–3 days, though patients usually need hospitalization for few more days)

four categories **(Table 8.9)** based on their mechanism of action.

EMERGENCIES IN SUBSTANCE USE DISORDER

Emergencies may arise in cases of substance users which may be due to drug overdose, severe withdrawal or accidents, and injuries occurring in intoxicated state (drunken driving).

The victims of emergencies related to substance use often arrive at an emergency setting in general hospital settings of various levels (primary to tertiary care). Hence, a routine enquiry regarding substance use preferably using the screening questionnaire to all trauma cases should be done. Routine drug screen should also be done in these cases. The physicians attending the emergency treatment setting should have knowledge of the signs and symptoms of intoxication and withdrawal of various psychoactive substances.

- *Drug overdose*:
  - *Cannabis intoxication (bad trip)*: Cannabis intoxication may be associated with dysphoria, restlessness, and fear and even panic attack which is known as "bad trip". For providing quick relief from psychotic excitement, quick parenteral antipsychotics are useful. Delirium rarely occurs in neurologically intact individuals. If psychotic symptoms persist beyond 1 or 2 hours, a psychiatrist should be consulted.
  - *Opioid intoxication*: Overdose of opioids (suicidal or accidental) is a medical emergency. The classic triad of opiate intoxication or overdose is—(1) pinpoint pupils, (2) depressed respiration, and (3) coma. In such cases, immediate intravenous naloxone (0.4 mg) can be lifesaving.
- *Severe withdrawal (e.g., DT)*: DT or impending DT is also an emergency (with mortality rates of 20–25% in untreated cases and 5–10% with treatment). The steps for management of DT are provided in **Box 8.3**.

PSYCHOSOCIAL INTERVENTIONS

Pharmacotherapy needs to be supplemented with a variety of psychological and social interventions. Brief therapies may include single-session counseling and motivational enhancement. In specialized treatment settings, therapies which are complex and time-consuming like family and marital therapy and network therapy may be carried out to promote abstinence and healthy lifestyle. Creating a strong patient-therapist relationship, therapeutic alliance, and better communication with the patient and family are other important tasks. Such approaches are very effective for enhancing treatment compliance.

Motivation to reduce or stop using substances is a dynamic, ever-changing process. The first step in the treatment of poorly motivated substance user is "motivation enhancement". The three critical elements of the variable nature of motivation are: that a person is (1) *Ready to change*, (2) *Willing to change*, and (3) *Able to change*. People may be able to change, but may not be willing, because of poor motivation. Thus, the purpose of therapist is to help the patient become ready, *willing*, and able for change. This style of counseling is needed not only for enhancing the motivation in initial phase, but during the long-term treatment also.

As described in the earlier section, all substance users are not *dependent user*, but may fall into the category of *harmful use*. There is evidence that many of the substance *harmful users* may not require very intensive treatment, but can be helped by less intense psychosocial interventions. One such category of interventions is—brief intervention (BI).

Brief intervention is mostly employed in the primary care settings and for providing help to the treatment nonseekers. These counseling sessions are short (5–20 minutes), focused and seek identification of problems (real or potential), and motivate the patient to take action. The sessions are based on motivation enhancement, as described above.

The nonjudgmental and nonconfrontational technique of motivational interviewing strives to deal with the specific problems that patients face at any particular stage. Through these techniques, patients are helped to start thinking differently about their drug use and considering whether a change of behavior will be beneficial for them.

Before achieving lasting recovery, patients may go through short cycles of abstinence → relapse → abstinence for a long duration. Patient, family members, and the therapists are required to have considerable patience during the process of treatment.

Once the substance user achieves abstinence, the goal shifts to maintaining the drug-free status. Relapse prevention, a psychological technique which discusses strategies, which help the patient maintaining the abstinence over time. The patient is made to understand that recovery and relapse are a process and lapsing to occasional drug use does not indicate failure of treatment. The patient is also taught to identify high-risk relapse factors and social pressures of drug use and trained to employ strategies to deal with them. Involving family and significant others in the treatment is encouraged.

Self-help approach is another treatment modality, where people with similar problems come together to form "self-help" groups for providing mutual help to each other. These voluntary, self-sufficient groups provide mutual assistance to all their members. Classical examples of self-help groups include "alcoholics anonymous (AA)" and "narcotics anonymous (NA)" which are active in many parts of the world. Such groups have also been developed for family members, friends, and children of drug and alcohol users.

Another approach, the "social correctional approach", looks at drug and alcohol use as a deviation from social norms for which correctional methods are applied in residential settings. Therapeutic community (TC) is the classic example of this concept. However, evidence regarding effectiveness of these approaches is very limited.

OUTCOME

Assessment of Outcome and Effectiveness of Treatment

Traditionally, treatment success has been measured by abstinence. Nowadays, overall improvement in functioning in various dimensions of the patient's life (familial, economical, and legal) is given more importance than abstinence alone. Research studies suggest that longer therapeutic contact, retention in treatment, and more comprehensive the treatment package, better is the outcome. Detoxification alone in isolation has been found not to change the outcome and in fact may be detrimental by increasing the risk of overdose in opioid dependence. Addition of psychosocial therapies to pharmacotherapy is associated with better outcome than pharmacotherapy alone.

Various parameters for assessment of outcome of substance use disorder treatment are as follows:

- Abstinence
- Reduction in habit size
- Retention to treatment
- Employment
- Stability in housing
- Decrease in crime
- Social support
- Perception of care.

PUBLIC HEALTH ASPECTS

Substance use is a major public health problem that affects the society at multiple levels. Every community is affected by drug use and addiction, directly or indirectly. This not only includes the direct healthcare costs, but also lost earnings and losses associated with crime and accidents.

Stigma and Discrimination

Stigma may pose as a barrier to a wide range of opportunities and rights for the people who use drugs, or are recovering from drug use problem. Stigma is defined as a set of negative beliefs that a society holds about a group of people. Individuals using substances may suffer from social rejection, labeling, and discrimination for their drug use. People who use drugs are less likely to get help than those with mental illness or physical disability. Unfortunately, negative, stereotyped views of substance use are also prevalent among healthcare professionals. Stigma is also a major impediment for treatment seeking and completion of treatment.

From a public health perspective, effective intervention strategies target the host (substance user), agent (drug and related factors), and environment (supportive environment). Such strategies can be incorporated within the various stages of "behavioral health continuum of care". This model consists of four stages: (1) Promotion, (2) Prevention, (3) Treatment, and (4) Recovery.

For implementation of various strategies, involvement of various agencies, communities, and stakeholders is needed. The components of effective treatment strategies are as follows:

- Provision of treatment in various settings (emergency, community, etc.)
- Outpatient treatment setting
- A referral system from primary to tertiary care settings

- Alliance and synergy with other health programs
- Utilization of community resources for effective control of environment.

CONCLUSION

Substance use disorders are biopsychosocial disorders with significant public health burden. All physicians are expected to be able to recognize and diagnose the common substance use disorders and provide basic interventions as well as referral to specialists, if required. Effective treatment strategies (both pharmacological as well as psychosocial) exist which can be employed to help a large number of patients suffering from substance use disorders, even in the general healthcare settings.

TAKE-HOME MESSAGES

- Substance use disorders are complex biopsychosocial conditions with a significant public health burden.
- Most commonly used substances in India are tobacco and alcohol. However, a significant number of people also suffer from cannabis, sedative, opioid, and inhalant use disorders.
- Every physician should possess the knowledge and skills to assess and treat/refer patients presenting with common substance use disorders. In all health settings, substance use history should be enquired into and if needed, brief interventions should be provided.
- Physicians should employ an empathetic attitude to patients presenting with substance use problems. A judgmental attitude should be avoided.
- Severe alcohol withdrawal is a medical emergency, which is often unrecognized. However, alcohol withdrawal symptoms can be effectively treated with benzodiazepines.
- Substance use disorders are chronic, relapsing conditions. Most patients require long-term treatment which involves combining pharmacotherapy and psychosocial approaches.
- Most patients of substance use disorders can be treated in the outpatient, non-specialist settings.

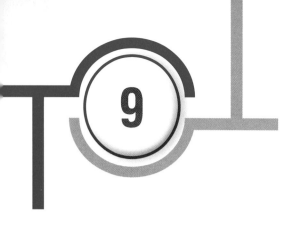

Schizophrenia and Other Psychotic Disorders

R Thara, Aarthi Ganesh, Vijaya Raghavan

INTRODUCTION

Psychotic disorders are a group of major mental illnesses where the person's ability to think rationally, make sound judgment, react appropriately, and communicate effectively, or maintain touch with reality is impaired. This leads to difficulty in maintaining his job and further to significant socio-occupational dysfunctions.

About 1% of the population worldwide suffers from psychotic disorders. These disorders most often first appear when a person is in his or her late teens, 20s, or 30s. However, we see them in children and elderly also. They tend to affect men and women about equally. All the psychotic disorders have certain symptoms in common, i.e., hallucinations, delusions, disorganized or incoherent speech, confused thinking, slowed or unusual movements, loss of interest in personal hygiene, loss of interest in activities, not being motivated to take up or maintain a job, problems at school or work and with relationships, difficulty in expressing emotions, mood swings or other mood symptoms, such as depression or mania.

The most important among psychotic disorders is schizophrenia. Others include acute and transient psychotic disorders, brief psychotic disorder, delusional disorder, schizoaffective disorder, schizophreniform disorder, shared psychotic disorder, substance-induced psychotic disorder, etc.

SCHIZOPHRENIA

Schizophrenia is a brain disorder that affects mental functions and behavior. It is often a chronic illness, which generally starts during adolescence and may persist for lifelong. The illness is associated with a variable course, and outcomes range from complete recovery to severe disability. The most prominent characteristics of schizophrenia are hallucinations, delusions, social withdrawal, and socio-occupational dysfunction. Because onset is usually in late adolescence or early adulthood, schizophrenia and related disorders are a leading cause of disability. There is no laboratory test pathognomonic for schizophrenia; it is diagnosed by the history and clinical presentation.

Historical Perspectives

A good number of historical writings refer to descriptions of the mentally unsound. The classic Indian text Atharvaveda in BC 1,500 termed insanity as *unmada*. Conditions such as *vatanmada, pithanmada*, and *kaphonmada*, corresponding to psychosis and depressive states, have been described by Ayurveda.

Benedict Morel, a French psychiatrist, had used the term "demence precoce" for patients whose illness began in the adolescence and who had a deteriorating course. Kraepelin observed his patients closely over many years and coined the term "dementia praecox" for this condition, which had its beginning in early adulthood, was characterized by hallucinations and delusions, and had a downhill course with intellectual deterioration. He differentiated these patients from those suffering from manic-depressive illness, which was characterized by episodic illness with periods of normal functioning in-between.

Eugene Bleuler in Zurich, Switzerland also found that not all such patients failed to improve. He coined the term "schizophrenia", or a group of "schizophrenic psychoses", which replaced "dementia praecox." He highlighted that in this disorder, there was a schism between the thought, emotion, and behavior of the patient.

Bleuler identified the fundamental or primary symptoms of schizophrenia, which has been summarized as four *A*'s of Bleuler **(Box 9.1)**—association, affect, autism, and ambivalence. He reported that the schisms resulted in disturbances in association, affective disturbances, autism, and ambivalence. Bleuler also identified the accessory or secondary symptoms—hallucinations and delusions.

Kurt Schneider was a German psychiatrist famous for his writing on the diagnosis and understanding of schizophrenia. He observed several patients with schizophrenia and made a statistical analysis of the symptoms. Following this, he described the first-rank symptoms of schizophrenia **(Box 9.2)**. These symptoms are not specific for schizophrenia but are definitely useful for making a diagnosis of schizophrenia. The other symptoms described can be referred in **Boxes 9.3 and 9.4**.

Epidemiology

Prevalence and Incidence

Understanding the prevalence of schizophrenia has implications for planning of policies and programs as well as studying epidemiology. The prevalence of schizophrenia at any point in time (point prevalence) is around 4.6, while lifetime prevalence is 4 per 1,000. There are no significant gender differences. It has always been held that the prevalence all over the

Box 9.3: Second-rank symptoms.

- Other disorders of perception
- Sudden delusional ideas/delusional notions
- Perplexity
- Depressive and euphoric mood changes
- Feelings of emotional impoverishment

Box 9.4: Third-rank symptoms.

- Other abnormal modes of expressions, e.g., disorders of speech
- Other motor manifestations

world is almost the same, though the rates have been found to be higher in developed countries and in the migrant population. It may also be higher in people living in deprived environments and some ethnic minorities. The incidence rate of schizophrenia all over the world is around 0.5 per 1,000. The debate whether it is different in the third world is ongoing with contradictory opinions.

Etiology

The etiology of schizophrenia is still largely obscure. Even though decades of research have not produced major breakthroughs, gradual progress has been made in identifying risk factors and etiologic process. While the debate on whether schizophrenia represents a single disorder or a syndromal diagnosis with heterogeneous etiologies is still unresolved. Many biological, psychological, and social theories have been proposed to understand this complex disorder.

Biological Theories

Genetics: A risk for schizophrenia has a definitive genetic basis and is inherited. Decades of twin and family studies have verified this genetic predisposition. It is established that the more closely one is related to an individual with schizophrenia, the greater is the risk for the illness. Worldwide,

the prevalence of schizophrenia in general population is around 1% and has remained stable. Monozygotic twins, who share identical genetic material, have 40–50% risk for developing the illness, while for dizygotic twins, the risk decreases to 17%. This indicates that various other factors such as environment have a significant role in the initiation and progression of schizophrenia. Similarly, the risk changes for other first-degree relatives. For example, while the risk is about 13% for children, it is about 9% for siblings. In a recent meta-analysis, it is observed that a close relative of a patient with schizophrenia has an average 10 times the baseline population risk of the disorder **(Fig. 9.1)**.

Association studies in schizophrenia suggest that schizophrenia is a complex multi-genetic disorder. Schizophrenia does not follow a classical Mendelian inheritance but a complex pattern of inheritance by multiple genes, each having a small effect. Many genes associated with the illness have been identified in different studies. Recently, genome-wide association studies (GWAS) has indicated several genes, which may have a role to play in the etiology of schizophrenia such as neuregulin 1 (*NRG1*), dystrobrevin-binding protein 1 (*DTNBP1*), and disrupted in schizophrenia 1 (*DISC1*).

Biochemical hypothesis: One of the major theories of schizophrenia is the biochemical hypothesis. This hypothesis is the result of the successful treatment of schizophrenia with antipsychotic drugs, which act on different neurotransmitters in the brain. This implicates that schizophrenia could be due to aberrant neurotransmission systems—in particular, aberrant dopaminergic, seroto-ninergic, and glutamatergic systems. But it is still unclear whether these changes in the neurotransmitters reflect primary rather

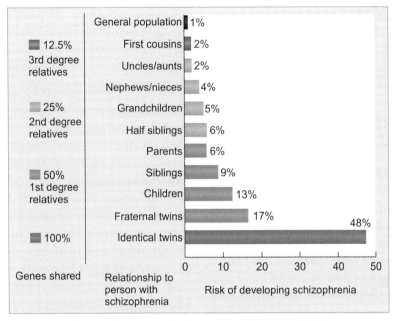

Fig. 9.1: Genetics and schizophrenia (*Gottesman, 1991*).

than secondary pathology, compensatory mechanisms, or environmental influences.

- *Dopamine neurotransmitter*: The classical "dopamine hypothesis of schizophrenia" postulates a hyperactivity of dopaminergic transmission at the dopamine D2 receptor in the mesencephalic projections to the limbic striatum. This is supported by a tight correlation between the therapeutic doses of conventional antipsychotic drugs and their affinities for the D2 receptor. Moreover, indirect dopamine agonists (e.g., L-dopa, cocaine, and amphetamines) can induce psychosis in healthy subjects. Many postmortem and positron emission tomography (PET) studies have strengthened the notion that dopamine dysregulation as a central feature in schizophrenia by showing increased dopamine D2 receptor levels in the brains of individuals with schizophrenia. Recently, presynaptic dopaminergic abnormality has been identified in schizophrenia, implying dysfunction in presynaptic storage, vesicular transport, release, reuptake, and metabolic mechanisms in mesolimbic dopamine system.

- *Serotonin neurotransmitter*: Serotonin (5-HT) is the next major neurotransmitter that has been implicated in the etiology of schizophrenia. The "serotonin hypothesis of schizophrenia" gets support from several observations of different studies. For example, serotonin receptors are involved in the psychotomimetic and psychotogenic properties of hallucinogens [e.g., lysergic acid diethylamide (LSD)]. Similarly, the number of cortical serotonin receptors (5-HT2A and 5-HT1A) is altered in the brain of schizophrenic patients. Moreover, clozapine, an antipsychotic drug used for the treatment of resistant schizophrenia, has its action through 5-HT2A and 5-HT1A receptors. Serotoninergic and dopaminergic systems are interdependent and may be simultaneously affected in schizophrenia.

- *Glutamate neurotransmitter*: Glutamate is an excitatory neurotransmitter, involved in various normal brain functions, and acts through N-methyl-D-aspartate (NMDA) receptors. Phencyclidine (PCP) and ketamine, both potent non-competitive antagonists of the NMDA subtype of glutamate receptor (NMDA-R), induce schizophrenia-like symptoms in healthy individuals and worsen some symptoms in schizophrenia. Decreased NMDA-R function is found in brains of individuals with schizophrenia. Postmortem studies of individuals with schizophrenia indicate abnormalities in pre- and postsynaptic glutamatergic indices. NMDA-R hypofunction in the cortical association pathways could be responsible for a variety of cognitive and other negative symptoms. Moreover, excitotoxicity attributed due to glutamate neurotransmitter and the consequence of neuronal damage is also found to contribute to schizophrenia.

Neurodegenerative hypothesis: Kraepelin called schizophrenia as "dementia praecox," with a notion that it is a progressive disorder with no recovery possible. Neurodegenerative hypothesis stems from this idea and focuses on the fact that schizophrenia is mostly characterized by a chronic and progressive course, resulting in biochemical changes that lead to different clinical syndromes, reflecting the loss of neurological function and subsequent deterioration of behavior. The finding that the psychosis almost always emerges in late adolescence or early adulthood when the prefrontal cortex is still passing through developmental stage, strengthens this hypothesis. The observation that this disorder shows a downhill course despite satisfactory treatment also supports the neurodegenerative hypothesis.

Neurodevelopmental hypothesis: The "neurodevelopmental hypothesis of schizophrenia" suggests that abnormalities of early brain development increase the risk for the subsequent emergence of clinical symptoms. Several lines of evidence have been identified to support this hypothesis such as abnormalities of early motor and cognitive development and histories of obstetrical adversity and lack of neurodegeneration in many postmortem brains of individuals with schizophrenia. In this neurodevelopmental model, schizophrenia may be associated with a subtle, early life static brain lesion that is caused by a combination of genetic and/or early environmental factors, which eventually interact with normal maturational processes of the brain to facilitate the emergence of psychotic symptoms. The relatively subtle childhood abnormalities may thus be a period-dependent expression of aberrant neural networks.

Schizophrenia may involve a two- or three-"hit" process in their pathophysiology. This hypothesis suggests that those individuals who are diagnosed with schizophrenia later in life may have their first pathogenic hit during early neurodevelopmental phase (first hit), because of genetic load, adverse embryonic events, or perinatal events; this may further be followed by a second and possibly a third hit arising from hormonal events, excitotoxicity, or free oxygen radical formation leading to further neurodegeneration of other brain regions. This hypothesis emphasizes that the pathophysiology of schizophrenia may thus be related to the developmental process, inclusive of neurite formation, synaptogenesis, neuronal pruning, and apoptosis.

Neuropathological changes in the brain: Neuropathological investigation in schizophrenia is seen as a "graveyard" for pathologist as no evidence of usual features of neurodegenerative diseases such as inclusion bodies, dystrophic neuritis, or reactive gliosis are seen. But subtle cytoarchitectural anomalies in entorhinal gray matter and in other corticolimbic regions and an abnormally high frequency of aberrant neurons in the white matter underlying prefrontal cortex, temporal, and parahippocampal regions are found in the brains of individuals with schizophrenia. Moreover, there is also a reduction in the volume of cortical neuropil without comparable neuronal loss, suggestive of quantitative and qualitative deficits in neuronal processes and synaptic connectivity in schizophrenia. Taken together, these subtle abnormalities point toward neurodevelopmental abnormalities in schizophrenia.

Electrophysiological changes in the brain: The electroencephalogram (EEG) was the first physiological technique used to examine brain activity in schizophrenia and it has now evolved into more robust methodologies such as visual and auditory event-related potentials (ERPs). The most prominent electrophysiological changes observed in schizophrenia are P50, antisaccade, mismatch negativity (MMN), P300, and gamma power and phase measures. In this, P300 has been extensively studied in schizophrenia, which has led to identification of two significant changes when compared with normal controls: P300 amplitude is reduced and there is increase in latency.

Structural and functional changes in the brain: Neuroimaging techniques have contributed significantly to the study of schizophrenia. Earliest neuroimaging findings have demonstrated that there are clear brain structural abnormalities associated with schizophrenia. Structural studies on the postmortem brains of patients with schizophrenia revealed ventricular enlargement and loss of temporal lobe gray matter, although the changes in the brain could be directly attributed due to the disease process or it may also be because of other associated variables such as extensive medication and dietary abnormalities, which might themselves alter brain anatomy.

Recent magnetic resonance imaging (MRI) research has identified brain characteristics associated with the early stages of schizophrenia. This includes deficits in temporal lobe (i.e., gray matter, superior temporal gyrus, and hippocampus), reduced whole brain volume, reduced prefrontal cortical gray matter volume, significant enlargement of lateral and third ventricles, and reduced thalamic volume. Volume reduction is also seen in the superior temporal gyrus, including bilateral Heschl's gyrus gray matter and left planum temporale gray matter, which could account for the deficits in language and thought processing in schizophrenia.

Studies using functional MRI (fMRI) have identified neural structures associated with observed cognitive problems associated with schizophrenia. These studies have highlighted the cortical prominence in cognitive functions and their deficits in schizophrenia. For example, fMRI analysis of working memory tasks revealed reduced activity in frontal areas of the brain such as the dorsolateral prefrontal cortex and the anterior cingulate cortex. Similarly, auditory hallucinatory states are associated with activation in the inferior and frontal insular, anterior cingulate, bilateral temporal cortex (with greater responses on the right), right thalamus, inferior colliculus, left hippocampus, and parahippocampal cortex.

Recently, magnetic resonance spectroscopy (MRS) has been used to measure in vivo metabolite levels in particular regions of the brain in schizophrenia. ^{1}H-MRS studies show increased levels of glutamine and glutamate in frontal lobe voxels, which are associated with illness duration and reduced by atypical antipsychotic drug treatment. Some, but not all, ^{1}H-MRS studies also indicate a decrease in neuronal cell mass in the hippocampal region and the frontal lobes. The results of ^{31}P-MRS suggest decreased synthesis and increased degradation of membrane phospholipids in prefrontal cortical regions and medial temporal lobe structures at certain phases of schizophrenia.

White matter dysconnectivity hypothesis: Recently, schizophrenia is hypothesized as a "disconnection" disorder and its symptoms are thought not to be due to a single, regionally specific pathophysiology but to abnormal interactions between regions. Evidence from postmortem brain tissues has shown that anatomical connectivity might be pathologically changed in schizophrenia. Major aberrant connectivity is observed from the prefrontal cortex (PFC) to other brain regions such as the parietal cortex, temporal regions, and regions in the default mode network.

Studies involving diffusion tensor imaging (DTI), a new and powerful tool to explore the anatomical connectivity in the human brain in vivo, have shown significant reductions in the left frontal and left temporal deep white matter. Fiber tracking showed that the main tracts involved are the cingulum bundle (CB), the left inferior longitudinal fasciculus, the left inferior fronto-occipital fasciculus, and the interhemispheric fibers running through the corpus callosum. These findings show the disrupted anatomical connections in the frontolimbic circuitry in schizophrenia. These abnormal functional interactions form the basis for several cognitive deficits in schizophrenia such as working memory, attention, and task shifting.

Neuroinflammatory theories: Recent research has highlighted the role of neuroinflammation in schizophrenia. High levels of proinflammatory substances such as cytokines have been described in the blood and cerebrospinal fluid of individuals with schizophrenia. Moreover, infection during early life could trigger immune activation leading to lifelong increased immune reactivity. For example, a large epidemiological study clearly demonstrated that severe infections and autoimmune disorders are risk factors for schizophrenia. Similarly, genetic studies have shown a strong association for schizophrenia with chromosome 6p22.1, a region related to the human leukocyte antigen (HLA) system and other immune functions. Another line of evidence demonstrates that chronic stress is associated with immune activation. Immune alterations influence the dopaminergic, serotonergic, noradrenergic, and glutamatergic neurotransmission. Further support for the inflammatory hypothesis comes from the therapeutic benefit of anti-inflammatory medication. Meta-analyses have shown an advantageous effect of cyclooxygenase-2 inhibitors in early stages of schizophrenia. Moreover, antipsychotic medications have intrinsic anti-inflammatory and immunomodulatory effects.

Neuroinfection theories: Prenatal exposure to influenza, elevated toxoplasma antibody, rubella, genital-reproductive infections, and other infections have been associated with an increased risk of schizophrenia among offspring. This is supported by animal models revealing that maternal immune activation causes phenotypes analogous to those found in patients with schizophrenia. Since the exposure to microbial agents is either preventable or treatable, interventions to diminish the incidence of infection during pregnancy have the potential to prevent an appreciable proportion of schizophrenia cases.

Neuroendocrine theories: Recent research has evidently shown that the environmental factors play an important role as risk factors for schizophrenia. Especially, the environmental stress acts through two biological pathways namely—hypothalamic–pituitary–adrenal (HPA) axis and the sympathetic nervous system. These have a profound impact on the course and outcome of schizophrenia. The evidence suggests individuals with schizophrenia can experience both hyper- and hypofunction of the HPA axis. Moreover, this could contribute to poor physical health and premature mortality suffered by people with schizophrenia, in particular the high rates of cardiovascular and metabolic disturbance.

Psychological Theories

Psychoanalytical theories: Schizophrenia is conceptualized to result from a regression to the oral stage of psychosexual development, when the ego has not emerged from the id. Since there is no distinct ego, individuals with schizophrenia lose contact with the world. Lack of interpersonal relations and libidinal attachment is attributed to their heightened sensitivity to criticism of their behavior. By trying to adapt to the demands of the id impulses as well as the necessity to have contact with some external stimulus, symptoms of delusions, hallucination, and other thought disorders are thought to develop.

Double bind theory: In 1956, Bateson reported clinical evidence suggesting possible pathogenic role of use of double bind communication by parents of schizophrenia patients. It is hypothesized that schizophrenia is a consequence of abnormal patterns of communication in the family. In a "double bind" situation, a person is given mutually contradictory signals by another person. This places the patient in an impossible situation, causing internal conflict. Emergence of schizophrenic symptoms represents an attempt to escape from the double bind.

Social learning theories: According to this theory, patients with schizophrenia do not respond appropriately to the social environment like their normal counterparts. They seem to have a specific deficit of social attention. This leads to patient appearing withdrawn, lack of formation of proper social associations, lack of understanding of one's own role, and difficulty in comprehending role behavior of others. Hence, they create their own social role to protect themselves from social expectations and demands. However, though a split occurs between their outer and inner selves, their hopes, aspirations, etc. in the inner self may still remain intact.

Social Theories

Place of birth and upbringing: There is robust evidence for linking place of birth and risk of schizophrenia. Those who are born and/or raised in urban regions have an increased risk of developing schizophrenia when compared to rural regions. Moreover, place of birth may be a proxy marker for the risk-modifying variables existing in the urban setup. For example, urban factors such as lead exposure, overcrowding, and high stress experienced more in the urban setting could be the underlying factors, which increase the risk of schizophrenia in urban setup.

Migration: In the recent times, markedly increased risk of schizophrenia has been observed in the migrant groups. In a meta-analysis, both the first- and second-generation migrants have shown an increased risk of developing schizophrenia.

Trauma and stress-related exposure: Stress has a major role in the etiology of schizophrenia. Stress experienced at different stages of life could act as a risk factor or trigger for the development of schizophrenia. For example, extreme prenatal maternal stress is associated with adverse health outcomes in the offspring

including schizophrenia. Similarly, there is a relationship between the unwantedness of pregnancy and risk of schizophrenia. A large body of research has shown that childhood trauma such as physical and sexual abuse and neglect is associated with a broad range of adverse consequences, including schizophrenia. Moreover, people who develop psychosis tend to have more life events before the start of the illness.

Classificatory Systems used in Psychiatry

There are two main classificatory systems used in psychiatry. The DSM-5 (Diagnostic and Statistical Manual of Mental Disorders-5) is primarily used in USA. The ICD-10 (International Statistical Classification of Diseases and Related Health Problems-10) is commonly used in other parts of the world **(Boxes 9.5 and 9.6)**.

Box 9.5: The International Classification of Diseases (ICD-10) diagnostic criteria for schizophrenia.

1. One very clear symptom (and usually two or more if less clear cut) belonging to any one of the groups listed as (a) to (d):
   a. Thought echo, thought insertion or withdrawal, and thought broadcasting.
   b. Delusions of control, influence, or passivity, clearly referred to body or limb movements or specific thoughts, actions, or sensations; delusional perception.
   c. Hallucinatory voices giving a running commentary on the patient's behavior, or discussing the patient among themselves, or other types of hallucinatory voices coming from some part of the body.
   d. Persistent delusions of other kinds that are culturally inappropriate and completely impossible, such as religious or political identity, or superhuman powers and abilities (e.g., being able to control the weather, or being in communication with aliens from another world).
   OR
2. *Symptoms from at least two of the groups (e) to (i):*
   e. Persistent hallucinations in any modality, when accompanied either by fleeting or half-formed delusions without clear affective content, or by persistent over-valued ideas, or when occurring every day for weeks or months on end.
   f. Breaks or interpolations in the train of thought, resulting in incoherence or irrelevant speech, or neologisms.
   g. Catatonic behavior, such as excitement, posturing, or waxy flexibility, negativism, mutism, and stupor.
   h. "Negative" symptoms such as marked apathy, paucity of speech, and blunting or incongruity of emotional responses, usually resulting in social withdrawal and lowering of social performance; it must be clear that these are not due to depression or to neuroleptic medication.
   i. A significant and consistent change in the overall quality of some aspects of personal behavior, manifested as loss of interest, aimlessness, idleness, a self-absorbed attitude, and social withdrawal.
3. The above should have been clearly present for most of the time during a period of 1 month or above.

Box 9.6: Differential diagnosis.

Medical and neurological conditions:
- Trauma
- Tumor-ICSOL (intracranial space-occupying lesion)
- Electrolyte imbalance
- *Substance induced:* Amphetamine, hallucinogens, alcohol, cocaine, and phencyclidine
- *Epilepsy:* Temporal lobe epilepsy
- Wernicke–Korsakoff psychoses
- *Infections*: Cerebral malaria, toxoplasmosis, neurocysticercosis, sleeping sickness, neurosyphilis (to assess immune status), SSPE, herpes simplex encephalitis, meningitis, HIV encephalopathy, and paraneoplastic encephalitis
- *Metabolic*: Hepatic encephalopathy, uremia, and acute intermittent porphyria
- *Endocrine*: Thyroid—hypo-/hyperthyroidism, Cushing's disease, hyperadrenalism, insulinomas, pheochromocytoma, and steroid-producing tumors
- *Nutritional deficiency:* Vitamin B1 deficiency and pellagra
- *Medications—common*: Steroids, antibiotics like ciprofloxacin, stimulants like amphetamines, dopaminergic drugs (L-dopa, amantadine), anticholinergic agents, antiarrhythmic drugs, antimalarial (chloroquine and mefloquine), ATT, antiviral, antihypertensive, anticonvulsants, antiarrhythmics, antihistamines, oral contraceptives, chemotherapy drugs (vincristine and vinblastine), opioids, sympathomimetics, interferon
- *Demyelinating diseases*: AML and MS
- *Basal ganglia disorders:* Wilson's disease, Huntington's disease, and Fahr's disease
- *Autoimmune disorders*: SLE—psychosis and seizures are diagnostic criteria. About 10–15% has psychotic symptoms secondary to brain involvement
- *Hashimoto encephalopathy with autoimmune thyroiditis*: Recurrent psychosis
- *Paraneoplastic limbic encephalitis:* Look for tumors
- *Storage disorders:* Tay–Sachs disease and Niemann–Pick disease

Other psychiatric conditions:
- Brief psychotic disorder
- Delusional disorder
- Atypical psychoses
- Mood disorders
- *Personality disorders*: Schizoid, schizotypal, borderline, and paranoid
- Schizoaffective psychoses

(AML: acute myeloid leukemia; MS: multiple sclerosis; SLE: systemic lupus erythematosus; SSPE: subacute sclerosing panencephalitis)

Subtypes of Schizophrenia

The subtypes of schizophrenia has been there in ICD-10, which is listed in **Box 9.7**. However, subtypes of schizophrenia have been removed from DSM-5 and the same is likely to be followed in ICD-11 which is to come in force from January 2022.

Clinical Presentation

The cardinal symptoms of schizophrenia can be broadly divided into two sets; positive and negative symptoms **(Table 9.1)**.

Positive Symptoms

Positive symptoms are the ones, which either appear de novo or are distortions/excesses of

Box 9.7: The International Classification of Diseases (ICD-10) schizophrenia subtypes.

- F20.0 Paranoid schizophrenia
- F20.1 Hebephrenic schizophrenia
- F20.2 Catatonic schizophrenia
- F20.3 Undifferentiated schizophrenia
- F20.4 Post-schizophrenic depression
- F20.5 Residual schizophrenia
- F20.6 Simple schizophrenia
- F20.8 Other schizophrenia
- F20.9 Schizophrenia unspecified

the normally present functions. It can manifest as suspiciousness, hallucinations, and hyperactivity. Positive symptoms occur due to aberrations in perception, hypervigilance, and misattribution of environmental cues.

Table 9.1: Cardinal symptoms of schizophrenia.

Positive symptoms	Negative symptoms
Delusions	Amotivation/anhedonia
Hallucinations	Alogia
Disorganized thinking	Asociality

Delusions: Delusions are firm, false, and fixed beliefs that are held despite information being given to the contrary. The delusions may be in the form of suspicions, which may be directed against one or many people. The person may feel persecuted and feel that someone is out to get him.

> *"My food tastes different.*
> *I think it is poisoned."*

> *"People are following me when*
> *I walk on the road."*

The person may react to these beliefs. He may feel very afraid or become very violent as if trying to protect himself from a persecutor.

Sometimes, the delusions are very grandiose and the person may imagine himself to be a great man or even God.

> *"I am the avatar of Lord Krishna."*

> *"I have been sent on a special*
> *mission to Earth."*

There may be other delusions referring to the individual's body, to physical or paranormal explanations.

> *"My nose is deformed."*

> *"My brain and other organs no longer exist."*

At times, the person is convinced that objects or people are controlling his thoughts and actions.

> *"My movements are being watched and*
> *controlled by a space satellite."*

Hallucinations: Hallucinations are perception in the absence of a stimulus.

The most common type of hallucination in schizophrenia is auditory hallucination, i.e., hearing voices when no one is around. This may be a single voice or multiple voices talking or calling to him, commenting, instructing, and, sometimes, telling them to do distressing things. He may respond to these voices and may be seen as if talking to him. A patient of schizophrenia may report—"I hear a female voice all the time, threatening to kill me."

Other types of hallucinations are visual, gustatory, tactile, or olfactory, which are generally uncommon in schizophrenia.

Disorganization: Disorganization refers to loss of normally present mutual relationship between different component parts of any mental function. It may manifest at the level of thought or behavior. Disorganization is considered a positive symptom. It may present itself as conceptual disorganization, incoherent speech, bizarre behavior, poor attention, inappropriate affect, and difficulty in abstract thinking.

Negative Symptoms

Negative symptoms basically refer to a reduction or absence of functions, which are normally present. It refers to lack of emotional responsiveness, motivation, socialization, speech, or movement. They include blunted affect, emotional withdrawal, social withdrawal, poor rapport with others, and stereotyped thinking. Primary negative symptoms are thought to be etiologically related to the core pathophysiology of schizophrenia, whereas secondary negative symptoms are secondary to either medications or due to depression. Lack of stimulation in impoverished institutional environments can lead to problems with motivation and initiation of productive activities.

Cognition

Cognitive impairment is now being consi-dered to be a core symptom of schizophrenia and not the result of other symptoms or treatment. Cognitive deficits present as impaired attention, poor concentration, and difficulty in carrying out routine activities as before. In some cases, nonspecific symptoms appear and there is a slow change in the person's normal routine, which is an indication of the onset of schizophrenia **(Box 9.8)**. These nonspecific symptoms are termed as prodromal symptoms. Some of the early symptoms are physical and some are behavioral. At times, a combination of these problems may be reported. The most common symptoms reported are sleep disturbances, confusion, reduced attention and concentration, depressed mood, deterioration in functioning, neglect of self-care, muttering or smiling to self, and reporting suspicious ideas. However, sometimes, a sudden development of abnormal behaviors may be the first manifestation of a breakdown.

Schizophrenia in Special Populations

Women

Women tend to have a later age of onset of symptoms. In females, the peak age of onset is from 25 to 32 years. This is thought to be due to the protective effect of estrogen.

Box 9.8: Prodromal symptoms.

- Sleep disturbance
- Reduced attention and concentration
- Reduced drive and motivation
- Depressed mood
- Anxiety
- Social withdrawal
- Suspiciousness
- Reduced role functioning
- Irritability
- Fear

Life events precipitating the onset seem to be more commonly reported by women. Women have a better prognosis and tend to present with more affective features. They are more likely to receive differential diagnosis of affective psychosis and appear to be more susceptible to acute reactive psychosis and schizophreniform disorders. They present as florid and abrupt onset psychotic states and tend to resolve with good outcome.

Elderly

Although most people with schizophrenia have an early onset of the disease, in a minority of patients, the illness first emerges during their middle years, or even after 65 years of age. This is a distinct subset of schizophrenia, which is often referred to as paraphrenia. It is estimated that up to 0.5% of people older than age of 65 years have schizophrenia.

Patients with paraphrenia present for the first time in old age with persecutory delusions, delusions of reference, grandeur, misidentification, auditory, and/or visual hallucinations and Schneiderian first rank symptoms. They tend to have less severe negative symptoms, less cognitive impairment, and a better prognosis. It is more common in women. Sensory deficits including auditory and visual impairment are common. Personality features of suspiciousness, sensitivity, quarrelsomeness, and unsociability are also associated with this disorder.

Children

Childhood-onset schizophrenia is a severe form of psychotic disorder that occurs at age of 12 years or younger. It is often chronic and persistently debilitating. Although the essential features of schizophrenia are the same in childhood also but it is harder to diagnose. Children experience less elaborate delusions and hallucinations than adults. Visual hallucinations are more common in children and should be distinguished from normal fantasy play. Symptoms such as disorganized speech and behavior, which are typically present in schizophrenia, also occur in many disorders of childhood onset (e.g., autism spectrum disorder and attention-deficit hyperactivity disorder). It is important to consider these more common disorders of childhood before attributing such symptoms to schizophrenia.

Course and Outcome

Course refers to the pattern of illness over a period of time, which includes periods of improvements or worsening of symptoms; outcome refers to the endpoint of the illness. In the earlier decades, people believed that people who developed schizophrenia had poor outcomes always, but researches done in subsequent years have clearly shown that this is not the case.

The various patterns of course are depicted in the **Figure 9.2**. Episode refers to the period of illness when the person is symptomatic, remission refers to the period when the patient is symptom free (full remission) or has a few symptoms persisting (partial remission).

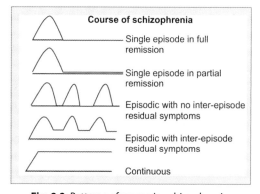

Fig. 9.2: Patterns of course in schizophrenia.

Most people get better with treatment. Some people with one episode of the problem may never have another attack. Many people, however, are likely to have one or more recurrences of the problem. In a small group of patients, especially those who do not respond to medication, the symptoms are likely to persist continuously. The various prognostic factors have been compared in **Table 9.2**.

Assessment of outcome in schizophrenia is multidimensional. Improvement in clinical symptoms and overall functioning of the person are generally considered while assessing outcome. Functioning includes both role functioning at work place, at home, studies, and social functioning. Sometimes, parameters such as quality of life and extent of burden on the caregivers are also taken into account.

International multisite studies have clearly revealed that substantial number of people with schizophrenia may have a favorable outcome and are able to get back to work, get married, and lead a meaningful life. Very broadly speaking, 30% of people diagnosed with schizophrenia have a favorable outcome, 30% have intermediate outcome, and the remaining 30% have a poor outcome. The longer the duration of untreated psychoses, the poorer is the outcome. Hence, the current emphasis is on early identification and intervention. Early intervention improves outcome and reduces disability. This would be possible only if more awareness regarding mental illness is created and people are educated about the illness. The need to treat the person early even when he is in the attenuated psychotic state is very important.

Availability of effective medicines, access to such medicines and to professional mental healthcare, improved community care and enhanced awareness about the illness seem

Table 9.2: Prognosis in schizophrenia.

	Good prognostic factors	Poor prognostic factors
Gender	Female	Male
Marital status	Married	Single
Mode of onset	Sudden onset of illness	Insidious onset
Premorbid status	Premorbidly well adjusted	Poor social and work functioning
Age and duration of untreated psychoses (DUP)	Late-onset and continuous treatment, less DUP, seek treatment early	Young onset and irregular treatment, longer DUP, delay in seeking treatment
Family support	Good family/social support	Poor family support
Employment status	Employed	Unemployed
Family history	Family history of mood disorders	Family history of psychoses, use of alcohol, cannabis, and other addictive drugs
Subtype	Paranoid/catatonic subtype	Other subtypes of schizophrenia
Symptom profile	Mood symptoms	Withdrawn, autistic

to have improved the outcome in a substantial number of persons with schizophrenia.

The famous International Pilot Study of schizophrenia (IPSS) showed that persons with schizophrenia in developing countries had a better outcome than those living in developed nations. This has since then been replicated in several other studies. Why is the outcome better in developing countries? There is still no categorical, final answer to this. It is, however, true that many more persons with schizophrenia in the third world countries have more and longer symptom-free periods. Significantly, fewer persons have continuous illness.

The SOFACOS (Study of Factors Affecting Course and Outcome in Schizophrenia) showed that two-thirds (67%) of people had a better outcome. Another study from Chennai with 25-year follow-up of 90 first episode schizophrenia patients showed that 68% of the out of the original 47 patients who could be assessed at the end of 25 years, were in partial or total remission and only 19% had a poor prognosis. Only five patients were continuously ill during the entire 25-year period. Greater family support and community tolerance, better job opportunities in the unorganized sectors of employment, especially in the rural areas, and ensuring regular intake of medicines by family members could all be playing a part.

Scales to Assess Symptom Severity

Positive and Negative Syndrome Scale (PANSS) for Schizophrenia (Kay et al., 1987): It is made of 30 distinct items organized into three independent subscales (positive, negative, and general psychopathology subscales) with scoring that ranges from 30 to 210 points. It is a "gold standard" in treatment studies of schizophrenia, as it is sensitive to change.

The Brief Psychiatric Rating Scale (BPRS) (Overall and Gorham, 1962): It is a widely used instrument for assessing the positive, negative, and affective symptoms of individuals who have psychotic disorders especially schizophrenia. It is a 24-item symptom scale, which has proven particularly valuable for documenting the efficacy of treatment in patients who have moderate-to-severe illness.

Management

Management of schizophrenia is a challenge for every clinician. There is no preventive measure for schizophrenia. The goals of care are to identify the illness as early as possible, treat the symptoms, maintain the improvement over a period of time, prevent relapses, and reintegrate the ill person in the community to lead a normal life.

There are no laboratory tests, which can diagnose schizophrenia. Different laboratory tests may be required, if any comorbid or contributory organic factors that are presumed to be present. Imaging studies are also done when organic causes are suspected.

Management can be broadly viewed as being short term and long term. Short-term treatment is for symptom management. The major modes of management are pharmacotherapy, psychosocial therapies, electroconvulsive therapy, and psycho-surgery. Medications are started and continued till symptoms remit and then patients are stabilized on a maintenance dose. Owing to poor insight into the illness, medication compliance is an issue faced by the family and treating psychiatrist. Families and patients are educated regarding illness, so that they can cope up with the same and help in preventing relapses. In selected cases, electroconvulsive therapy and psychosurgery may be used. Long-term goals are aimed at reintegrating the patient into the community and at assisting the person in regaining educational or occupational functioning at the earliest.

Drug treatment is a very important component of intervention and must be adhered to, if the patient has to maintain consistent improvement. The most commonly used drugs in the treatment of schizophrenia are known as antipsychotics, neuroleptics, or major tranquilizers. They are further subdivided into two types—typical antipsychotics or first-generation antipsychotics (FGA) and atypical antipsy-chotics or second-generation antipsychotics (SGA). The former has been in use for last about half a century and the latter has been in use mostly for last 2–3 decades. The former are mostly dopamine antagonists (DAs) and latter ones are serotonin–dopamine antagonists (SDAs).

The use of antipsychotic drugs is aimed mostly at controlling the acute symptoms of the illness, suppressing distortions in perception and thinking, and also ameliorating some of the symptoms of the chronic state, such as apathy and social withdrawal. Occasionally, ECT (electroconvulsive therapy) is advised during an acute phase of schizophrenia, but usually in conjunction with drugs **(Tables 9.3 and 9.4)**.

Typical/First-generation Antipsychotics

These include phenothiazines, butyro-phenones, and thioxanthines, which act by blocking the D2 (dopamine) receptor predominantly. There is reliable evidence that in the acute phase of the illness, these drugs are effective in controlling the positive symptoms (delusions, hallucinations, and thought disorder). About 60–75% of patients improve in 6–12 weeks of regular medications.

The common drugs used extensively even now in many developing countries are chlorpromazine, haloperidol, and trifluoperazine. These form the mainstay of treatment, especially in rural areas, where availability of medicines is much less than that in urban areas. They may have certain short- and long-term side effects. Despite

Table 9.3: Antipsychotic classification based on receptor profile.

First-generation antipsychotics (dopamine antagonist): FGA (DA)

Phenothiazines	Chlorpromazine, trifluoperazine, thioridazine, triflupromazine, prochlorperazine, and fluphenazine
Butyrophenones	Haloperidol and trifluperidol
Thioxanthenes	Flupentixol, thiothixene, and zuclopenthixol
Diphenylbutylpiperidines	Pimozide and penfluridol
Dibenzoxazepines	Loxapine
Indolic derivatives	Molindone

Second-generation antipsychotics (serotonin dopamine antagonist): SGA (SDA)

Thio-benzodiazepines	Olanzapine
Dibenzothiazepines	Quetiapine
Dibenzodiazepines	Clozapine
Benzisoxales	Risperidone
Benzisothiazolyl	Ziprasidone
Phenylpiperazine	Aripiprazole
Benzamide	Amisulpride

Table 9.4: Antipsychotic classification based on potency.

Low potency	Antipsychotic effect is seen at a higher dose in mg terms; has lower propensity for extra pyramidal effects, e.g., Chlorpromazine
High potency	Antipsychotic effect is seen at a lower dose in mg terms; has greater propensity for extra pyramidal effects, e.g., Haloperidol and risperidone

side effects, the low cost, wider availability, and years of experience in using these drugs make them still suitable for any psychiatric patients, especially in developing countries.

Atypical/Second-generation Antipsychotics

Drugs belonging to this group are chosen preferentially these days, principally because of their less severe dramatic side effects; they also have the advantage of being more effective against negative symptoms. These include drugs like clozapine, olanzapine, risperidone, aripiprazole, and quetiapine. They have a different side effect profile and also most of them are tolerated better than the drugs of typical group. Their high cost, however, limits their use in most developing countries.

Depot Injection

Apart from being available as tablet and liquid forms, some antipsychotics are also available as injections. Injections may be either in the immediate-release form or depot form. Depots are slow-release formulations of antipsychotics, administered through injections about once every 2-6 weeks. Because of the convenient dosage schedule, many patients can be made compliant much more conveniently with depot injections than with tablets; however, the usual side effects remain. Depot injections of both the first- and second-generation antipsychotics are available. They differ in cost and side effect profile.

Treatment in Acute Phase

Antipsychotic medications have proven efficacy in symptom reduction in acute phase of illness. In choosing an antipsychotic medication for this phase, consideration of tolerability is the key factor. Generally, a rapid phase of improvement lasting for a week to 10 days is followed by a slower phase of improvement continuing for several weeks. Positive symptoms respond better as compared to negative symptoms.

Maintenance

The need for maintenance treatment in schizophrenia is a norm rather than an exception. Intermittent treatment results in increased rates of relapse and need for higher dose of medications for symptoms to remit. Low dose of medicines is often required as maintenance dose for long and variable period, sometimes even for whole life, usually based on the duration of illness. Hence, the emphasis on early diagnosis and intervention is very important.

Role of Electroconvulsive Therapy

Indications for ECT in schizophrenia are:
- Acutely suicidal
- Catatonia
- Treatment refractory schizophrenia
- Schizophrenia with predominant depressive symptoms
- Violent behavior

Side Effects of Antipsychotics

It is very important to be familiar with the side effect profile of various antipsychotics,

because they often require to be taken care of during long periods of treatment of a psychiatric patient. The choice of antipsychotic is also very largely influenced by their side effect profile, because most antipsychotics have equal clinical effectiveness, but have a different side effect profile. Given below is the common side effects produced by antipsychotics.

- *Sedation*: It is a common early side effect of generally low-potency antipsychotics. It is helpful in patients having symptoms of insomnia and agitation.
- *Anticholinergic side effects*: Individuals vary as regards the intensity and location of this side effect. This includes dryness of mouth, constipation, urinary hesitancy, visual blurring, and tachycardia.
- *Dystonia*: It is a reversible extrapyramidal side effect. It is intermittent, spasmodic, or sustained involuntary contractions of axial muscles, mostly of neck, and trunk. It is a cause of intense distress to patient and family.
- *Akathisia*: It refers to a feeling of internal subjective motor restlessness, which manifests generally as continuous pacing by the patient and inability of the patient to keep still. It can also present as tension, nervousness, or anxiety.
- *Other extrapyramidal side effects (EPS):* These may present as rigidity, brady-kinesia, tremor, masked facies, shuffling gait, stooped posture, and sialorrhea.
- Weight gain is another important side effect. The US-FDA defines weight gain as more than 7% increase in total body weight relative to baseline. Abdominal adiposity is typical of antipsychotic associated weight gain. It possibly occurs due to increased levels of serum leptin and imbalance between energy intake and expenditure.

- *Metabolic side effects*:
  - Diabetes and impaired glucose tolerance—possibly occur due to increased plasma lipids, weight gain, leptin, and/or insulin resistance in various combinations.
  - *Dyslipidemia* is an established risk factor for cardiovascular disease, which may appear as side effect, independent of weight gain.
  - *Metabolic syndrome*: It refers to simultaneous appearance of a cluster of features such as obesity, hypertension, hyperglycemia, and dyslipidemia in variable combinations, which is associated with increased chances of adverse health consequences, including cardiac and other vascular events. An easy screening tool for metabolic syndrome is by the measurement of waist circumference and of fasting blood glucose levels.
  - *Hyponatremia* may be because of syndrome of inappropriate antidiuretic hormone (SIADH) secretion or due to water intoxication.
- *Hypertension*: Slow and steady rise of blood pressure over time may be seen.
- *Hyperprolactinemia*: Often it remains asymptomatic but may cause menstrual disturbances, gynecomastia, galactorrhea, sexual dysfunctions, and reductions in bone mineral density and possibly increased risk of breast cancer.
- *Tardive dyskinesia* is an involuntary neurological movement disorder of oro-bucco-lingual and facial muscles; sometimes, muscles of extremities may also be involved. It is generally a chronic condition associated with long-term use of antipsychotics.
- *Neuroleptic malignant syndrome* is a potentially life-threatening reaction to neuroleptic medication characterized by symptoms of high fever, confusion, rigidity, altered blood pressure, sweating, palpitations, etc. Complications may include rhabdomyolysis, renal failure, seizure, or death.

Challenges Faced by Clinician

Choice of antipsychotic medication: CATIE (Clinical Antipsychotic Trials of Intervention Effectiveness) conducted in US was a study designed to examine fundamental issues about second-generation antipsychotic (SGA) medications (olanzapine, risperidone, quetiapine, and ziprasidone), their relative effectiveness, and their effectiveness as compared to a first-generation antipsychotic (FGA)—perphenazine. The UK CUtLASS study (Cost Utility of the Latest Antipsychotic Drugs in Schizophrenia Study) compared the classes of drug, i.e., first-generation versus second-generation drug other than clozapine and other second-generation drug versus clozapine. The primary outcome was quality of life at 1 year and symptoms were the main secondary outcome. The results of both the studies were not what was expected. Both studies showed that the newer drugs were no more effective or better tolerated than the older drugs. Clozapine outperformed other second-generation drugs. Other studies comparing the SGAs and their extrapyramidal side effects have shown that extrapyramidal syndrome remains clinically important even in the era of second-generation antipsychotics. The incidence and severity of extrapyramidal syndrome differ among these antipsychotics, but the fact is that these drugs have not lived up to the expectation regarding their tolerability.

There is no single antipsychotic that is best for every schizophrenia patient, as individual responses differ markedly. Treatment has to be tailor made. More often than not, the side effect profile is taken into consideration before prescribing antipsychotics.

Poor drug compliance: This is a common issue faced by the treating clinician. Not taking medications as prescribed or in the prescribed dose constitutes poor drug compliance. Poor drug compliance can be due to lack of insight, distressing side effects, polypharmacy, financial constraints, poor social support, or simply inadequate health information. At times even the family does not understand the implication of regular medications. This results in frequent exacerbations and relapses.

How to deal with poor drug compliance?
- *Avoid polypharmacy*: The clinician can reduce the number of medications while keeping in mind the dose required for the patient. Polypharmacy can lead to increased side effects and financial burden on families often resulting in poor compliance. At times, patients/families end up choosing one/two out of the whole prescription and mostly the main antipsychotic is left out.
- *Dose timing*: Once a day dosing is ideal, many patients complain about having to take medicines all three times in a day.
- *Pillboxes*: Medicines can be sorted out and kept in pillboxes, so that family can keep a check on the medicines being consumed. However, this is not a foolproof method as patients can take the drugs and discard them instead of consuming them.
- *Depot injection*: Depot injections are a proven method to ensure compliance by the uncooperative patients. Fortnightly or monthly injections are preferred to daily dose of medicines. Clinicians have to be watchful about the increased propensity of such injections to cause EPS.

- *Psychoeducation*: Educating families/ caregivers and the patient regarding the illness and need for continued medications helps in better compliance. Though structured sessions can be conducted, the same can also be done on a regular outpatient basis to empower them with valid information to improve the outcome by augmenting compliance.

Psychosocial Rehabilitation

Psychosocial rehabilitation (PSR) is a process that facilitates the opportunity for individuals who are impaired or disabled by a mental disorder to reach their optimal level of independent functioning in the community (WHO).

In the pre-independence era, the emphasis was on custodial care in lunatic/ mental asylums. Gradually, the asylums became mental hospitals and the focus was on curative care. The current thinking favors decentralization of facilities and services for treatment, moving toward general hospital psychiatric care and on rehabilitation, and recovery and reintegrating the individual into the society. Psychiatric residential facilities are both Government run and by private personnel. Rehabilitation has several facets. Rehabilitation of an individual with schizophrenia has to be recovery oriented. It has to focus on the real world and focus on strengths of the person. It should include skills training, environmental modification, and support. It is a multidisciplinary approach and should ensure continuity of services.

Strategies in PSR: Important strategies of PSR include social skills training, group therapy, cognitive retraining, and vocational rehabilitation.
- *Social skills training*: Patients with schizophrenia have difficulty in interacting

with others. They have difficulty in perceiving social cues and reacting appropriately. Social skills training is specifically designed to address these issues. It is a structured learning approach to acquire skills relevant to individual and the demands of his environment.

- *Cognitive retraining*: As mentioned earlier, cognitive deficits accompany schizophrenia. These deficits affect performance of day-to-day routine activities or at work place. Cognitive retraining is a structured technique usually using computer-based programs where in the global functioning is improved by amelioration of cognitive deficits like impaired attention, difficulty in planning, execution, and decision making.

- *Vocational rehabilitation*: The aim here is to rehabilitate an individual to secure employment. Supported employment models are more successful than prevocational training and then placing an individual in a job. The concept of token economy, a form of positive reinforcement wherein an individual is successfully rewarded for any progress he makes in the work assigned, works well in supported employment.

OTHER PSYCHOTIC DISORDERS

Schizoaffective Disorders

Jacob Kasanin introduced the term schizo-affective disorder to designate a condition, which had symptoms of both schizophrenia and mood disorder simultaneously or within a few days of each other, within the same episode of illness. Premorbid functioning is good in these patients and often the illness is preceded by a specific stressor. Family history of mood disorder is more common among these patients. The clinical course is often characterized by periodic and sudden onset of symptoms, which show relatively high degree of remission after several weeks. Illness is more common in women than in men.

Various types of this disorder are:

- *Schizoaffective disorder*: Manic type, where schizophrenic and manic symptoms (a disorder marked by periods of excessive energy and elevated mood) coexist.
- *Schizoaffective disorder*: Depressive type, here schizophrenic and depressive symptoms (a disorder where the person is sad and has low level of energy) coexist.
- *Schizoaffective disorder*: Mixed type, here schizophrenic symptoms coexist with mixed mood state.

Antipsychotics are the mainstay of treatment, although mood stabilizers are also commonly used. Predominant schizophrenic symptoms predict poor prognosis and predominant mood symptoms predict good prognosis.

Acute and Transient Psychotic Disorders

These disorders, described in ICD-10, present with acute onset of delusions, hallucinations, and other psychotic symptoms. The onset is associated with stress in a substantial number of patients. Another salient episode of such episodes is their tendency to recover completely within 2–3 months and only a small percentage develop persistent and disabling symptoms. Antipsychotics are the treatment of choice.

The CAPS (Cross-cultural Study of Acute Psychosis) conducted in 14 centers across seven countries showed that a large proportion of acute psychoses (41.2%) patients showed schizophrenic symptoms, whereas 20% showed affective symptoms; about 41.7% showed evidence of stress close to the onset of illness and close to two-thirds of patients remained well with no relapse at 1 year. A 20-year follow-up of this cohort showed that 82% had excellent outcome with no relapse and no residual symptoms. The Chandigarh Acute Psychosis Study was another major study of acute onset psychoses. This study showed that only 60% cases of acute psychoses met the criteria for schizophrenia and MDP. The remaining 40% cases were nonschizophrenic and nonaffective and could be considered as acute psychoses. These cases had greater frequency of association with stress and presented with undifferentiated symptomatology. A 5-year follow-up of these cases found that majority (75%) had good outcome in the form of complete recovery and no residual symptoms.

Brief Psychotic Disorder

This entity described in DSM-5, refers to sudden and short periods of psychotic behavior, often in response to a very stressful event, such as a death in the family. Recovery is quick, usually less than a month. It is akin to reactive psychoses, which is a diagnosis often made by clinicians. Proposed by Karl Jaspers, this brief psychotic illness occurs in response to stress, is acute in onset, the content of the psychotic experience is non-bizarre, and often reflects the stressful precipitating life event. It lasts for less than a month and symptoms remit once the stressor is removed. This condition is very similar to 'Acute and Transient Psychotic Disorders, described earlier.'

Schizotypal Personality Disorder

It is a disorder characterized by eccentric behavior and anomalies of thinking and affect, which resemble those seen in schizophrenia though there are no characteristic schizophrenic anomalies. Brief episodes of psychosis (quasi-psychotic episodes) may occur in times of stress, but they do not persist. Schizotypal patients have odd thinking, appear odd, have eccentric behavior, and may show ideas of reference, magical thinking, and unusual perceptions. They have considerable deficits in social skills and cognition. Once the disorder appears, it has a chronic course. Patients treated with antipsychotics have better outcome. Hoch and Polatin proposed the concept of pseudoneurotic schizophrenia, which described a subgroup of patients with predominant anxiety features. They had features of pananxiety, pansexuality and panneurosis, which are supposed to have masked a latent psychotic disorder.

Delusional Disorder

Delusional disorder presents with delusions, which are non-bizarre in nature and last for at least 1 month. Delusions are usually single and revolve around a single theme. These are delusions, which involve real-life situations that could be true, such as being followed, being spoken about (referential delusion), being conspired against (persecutory delusion), or belief that one's spouse is unfaithful (delusion of infidelity—Othello syndrome) belief of having a disease (hypochondriacal delusion). Other somatic delusions are delusional parasitosis (where they believe that they are infested with insects either externally or internally), delusional dysmorphophobia (conviction that body part is misshapen), and olfactory reference syndrome/delusion of foul odor (where the person believes that he/she emits foul odor), De Clerambault syndrome or erotomanic delusion is the delusion of having secret lovers. Person believes that a suitor usually of a high socioeconomic status is deeply in love with him/her.

As mentioned already, delusions are fixed, firm, and false beliefs, which extend to all spheres of life and persist, despite all evidences point to the contrary. This disorder generally begins around 40 years of age with a female preponderance. It is typically characterized by the absence of disorganization in thinking (formal thought disorder), which occurs in schizophrenia, and the frequency of hallucinations (auditory) is less. The socio-occupational functioning is not affected in majority of the patients. Treatment is with antipsychotics, though the response to treatment is variable. Hallucinations respond quickly while delusions may remain fixed.

Schizophreniform Disorder

It is a concept given by Gabriel Langfeldt. Schizophreniform disorder is similar to schizophrenia except that the symptoms last at least 1 month but less than 6 months. Relatives of patients with this disorder are more likely to have mood disorder than relatives of patients with schizophrenia. Treatment is with antipsychotics. About 60–80% of patients with this disorder go on to develop schizophrenia.

Shared Psychotic Disorder

First described by Lasegue and Falret, shared psychotic disorder is characterized by transfer of delusions from one person to another. One person develops the delusion, which is induced into the other. The delusion generally disappears in the latter when they are separated. Almost invariably, the concerned people have a very close relationship, living together for a long time in relative social isolation. The individual who first develops the delusion (primary case) is the influential member, dominant and the person who in whom it is induced (secondary case), is generally more passive and may have below normal intelligence. Based on the number of people involved, it is termed *folie a deux* (two people usually husband and wife, mother and child), *folie a trois* (three persons), *folie a quatre* (four persons), and *folie a famille* (whole family). Rarely, *folie a simultanee* occurs, wherein two persons become psychotic at the same time independently and mutually induce and share features. Treatment is with antipsychotics.

Culture-bound Syndromes

Culture refers to the meaning, values, and norms for behavior that are learned and transmitted within social groups. It includes subjective dimensions like feelings, values, ideas, and objective dimensions including beliefs, traditions, laws, and rituals.

Culture-bound syndromes are culturally based signs and symptoms of mental distress or maladaptive behavior that present as a disorder. They are recurrent and show culture-specific patterns of aberrant behavior. A few examples of relatively common culture-bound syndromes seen in India are Dhat syndrome and Koro. Dhat syndrome is a neurotic disorder seen in Indian subcontinent, where there is morbid preoccupation with health consequences of loss of semen through any process either with urine or masturbation or nocturnal emission. It is more common in young males who present with intense anxiety and somatization symptoms. Koro is characterized by acute-onset morbid anxiety regarding the hyperinvolution of genitalia leading to death. They believe that the genitalia are gradually reducing in size and are being retracted into the body and they would die soon as a consequence. It is more commonly seen in Northeast India.

People living in the same cultural milieu can provide information, if the person is exhibiting behavior not seen in a particular cultural setup. Medications provide moderate relief. Family support and use of indigenous healers when available are helpful.

Substance-induced Psychotic Disorder

This condition is caused by prolonged and excess use of or withdrawal from some substances, such as alcohol, cannabis, and cocaine, which may cause hallucinations, delusions, or disorganized speech.

Psychotic Disorder due to a Medical Condition

Hallucinations, delusions, or other symptoms may be the result of another medical illness that affects brain function, such as a head injury, a brain tumor, a metabolic condition, or an endocrinopathy.

CONCLUSION

Schizophrenia is a major relatively common disorder of the mind. In all likelihood, it is a group of disorders. It begins most often during late adolescence and early adulthood, often has a chronic course, and may lead to severe disability in some. The etiology appears to be multifactorial with both genetic and environmental factors contributing to it. It is important for all medical practitioners to be familiar with the signs and symptoms of this disorder, so that early detection is made and prompt treatment can be instituted. Management entails a combination of medicines and psychosocial measures. It also includes rehabilitation and reintegration of the patient in the community.

TAKE-HOME MESSAGES

- Schizophrenia and other psychotic illness are characterized by altered thinking, loss of touch with reality, poor judgment, and insight.
- In this illness, levels of dopamine, glutamate, and GABA are altered. Patients with schizophrenia exhibit positive and/or negative symptoms.
- Positive symptoms include delusions/hallucinations/thought disorder/disorganized behavior, and respond better to medications.
- Alogia, anhedonia, amotivation, and asociality form the negative symptoms.
- Course and outcome vary in schizophrenia, about 30% show good improvement with medications.
- Oral and depot forms of antipsychotics are available; the latter being preferred in uncooperative patients.
- Along with medications, psychosocial rehabilitation is important in managing patients with schizophrenia, which deals with reintegrating them into the society.

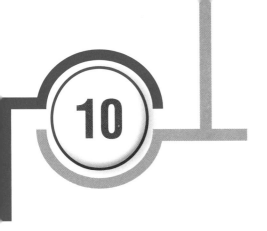

Nishant Goyal, Vinod K Sinha, Vidya KL

Depressive Disorders

INTRODUCTION

Depression is a common but highly treatable psychiatric disorder that can affect anyone. About one in 20 people gets depressed every year. Depression is not reflective of a character flaw, nor is it a sign of personal weakness. Depression is an eminently treatable clinical condition. Unfortunately, many persons with depression do not share their suffering and symptoms either with a doctor or their family members. This is very regrettable since effective treatments are available for depression, and most people with depression can begin to feel better with treatment within a few weeks. Talking with a doctor about how they are feeling is the depressed person's first important step toward getting better.

WHAT INCLUDES DEPRESSION: AN OVERVIEW

Depression is a mental disorder that is characterized by changes in mood, thoughts, behavior, and physical health. It is a common but serious disease that can take away a person's ability to enjoy life and cause decline in his capacity to undertake even the simplest of daily tasks. It may also be recurrent and life-threatening. According to the World Health Organization (WHO), unipolar depression is one of the leading causes of disability-adjusted life year (DALY) and approximately 300 million people worldwide are said to suffer from this mental disorder. As described in the Diagnostic and Statistical Manual of Mental Disorders, 5th edition (DSM-5), the hallmark of major depressive disorder (MDD) is the occurrence of depressed mood (dysphoria) and loss of interest in activities that were rather pleasurable in the past (anhedonia) for a duration of at least 2 weeks. These symptoms must also be accompanied by at least four of the following manifestations such as changes in appetite or weight, sleep patterns, altered psychomotor activity, feelings of worthlessness or guilt, difficulty concentrating or making decisions and recurrent thoughts of death or suicidal ideation. Even though there are plenty of drugs developed for the management of depression, one of the challenges in dealing with this disease is that a significant percentage of patients taking antidepressants fail to attain full remission. Some patients also develop treatment resistant depression in which the patients fail to respond to the available drugs or other therapeutic approaches.

TYPES OF DEPRESSIVE DISORDERS

Depression is a heterogeneous disorder often mistaken for a single clinical entity. There are indeed diverse forms of depression that can range from being mild to extremely severe, including conditions like psychotic depression in which the patients show symptoms of hallucinations and delusions. Diagnosis of this disorder gets complicated also because of its very high comorbid association with other mental conditions such as anxiety disorders, including panic agoraphobia syndrome, severe phobias, generalized anxiety disorder, social anxiety disorder, post-traumatic stress disorder (PTSD), obsessive–compulsive disorder (OCD), and somatic symptoms of various kinds. This comorbidity is more commonly seen in elderly patients. The different types of depression are described in the following text.

Recurrent Depressive Disorder

Patients with this type of depressive disorder typically show dysphoric mood and anhedonia accompanied by physical changes such as weight loss or gain, increased or decreased appetite, alteration in sleep pattern, and sustained fatigue. Disturbances in cognitive and executive functions are also manifested by lack of concentration and coherent thinking as well as morbid preoccupation with thoughts of death and suicide. Majority of these symptoms normally are present nearly every day and result in significant distress and impaired social life and occupational performance.

Dysthymia

Dysthymia is also known as persistent depressive disorder. Patients display depressed mood or sadness that persists for the majority of the duration of the day for a minimum of 2 years in adults and 1 year in children and adolescents. Majority of these patients do not meet the full criteria for MDD. However, there are instances where patients meet full criteria in which they are diagnosed along with MDD.

Melancholic Depression

There is an almost absolute lack of ability to experience pleasure. Psychomotor retardation and early morning worsening of mood is also clearly present in this subset of patients. This type of depression is seen more commonly in the elderly, in patients with more severe forms of depression and psychotic depression.

Seasonal Affective Disorder

Seasonal affective disorder (SAD) is a type of depression described as recurring annually during fall or early winter. This "winter blues" or SAD is characterized by low mood, feelings of guilt and worthlessness, and increased irritability, symptoms shared with other depressive disorders. Additionally, patients show a significant increase in appetite and craving for foods high in carbohydrates, which result in weight gain.

Postpartum Depression

Postpartum depression (PPD) presents with a heterogeneous group of depressive symptoms that affects mothers around the postpartum period. These symptoms may surface before or after giving birth. Half of the "postpartum" episodes begin before the time of delivery. Thus, they are referred to collectively as "peripartum" episodes. According to DSM-5, mood swings and anxiety symptoms during pregnancy, as well as the "baby blues" increase the risk for a postpartum major depressive episode.

Psychotic Depression

Psychotic depression is a type of depressive disorder, which is very severe and accompanied by psychotic symptoms. It is commonly seen as a combination of psychosis and depression that is not separable into either of the two. Symptoms include psychotic features such as hallucinations or delusions. Other than its severity, psychotic depression is associated with prolonged course, poor response to available drugs, and higher relapse rate.

EPIDEMIOLOGY OF DEPRESSIVE DISORDERS

Recently conducted world mental health surveys indicate that 10–15% people experience major depression in their lifetime and about 5% suffer from major depression in any given year. Lifetime prevalence of all depressive disorders taken together is over 20%, that is, one in five individuals. In Indian context, a recent large sample survey with rigorous methodology reported an overall prevalence of 15.9% for depression, which is similar to western figures. The National Mental Health Survey conducted in 2015–2016 found that the weighted prevalence of depression for both current and lifetime was 2.7% and 5.2%, respectively, indicating that nearly 1 in 40 and 1 in 20 suffer from past and current depressions, respectively. Depression was reported to be higher in females, in the age group of 40–49 years and among those residing in urban metros. Equally high rates were reported among the elderly (3.5%). The average age of onset for major depression is 24 years as per the recent epidemiological research, though it can begin at anytime throughout the lifespan. One of the consistent findings across almost all research studies is that women are twice as likely to have depression compared to males. Depression is much more likely among people, who are unmarried, widowed, divorced or separated, or without close interpersonal relationships. Those residing in nuclear families and urban areas are possibly at a higher risk. Elderly age and presence of medical disorders pose an even higher risk of depression. Depression is a major contributor to the global burden of disease and affects people in all communities across the world.

ETIOLOGY AND PATHOPHYSIOLOGY OF DEPRESSIVE DISORDERS

There is no simple answer to what causes depression. Depression can strike people of any age, gender, race, or social background. Most experts believe that a combination of genetic, biological, and environmental factors interact to produce symptoms of depression. Even though there are numerous studies attempting to shed light on the pathophysiology of depression, it still remains elusive. This is in fact the major reason for the slow-paced drug development against this disease. There are diverse theories on the pathogenesis of depression, most based on measurement of indirect markers, postmortem studies, and neuroimaging techniques. They are enumerated as follows:

- *Neural circuitry of depression*: Various structural and functional studies report abnormalities in the areas of the brain that are responsible for the regulation of mood, reward response, and executive functions. Reductions in gray matter volume and glial density in the prefrontal cortex and the hippocampus, as well as a decrease in locus ceruleus (LC) neuron density are reported widely. The decline in hippocampal function, which is believed to have an inhibitory effect on the hypothalamic–pituitary–adrenal (HPA) axis, could possibly be responsible for the hypercortisolemia seen in depression. The mesolimbic dopamine system that consists of the nucleus accumbens (NAc) and the ventral tegmental area (VTA) also are believed to play a role in the pathogenesis of depression. These brain regions mediate the reward response to pleasurable stimuli such as food, sex, and even drugs. Therefore, a peculiar lack of pleasure in depressed patients can possibly be explained as a dysfunction in this brain reward circuit.

- *Stress response circuits*: Chronic stress and hyperactivity of the HPA axis causing chronic hypercortisolemia have been hypothesized to play a prominent role in the occurrence of depression and even in recurrence after complete remission. About 50% of people with clinical depression have an excess of the hormone cortisol in their blood. Chronic stress has been shown to alter the expression of genes regulating antioxidant systems, such as superoxide dismutases (SODs), catalase, glutathione peroxidase, glutathione reductase, and NADPH oxidase, thereby subjecting the body tissues to higher level of oxidative stress.

- *Genetic vulnerability and environmental interaction*: According to the WHO, 50–75% of children are likely to suffer from depression if both parents also have the illness. There are compelling observations that in order for depression to surface, the genetic predisposition has to undergo a complex gene–environment interaction that also alters an individual response to stressful life situations. A genetic polymorphism with allelic variation in the promoter region of the gene encoding the serotonin transporter (5-HTT) has been shown to put carriers at a greater risk of developing depression in response to stressful life events. This allele has also been related with poorer outcomes after antidepressant pharmacological and nonpharmacological treatments. The rate-limiting enzyme in serotonin biosynthesis, tryptophan hydroxylase (TPH), is encoded by two distinct genes *Tphl* and *Tph2* and has been proposed to play a role in pathogenesis of depressive disorders and suicide. Studies also suggest a complex interaction exists between the polymorphisms in genes encoding for brain-derived neurotrophic factor (BDNF) and 5-HTT to bring about a depressed phenotype.

- The biogenic monoamine theory:
  - *The serotonin hypothesis:* Subset of depressed patients has been reported to have a lowered level of 5-hydroxyindoleacetic acid (5-HIAA), a metabolite of 5-HT in the cerebrospinal fluid (CSF), which has been related to aggressive behavior and increased suicidal intent and impulsivity. The plasma level of the amino acid precursor of 5-HT, i.e. Tryptophan, has been found to be decreased in patients of depression and depressive symptoms can be induced in patients who are susceptible to depression by depleting this amino acid. Moreover, positron emission tomography (PET) imaging studies have reported a decrease in density of 5-HT1A receptor subtype among depressed patients in different regions of the brain. There is also evidence for decreased availability of 5-HTT in midbrain and brainstem regions.
  - *The catecholamine hypothesis:* Some symptoms of depression including anhedonia and psychomotor retardation are better explained by a derangement in the brain dopamine (DA) systems. These systems include the substantia nigra, basal ganglia motor system and the reward circuitry involving the NAc and VTA. There is

a diminished DA activity in the NAc specifically which corresponds to the inability to experience pleasure which is one of the hallmarks of depression. The concentration of the DA metabolite homovanillic acid (HVA) in CSF of depressed patients is also reported to be lower.

- *Inflammation and depression*: Many pro-inflammatory marker levels are reported to be elevated in depressed patients. Examples of these markers are C-reactive protein (CRP), interleukins (IL-6 and IL-1), and tumor necrosis factor alpha (TNF-α). An increase in generation of reactive oxygen and nitrogen species, leading to damage by oxidative and nitrosative stress (ONS), including lipid peroxidation, and damage to deoxyribonucleic acid (DNA) and proteins is also seen. Even though a complete understanding of the mechanisms involved remains obscure, an increase in pro-inflammatory cytokines results in a lack of neuronal plasticity and eventual neurodegeneration.

- *Neurotrophic hypothesis:* Significant atrophy of certain prefrontal cortex areas and hippocampus observed in depression as well as decreased levels of nerve growth factors (NGF) such as BDNF has led to the neurotrophic hypothesis. The expression of BDNF is halted by chronic stress and normal level of this growth factor is attained after a successful treatment with antidepressants. This is consistent with the fact that antidepressants take at least 2–3 weeks to elicit their actions, possibly through causing a longer-lasting neuroadaptive changes in the brain rather than a simple increase in the level of neurotransmitters. Vascular endothelial growth factor (VEGF) is another NGF that promotes proliferation of neuronal

cells in some brain regions such as the hippocampus. It achieves this by activating intracellular signaling cascades that involve mitogen-activated protein kinase (MAPK) pathway. This signaling pathway has also been postulated to underlie the late antidepressant response of currently available drugs.

- *Neuropeptides and depression*: There is increasing evidence that neuropeptides are involved in the modulation of stress-related behaviors and mood by acting on neurokinin type-1 (NK-1) receptors. Substance P (SP) is one of these neuropeptides known for its widespread distribution in the brain and its colocalization with 5-HT and norepinephrine (NE) neurons. Elevated CSF SP concentrations have been reported in depressed patients and patients with PTSD after exposure to a stressful stimulus.

- *Hormones and depression*: Boys and girls, during their childhood years, develop depression at equal rates. When they reach adolescence, the likelihood of girls becoming depressed increases. The National Alliance on Mental Illness reports that by the time they become adults, women are twice as likely as men to develop major depression.

  - *Estrogen involvement*: Increased female susceptibility to depression mostly overlaps periods of low estrogen levels in the menstrual cycle, postpartum and after the onset of menopause. Animal studies indicate mood-enhancing actions of estrogen as well as their synergy with monoaminergic drugs. Estrogen enhances mood by increasing the rate of degradation of monoamine oxidase (MAO) and of intraneuronal 5-HT transport, causing an overall increase in 5-HT availability in the synapse. In addition to enhancing serotonergic neurotransmission, estrogen is also believed to have modulatory effect on hippocampal neurogenesis, BDNF signaling, and HPA axis function.

- *Thyroid hormones*: Hypothyroidism has been found to show observations similar to depression, in that it also impairs hippocampal neurogenesis, which gets resolved with hormone replacement. Animal studies also reveal that thyroid hormone causes an increase in serotonergic neurotransmission, which supports the fact that TH supplementation has been beneficial in management of refractory cases of depression.

- *Vasopressin and depression*: Arginine vasopressin (AVP) is a hypothalamic hormone that seems to influence some key symptoms pertaining to a major depressive disorder. Its level is reported to be elevated in patients suffering from this mental disorder. AVP has been linked to play a role also in the regulation of stress response by synergizing with corticotropin-releasing factor (CRF) at the level of the pituitary to influence the release of adrenocorticotropic hormone (ACTH). Elevated AVP concentrations have been found to be associated with psychomotor retardation in patients with major depressive disorder.

■ *Implications of the circadian rhythm in depression:* Melatonin, a hormone secreted by the pineal gland in a circadian fashion, regulates the rhythm of various other biological parameters such as body temperature, cortisol secretion, and sleep cycles by acting on receptors in the suprachiasmatic nucleus (SCN) of the hypothalamus. Delayed circadian rhythm in patients with depression has been linked to diminished level of melatonergic signaling in the brain. Patients may present with delayed onset of sleep, difficulty in maintaining sleep, and early morning awakening. This has shown the way to the discovery of a new antidepressant agent, agomelatine, which acts on melatonin and serotonin receptors on the SCN. Disruption of circadian rhythm has also been proposed as a mechanism that makes an individual susceptible to depression.

DIAGNOSTIC CRITERIA AND CLINICAL FEATURES

The diagnosis of depression is based on a set of specific signs and symptoms. A healthy person experiences a variety of mood states including transient feelings of sadness. Depression as a clinical entity is different from everyday mood fluctuations and short-lived emotional responses to situations. It is important to differentiate clinical depression from these more ubiquitous transient negative mood states. In contrast to normal sadness, a clinically depressed state is more intense and pervasive as well as sustained for most of the time over several days, weeks, or months. It is usually accompanied by an intense guilt or hopelessness for future and may be accompanied by suicidal ideation or thoughts of self-harm. Impairments of various bodily functions, e.g., appetite, changes in sexual drive, and sleep disturbances are common. All of these begin to interfere with familial, social, and occupational functioning. Many a times, a person may not report sadness of mood, but instead may describe it as irritability, being down, feeling blue or simply being unable to cry or experience emotions. Anxiety symptoms may commonly occur, e.g., feeling palpitations, restlessness, etc. Indian patients with depression appear to have a high prevalence of physical or somatic symptoms compared to western population. Somatic symptoms such as body aches or vague pains are one of most common manifestations of depression in India. These have been considered to be a depressive-equivalent symptom, more often seen in Asian cultures.

The ICD (International Classification for Diseases) 10 criteria for depressive episode include:

- At least two of following should be present for a minimum 2 weeks:
  - Depressed mood to a degree that is definitely abnormal for the individual, present for most of the day and almost every day, largely uninfluenced by circumstances
  - Loss of interest or pleasure in activities that are normally pleasurable
  - Decreased energy or increased fatigability.
- Additional symptoms, two or more of the following:
  - Loss of confidence and self-esteem
  - Self-reproach or excessive and inappropriate guilt
  - Recurrent thoughts of death or suicide, or any suicidal behavior
  - Diminished ability to think or concentrate
  - Change in psychomotor activity (agitation or retardation)
  - Sleep disturbances
  - Change in appetite with corresponding weight change.

Assessment and Diagnosis of Depressive Disorders

Evaluation

History and examination: Diagnosis of depression is based primarily on information obtained from detailed history and mental status examination. In addition to features of depression, any signs and symptoms of anxiety, somatoform disorders, or use of alcohol or any other substance, which mask depressive symptoms, should be explored. Presence of psychosocial stressors or precipitating factors if any should be elicited. Mental status examination usually reveals decrease in psychomotor activity, increased reaction time, and depressed affect with depressive cognitions such as ideas of helplessness, worthlessness, and hopelessness. Suicidal ideas and plans may be present. Mood congruent psychotic features such as delusion of guilt and nihilism may be present in psychotic depression.

Screening and severity rating scales: Two brief screening instruments have been found to be quite useful for screening depression in medical settings. These are available free of cost in public domain:

- *Patient Health Questionnaire depression module (PHQ-9):* It is a self-administered 9-item scale, each item rated between 0 and 3 based on frequency. Sensitivity and specificity are both 88%, with a cutoff score of 10.
- *Patient Health Questionnaire-2 (PHQ-2):* A 2-item version similar to the PHQ-9 that enquires about the frequency of depressed mood and anhedonia over the past 2 weeks:
- Following two depression-screening tools specifically address the problem of transdiagnostic symptoms (symptoms which may overlap between medical disorder and depression) by excluding the somatic content or physical symptoms to enhance usefulness in persons with physical illness.
  - Beck Depression Inventory-Primary care (BDI-PC) (7-item)
  - Hospital Anxiety and Depression Scale (HADS) (7-item)

To assess the severity of depressive symptoms, HAM-D (Hamilton rating scale for depression) and Beck depression inventory are popularly used in both clinical as well as research settings.

Laboratory investigations are rarely needed to diagnose depression. However, hemoglobin, thyroid function tests, and vitamin B_{12} levels can be checked depending on the need of the case to rule out common medical conditions, which can cause/mimic depression.

Differential Diagnosis

Adjustment disorder occurs when an individual is unable to adjust to or cope with a particular stress, a major life event or a continuing stress. The symptoms include features of anxiety and/or depression but do not meet the criteria of a full syndrome. The symptoms have a tendency to generally resolve once the person is able to adapt to the situation or is removed from the stress.

Grief and bereavement: Grief is a natural response to loss and bereavement refers to the state of loss. Differentiation of depression from uncomplicated grief is based on symptom severity and length.

Premenstrual dysphoric disorder is distinguished by the prompt remission of symptoms with the onset of menstrual flow and characteristic association of symptoms with menstrual cycle.

Bipolar depression has predictors such as childhood-onset depression, presence of psychotic symptoms, acute onset, family history of bipolar disorder, agitation, and racing of thoughts.

Generalized anxiety disorder is distinguished from an agitated depressive episode by the relative absence of such symptoms as fatigue, loss of interest, guilt, and middle insomnia or early-morning awakening.

Secondary depression may result from Cushing's syndrome, hypothyroidism, long-standing epilepsy, Parkinson's disease, dementia, drugs such as beta-blockers, calcium channel blockers and opioids, and alcohol.

Obsessive–compulsive disorder is often accompanied by depressive symptoms, yet here the obsessions and compulsions generally precede the onset of depressive symptoms.

Psychotic disorders: Depression may present with delusions and hallucinations, which are typically mood congruent, involving themes like guilt, self-depreciation, punishment, and fatal illnesses. They resolve usually with resolution of depression. Severe depression may also result in loss of functioning, poor self-care, and social isolation secondary to depressed mood, which should not be confused with the negative symptoms of schizophrenia.

TREATMENT OF DEPRESSION

Treatment options for major depression include medications, psychotherapy, and electroconvulsive therapy (ECT). The most effective medications for major depression are antidepressants.

Several psychotherapeutic approaches are effective for depression, including cognitive behavioral therapy (CBT), and interpersonal therapy. These can be provided either alone or in combination with medications especially in mild-to-moderate depression. CBT works by helping people identify and challenge inaccurate and self-defeating thinking that contributes to depression. It encourages them to become involved again in enjoyable activities, and learn skills for having more rewarding interactions with other people. Interpersonal therapy helps people to work through their problems in current relationships while exploring the underlying causes for current behavioral patterns. Family psychoeducation can also be an effective treatment for major depression.

Medication is often prescribed for managing moderate-to-severe depression. Antidepressant medications work by adjusting mood-related brain chemicals such as serotonin and norepinephrine to normal levels. There are several types of antidepressants including selective serotonin reuptake inhibitors (SSRIs), tricyclics, and monoamine oxidase inhibitors (MAOIs). SSRIs are common initial choice to treat depression in view of their ease of use, more tolerable side effects, superior safety profile, and overall efficacy. There are no clinically significant differences in efficacy among antidepressants, but there are some clinical factors that are important to consider when choosing a medication, e.g., past response, adverse effect profile, comorbid conditions, drug–drug interactions, cost, availability, etc. Fluoxetine is the most economical and effective medication, which may be preferred in an otherwise healthy adult with depression. Escitalopram is preferred over fluoxetine in patients with multiple other medications/medical illnesses because of low propensity to cause drug interactions. More sedating SSRIs, e.g., paroxetine may be preferred in patients with marked anxiety and insomnia. Sertraline has been more extensively studied in patients with cardiac conditions and poststroke depression. Generally, it is advisable to start at a lower dose and increase gradually (start low, go slow); however, patients must be given adequate dose of SSRI to ensure a remission of symptoms. Medication usually takes 4–6 weeks for improvement in clinical symptoms. Physician should emphasize on frequent follow-up visits during the initial few weeks to monitor for depressive symptoms and adverse effects, if any.

In view of the chronic and recurrent nature of depressive disorders, treatment should be continued for at least 6–12 months after the remission of depressive episode is achieved. This continuation phase of treatment is important for minimizing the risk of future recurrence. In cases of multiple episodes and strong family history, maintenance treatment should be considered for longer period of time.

Antipsychotic medications, especially second-generation ones, are effective in psychotic depression along with anti-depressant medications.

Electroconvulsive therapy is indicated and effective for those who are extremely depressed, suicidal, or with catatonic features. It can be lifesaving in many severe cases of depression. Other somatic treatments such as vagal nerve stimulation and rTMS (repetitive transcranial magnetic stimulation) are being tried in resistant cases of depression.

ASSOCIATION OF DEPRESSIVE DISORDERS WITH SUICIDE

Suicide is clearly associated with the presence of depression. The feeling of hopelessness appears to be more important than other indicators of severity in assessing the risk. Surprisingly, the risk is variable and not consistently elevated in association with psychotic depression. Comorbid anxiety, substance abuse, and personality disorders are established adverse prognostic indicators. The operative word for risk assessment is "early." The chances of suicide are increased, shortly after the diagnosis of depression, earlier in the lifetime course of the illness, during the first few months after the initiation of therapy, earlier in the course of hospitalization and in the first month or 2 months after discharge from inpatient care.

ASSOCIATION OF DEPRESSIVE DISORDERS WITH SUBSTANCE ABUSE

Depression exists in 30–40% of people with a substance use disorder. Among people with mood disorders, about one third also have comorbid substance use disorders. Drug and alcohol use worsens the symptoms of major depression and can increase the risk of relapses of depression, including suicidal thinking and suicide attempts. Mood disorders rarely improve while people are addicted to alcohol or drugs. Even with treatment, active alcohol and drug use can compromise the potential benefits of antidepressant therapy. Major depression may be difficult to diagnose during the initial phases of abstinence or early recovery because negative feelings and depressed mood occurs in almost every patient during this phase. Therefore, in this situation, people with major depression are likely to go undetected and thus remain untreated. People with untreated major depression are at greater risk for suicide during early recovery, and they are also more likely to leave treatment early and relapse. Sometimes, the symptoms of major depression appear only after a period of abstinence.

COURSE AND PROGNOSIS

If untreated, a depressive episode may last between 6 and 12 months and with treatment, most of the episodes resolve over a few weeks. Depression may be a chronic and recurrent illness in at least one half to two thirds of the patients who usually have the next episode in less than 5 years. With time, a person may start to have more frequent episodes, which last longer. There may be average of five to six episodes of depression in lifetime, though it varies from person to person. Untreated depression increases a person's risk for future episodes of depression. Good prognostic factors are milder episodes, good social support, stable familial and social functioning before onset of depression, and absence of a comorbid medical or psychiatric disorder. Early onset, coexisting medical illness, substance use or anxiety disorder, and multiple episodes or poor functioning in the premorbid period are likely to have a poorer prognosis.

DEPRESSION IN PRIMARY CARE SETTINGS AND REFERRAL

Patients with mild-to-moderate depression, nonpsychotic or somatized depression can be managed in primary care settings by general physicians. Unless specifically screened, depression may remain under-recognized and untreated in primary care/medical settings. For patients with mild or subthreshold depression, treatment may entail psychological support, problem-solving, exercise, informal counseling, or formal psychosocial interventions.

During screening or follow-up of the patient, following situations require a referral to a psychiatrist for management:

- Risk of suicide
- *Severe depression*: Presence of all or almost all depressive symptoms listed in diagnostic criteria, extreme psychomotor retardation, etc.
- Presence of psychotic symptom, e.g., delusions and hallucinations
- Nonresponse to treatment and chronic resistant depression
- Presence of multiple comorbidities, e.g., depression, alcohol abuse, diabetes, etc.
- Presence of multiple and complicated polypharmacy
- Presence of significant individual, marital and/or family stressor, needing a more intensive psychotherapy

- Special population groups, e.g., adolescent depression or pregnant women
- Diagnostic difficulty or suggestion of a possible hypomania/manic episode in the past or family history.

CONCLUSION

Depression is one of the most common mental disorder which is showing gradual trend of increasing prevalence on a global scale. Within a decade, it is likely to become number one disorder afflicting mankind in terms of measures of burden of disease. It is a cause of severe dysfunction at times at the personal, social, and occupational levels. It is also the most important cause of suicide in all age groups. It may occur alone or be associated with several other medical and psychiatric comorbidities. Substance abuse is a common co-occurrence, which complicates the management of such cases. It is important for all medical practitioners to be sensitized to the signs and symptoms of depression and simultaneously develop skill to detect it early. Fortunately, effective antidepressant drugs are available, even though they take a few weeks' time to start showing clinical effect, provided they are given in proper dose for adequate duration. Psychotherapeutic interventions are also very important especially for cases of mild-to-moderate severity. Combination of drugs with psychotherapy shows better result. Electroconvulsive therapy is also one of the most effective interventions, which is generally used in cases of severe and nonresponding depressions.

TAKE-HOME MESSAGES

- Depression is a common mental disorder. Globally approximately 300 million people of all ages suffer from depression.
- Depression is the leading cause of disability worldwide and is a major contributor to the overall global burden of disease.
- Women are affected almost twice as often as men.
- Comorbid anxiety disorder, somatoform disorder, and substance use disorders are common.
- Early recognition and timely management serve to reduce the disability and even the risk of suicide.
- Apart from antidepressant medications, psychotherapy and somatic treatments such as ECT play a significant role in the treatment of depression.
- Severe depression, presence of psychotic features, risk of suicide, multiple comorbidities, and treatment-resistant depression need referral to a psychiatrist.

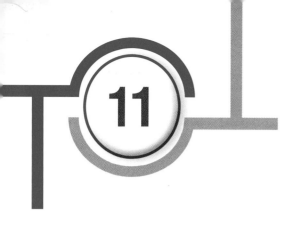

Bipolar Disorders

Om Prakash Singh, Sucharita Mandal

INTRODUCTION

"It is both a blessing and a curse to feel everything so deeply." **—David Jones**

Defining characteristic of humans is their emotion, which includes mood and affect. Mood can be defined as a sustained and pervasive emotion or feeling tone that influences a person's behavior and colors his perception of the world. Affect has been defined as observable expressions, verbal, and nonverbal, which are reflective of an emotional state. Mood has to be reported while affect can be observed. Mood states can be described as anger, fear, happy, sad, surprise, disgust, and many others.

"Disorders of mood" also known as "affective disorders" include depression, bipolar disorder, and others. Bipolar disorder would be discussed in this chapter. Bipolar disorder is a disorder of mood where patients have recurrent episodes of depression and mania. The patient experiences a distinctive qualitative change in their mood during such episodes.

HISTORY

La folie circulaire was a condition described by Jean-Pierre Falret in 1854. In this condition, patients experience alternating moods of depression and mania. A similar condition was described as *cyclothymia* in 1882 by Karl Kahlbaum.

Emil Kraepelin, in 1899, described *manic-depressive psychosis* which was same as described previously by Jean-Pierre Falret and Karl Kahlbaum. Kraepelin observed the absence of a deteriorating course in manic depressive psychosis and hence he categorized mental illnesses in two distinct categories namely *dementia precox* and *manic-depressive psychosis*. Following Kraepelin, Karl Leonhard in 1957 added to the definition of manic-depressive illness incorporating both unipolarity and bipolarity as separate entities. He maintained Kraepelin's emphasis on the cyclical and recurrent nature of these disorders. As far as official nosologies are concerned, this condition finds its first mention in Diagnostic and Statistical Manual of Mental Disorders-I (DSM-I) as "manic-depressive reaction" in 1952. Later it was also known as manic-depressive disorder or manic-depressive psychosis.

EPIDEMIOLOGY

Recent surveys have shown that the cross-national lifetime prevalence of bipolar affective disorder-I (BPAD-I) is 0.6%, of BPAD-II is 0.4% and of subthreshold bipolar disorders are 1.4%. National Mental Health Survey, India, 2016 has found the prevalence of bipolar disorder to be 0.3%.

Bipolar-I disorder has an equal prevalence among men and women.

Manic episodes are more common in men. Bipolar-II disorder, mixed episodes, and rapid cyclers show a higher prevalence in females.

CLASSIFICATION

According to ICD-10

For diagnosis of Bipolar disorder according to International Statistical Classification of Diseases and Related Health Problems-10 (ICD-10), it requires the occurrence of at least two episodes, one being mania and the other being either mania or depression. Symptom severity of manic episodes is specified by the presence or absence of psychotic symptoms. Severity of depressive episodes is specified as mild, moderate, or severe with or without psychosis.

A single manic episode is not labeled as bipolar disorder. A single manic episode is specified on the basis of severity as from hypomania to mania with psychotic symptoms.

According to DSM-5

Diagnostic and Statistical Manual of Mental Disorders-5 enlists various specific subtypes of bipolar disorder. Diagnosis of bipolar-I disorder requires the presence of mania characterized by persistent irritable or elevated mood, increased activity level for at least 1 week and symptoms should be severe enough to cause hospitalization. Presence of a depressive episode or psychosis is not required for fulfilling the criteria.

Bipolar-II disorder requires the presence of hypomanic episode and a depressive episode. Features of hypomania are similar to mania but attenuated to some extent and do not cause marked impairment in functioning. Duration for hypomania is at least 4 consecutive days.

Cyclothymia requires the presence of chronic fluctuation of mood from hypomania like symptoms to depressive symptoms and this fluctuation would be persistent for 2 years. The episodes would not meet criteria for hypomania or depression and would be of less severity and duration.

Change of mood due to any underlying medical condition is classified as bipolar disorder due to other medical condition. Presence of manic symptoms with substance abuse is classified as substance-induced bipolar disorder.

The symptom severity and description of remission are specified along with the diagnosis. Additional specifiers are used to describe like presence of mixed symptoms, rapid cycling (more than 4 episodes per year), melancholic symptoms, atypical symptoms, mood-congruent and incongruent psychotic features, and catatonic symptoms.

CLINICAL FEATURES

The age of onset for bipolar disorder ranges from 8 to 50 years or even older, with a mean age of 30 years. In many patients, the onset of depression at young age may evolve later on to developing mania. Manic and depressive episodes often alternate and are recurrent. Intermediate period is clinically symptom free. The course of manic or depressive episode depends on the variant of bipolar disorder. Bipolar-I disorder has more of manic episodes than depressive ones. Bipolar-II disorder has more of hypomanic episodes and prolonged depressive episodes.

Mania

An episode of mania is characterized by persistent elevated or irritable mood for at least 1 week causing significant impairment in social and occupational functioning.

Hypomanic episode is similar to a mania except that it does not cause significant impairment in social and occupational functioning.

- *Attitude and appearance*: Patients are usually flamboyant, might display over grooming inappropriate to the situation concerned.
- *Psychomotor activity*: There is increased energy and activity which can be called as "the sign" of mania. Patient feels overtly energetic and active. There is ceaseless energy to interact with surrounding people and might engage in tasks previously not amenable to the patient.
- *Mood:* The typical manic mood would be of euphoria. Patient feels very happy with or without reason. They typically have speech which is characterized by rhyming, punning, singing, and cracking jokes. When the severity of mania increases, mood becomes unstable or *labile*. Labile mood refers to spontaneous change of a happy state to a tearful and crying one. Sometimes patients also display extreme irritability and aggression instead of euphoria.
- *Speech*: There is rush of ideas and is evident in the speech of patient. It seems as if the patient has to complete his speech within a limited period of time and the "speech is pressured." *Flight of ideas* is used to denote rapidly produced speech with abrupt shifts from topic to topic. Association between the shifts is through rhyming, punning, etc. In severe mania, these associations are lost and the speech has loosening of association rendering it incoherent.
- *Impulsive behavior*: Impulsive behavior with lack of judgment is seen in these patients. Patients might indulge in spending spree, start new business undertaking, leaving current job for prospect of a better job. Gambling or indulgence in substance abuse can also be seen. Disinhibition is also seen in manic patients. Patients might be involved in sexually promiscuous behavior.
- *Lack of insight and poor judgment:* Patient has expansive ideas and increased self-esteem. Lack of insight along with poor judgment leads them to engage in harmful activities.

In severe mania with psychotic symptoms, patients often have *grandiose delusions* like delusion of being a millionaire and delusion of being God.

Delusions of reference and persecution are secondary owing to the belief that others are observing or following them out of jealousy for their special abilities.

Hallucinatory voices congruent with their euphoric mood and grandiose self-image might also be present, e.g., hearing voices singing in praise of them.

- *Sleep disturbances*: There is decreased need for sleep. In spite of the patient sleeping only a few hours, he feels very energetic the whole day. Sometimes the sleeplessness coupled with increased activity leads to physical exhaustion.

Depression

The depressive episode of bipolar disorder is similar to that of unipolar depression. There are a few differences by which we can attempt to distinguish between bipolar and unipolar depression **(Table 11.1)**.

The cardinal sign of depression is usually sadness of mood and loss of interest and pleasure in almost all activities.

- *Appearance*: Patient appears slow in action, speech is also slowed. Gaze is mostly downcast. Due to self-neglect, personal hygiene might not be maintained.

Table 11.1: Differentiating features between bipolar and unipolar depression.

Features	Unipolar	Bipolar
Age of onset	Late age of onset	Early onset—adolescence
Onset	Insidious	Often abruptly
Duration of episodes	Long (>6 months)	Short (3–6 months)
Recurrence	Few	More
Psychomotor activity	Agitation > retardation	Retardation > agitation
Sleep	Decreased	Increased
Psychotic symptoms	Less likely	More likely
Postpartum onset	Less common	More common
Family history	Less density	High density
Hyperthymic traits	Less	More
Response to treatment	Slow	Fast
History of mania	No	Yes
Atypical symptoms	Less	More
Suicidality	Less	More

Source: Sadock, Benjamin J, Virginia A. Kaplan & Sadock's Synopsis of Psychiatry: Behavioral Sciences/clinical Psychiatry. 11th edition, Philadelphia: Wolters Kluwer, 2015.

- *Psychomotor activity*: The psychomotor activity is reduced unlike mania. Social interaction is reduced, remains withdrawn to self. Posture is slumped and walking is also slow. This slowing is pervasive in all situations. Attention is disturbed. In some cases, patient might complain of agitation or restlessness. Irritability is present and patient becomes easily annoyed on slight provocation.
- *Mood*: Mood is typically low or sad in these patients. This sadness is persistent; however, diurnal variation may be found. The depressed patient usually feels very sad during morning hours and as day passes, he feels better.
- *Anhedonia*: Many patients lose their capacity to experience emotions and pleasure, they feel their emotions have become blunt. They lose interest in activities which they previously found to

be enjoyable. There is loss of interest in daily activities leading to social withdrawal and even loss of job. Sometimes due to severe anhedonia, patient might give up all activities including activities of daily living, leading to stupor or catatonia.
- *Pseudodementia*: Slowing is seen in all functions of a depressed person. The attention and concentration of a person also get slowed which might be expressed as memory impairment and confusion. This memory impairment is reversible as depression gets better with treatment.
- *Speech and thought disturbances*: Speech of depressed patients is slow; response to a question is also prolonged. Apart from slowness, these patients also have decreased speech output. Patient usually has negative thinking about himself and his surroundings. Feelings of hopelessness, worthlessness, and

feelings of guilt ensue. These feelings lead to development of suicidal feelings. In severe cases, psychotic symptoms might be present in having delusion of guilt or nihilism. Auditory hallucination of derogatory nature might also be present.

- *Sleep and appetite disturbances*: Sleep is usually disturbed. Patient feels difficulty in falling asleep. Early morning awakening is typically found in most of the patients. Appetite is usually decreased. Chronic appetite loss might lead to weight loss. In cases of "atypical depression," sleep is increased and appetite also increases. Patient might binge on food leading to weight gain.

COURSE AND PROGNOSIS

As stated earlier, bipolar disorder has got an early age of onset. An average manic episode lasts for around 3 months while a depressive episode lasts from 4–6 months or even longer. Of persons who have a single manic episode, 90% are likely to have another. There are patients who have four or more episodes in a year. These are *rapid cyclers*. Factors associated with rapid cycling include the use of antidepressants [especially tricyclic antidepressants (TCAs)], low thyroxine levels, female gender, and bipolar-II pattern of illness. The incidence of bipolar I disorder in children and adolescents is about 1%, and the onset can be as early as age 8 years. Prognosis in these patients is poor.

ETIOPATHOGENESIS

Research into the cause and etiology of bipolar disorder has been going on. Several years of research are now pointing the etiology to mainly have neurobiological roots. However, psychodynamic and cognitive theories have also been given, which are utilized sometimes in psychotherapy.

Psychological Theories

- *Psychoanalytic theory:* Major theories were given by Freud and later expanded by Karl Abraham. Depression is theorized to result from emotions directed against introjected lost object. Because the lost object is regarded with a mixture of love and hate, feelings of anger and aggression are directed inward at the self. The ego suffers a breakdown of self-esteem and worthlessness and hopelessness follows. All these happen at the level of unconscious mind. In *mania*, there is denial of painful aspects of reality. Denial is a subconscious defense mechanism of brain. Most theories of mania view manic episodes as a defense against underlying depression.

- *Cognitive theory*: Aaron T Beck was the main proponent of this theory. According to this theory, depressed patients tend to have negative cognition about (1) themselves, (2) their environment, and (3) the future. These negative thoughts are irrational "automatic thoughts" which are self-deprecatory. These negative ideas create hopelessness, worthlessness, and helplessness, eventually leading to depression. Cognitive theory has had less to say about manic than depressed states. Mania may be viewed as the mirror image of depression, wherein overvalued positive ideas ("I am special" or "I am the greatest") automatically arise, distorting reality, but this time in the opposing direction.

Genetic Hypothesis

There is no evidence for Mendelian inheritance for psychiatric disorders. A child of an affected parent has a tenfold increased risk of developing bipolar disorder. Twin studies estimate heritability of 0.7–0.8. Earlier-onset bipolar disorder appears to be associated with increased familial risk. Linkage studies have identified two genes 13q and *22q* as contributory for the disorder.

Environmental Factors

Some environmental factors have also been implicated in causation of bipolar disorder. Offsprings exposed *in utero* to maternal smoking exhibited a twofold greater risk for bipolar disorder in adulthood. Stress has also been found to be associated with relapses in bipolar disorder.

Biochemical Theories

Several theories of monoamines have been propounded from time to time in the causation of depression and mania. Norepinephrine and serotonin are implicated in the causation of depression. Whereas, dopamine has also been found to be involved in recent studies. However, this simplistic model of increase in mania and decrease in depression of amines at the synaptic level is now considered incomplete and various postsynaptic events are being described as important. They are triggering of second messenger systems, alteration of receptor function and subsequent modulation of excitation potential of membrane, etc. Mood stabilizers have been shown to exert their effect by modulation of G-proteins and gamma-aminobutyric acid (GABA).

Brain Imaging

Brain imaging studies have found results which are positive but not consistent and not exclusively seen in bipolar disorders. These findings have also been found in depression.

Abnormal hyperintensities in periventricular regions, basal ganglia, and thalamus are the findings. Ventricular enlargement and sulcal widening also have been reported in some studies. These studies are still at the research level.

MANAGEMENT

Bipolar disorder is a recurrent disorder and studies have confirmed that there are residual deleterious effects with every episode of mania or depression. Patients usually seek help during depression phase as insight is usually preserved during this phase. Clinicians should have an index of suspicion for possible bipolarity while treating cases of depression. Past history of mania, hyperthymic traits, substance abuse, or a positive family history of bipolar disorder should raise the suspicion index. Atypical features of depression and depression with psychotic symptoms should also be clarified. Patients put on regular antidepressant treatment might "switch" to mania or alternatively a manic episode might appear spontaneously. Cognitive impairment and poor response to pharmacotherapy may be seen with increased age and disease progression. Therefore early intervention and maintenance treatment to prevent recurrence is advised. Pharmacotherapy is needed for acute phase stabilization as well as for maintenance treatment. Certain psychosocial issues and occurrence of stress has been shown to be associated with relapses. Psychotherapeutic interventions are used to take care of such factors.

PHARMACOLOGICAL TREATMENTS

An acute episode of mania or depression in bipolar disorder needs stabilization as well as restoration of mood state and hence pharmacotherapy is needed.

As stated earlier to prevent recurrence of episodes, maintenance treatment with pharmacotherapy is also required.

Acute Mania

Treatment of acute mania should have certain goals:

- Patient's history of any psychiatric illness should be evaluated completely.
- Hospitalization is indicated when patient is suicidal, homicidal, or not willing to take medicines.
- While treatment, patient should not only be stabilized for the current episode but also measures should be taken for prevention of recurrence of further episodes **(Flowchart 11.1)**.

Various Drugs which can be used in Bipolar Disorder

Lithium

It has been the conventional drug of choice for acute and maintenance treatment of bipolar disorder. There is robust evidence for efficacy of lithium in treating acute mania though a period of 1–2 weeks is required for an appreciable response. For augmentation, typical or atypical antipsychotics or other anticonvulsants can be added along with short-acting benzodiazepines.

In acute phase, lithium is started to reach a blood level between 0.8 and 1.2 mEq/L. This level is measured after 5 days of starting of lithium and 12 hours post dose. However, efficacy might be seen in lower doses in elderly patients. In maintenance treatment of bipolar disorder, lithium level is maintained between 0.6 and 0.8meq/L. Symptoms of lithium toxicity occur when level is $\geq$1.5 mEq/L, which is when intervention should be done. Clinical monitoring for signs of lithium toxicity should be done and precautions need to be taken. Precautions include stable intake of salt, reduction, or cessation of lithium in case of diarrhea and vomiting and not combining it with drugs which can increase lithium level such as diuretics, acetyl salicylic acid, certain antihypertensives and antibiotics.

Anticonvulsants

- *Carbamazepine:* Carbamazepine is primarily used as an anticonvulsant.

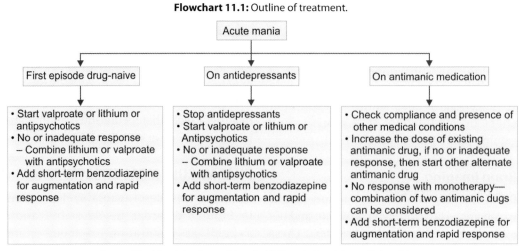

Flowchart 11.1: Outline of treatment.

Acute mania

First episode drug-naive	On antidepressants	On antimanic medication

• Start valproate or lithium or antipsychotics
• No or inadequate response
  – Combine lithium or valproate with antipsychotics
• Add short-term benzodiazepine for augmentation and rapid response
	• Stop antidepressants
	• Start valproate or lithium or Antipsychotics
	• No or inadequate response
	  – Combine lithium or valproate with antipsychotics
	• Add short-term benzodiazepine for augmentation and rapid response
		• Check compliance and presence of other medical conditions
		• Increase the dose of existing antimanic drug, if no or inadequate response, then start other alternate antimanic drug
		• No response with monotherapy—combination of two antimanic dugs can be considered
		• Add short-term benzodiazepine for augmentation and rapid response

Source: The Maudsley Prescribing Guidelines in Psychiatry, 13th edition.

Its efficacy as mood stabilizer is also established in acute mania. Dose should be given to reach a plasma level of at least 7 mg/L. Efficacy of carbamazepine is generally less than lithium in the *prophylaxis* of bipolar illness.

- *Sodium valproate:* Sodium valproate is primarily used as an anticonvulsant. Later studies have established its efficacy in treatment of mania. Valproate given in a loading dose of 20 mg/day has a rapid antimanic action. Efficacy of valproate in controlling manic symptoms is equal to lithium.
- *Oxcarbazepine:* Oxcarbazepine is another antiepileptic, which has found increasing acceptance and a very useful place in the management of mood disorders. It is an effective mood stabilizer and can be used either alone or as an add-on with other mood stabilizers.
- *Antipsychotics:* Atypical antipsychotics are preferred. Typical antipsychotics have also been used effectively in acute mania. Efficacy is increased when given along with mood stabilizer. Olanzapine, risperidone, quetiapine, aripiprazole and asenapine have been evaluated extensively and have been found to be effective in acute mania. In certain studies, olanzapine was found to be of equal efficacy as valproate or lithium.
- *Benzodiazepines:* Short-term addition of benzodiazepines is useful in controlling acute agitation, sleep disturbances, and aggressive behavior. This is usually administered along with mood stabilizers or antipsychotics.

Bipolar Depression

Patient presenting with depressive phase of bipolar disorder has also to be treated aggressively as there is increased suicidality, catatonic symptoms, or psychotic symptoms in this phase. Only a few drugs have proved their efficacy in bipolar depression.

Antidepressants are particularly not helpful in this phase due to the propensity to cause "switch" to mania or hypomania. Moreover, it has been seen that many bipolar depressed patients do not respond to antidepressants alone. CANMAT guidelines (Canadian Network for Mood and Anxiety Treatments, 2013) have suggested first-line treatment with lamotrigine or lithium or quetiapine. Lamotrigine is an anticonvulsant which has been seen to have better results when compared with lithium or valproate. Antidepressants can be used along with mood stabilizers. A combination of olanzapine and fluoxetine has been approved by US Food and Drug Administration (FDA) for treatment of bipolar depression. Electroconvulsive therapy is also advised as a second-line treatment where treatment with drugs has not worked.

Maintenance Treatment of Bipolar Disorder

This is required to prevent future recurrence of any manic or depressive episode. Lithium is still considered as the best of the lot in preventing the future episodes. Studies have found that prophylaxis with valproate as monotherapy was relatively less effective than lithium or the combination of lithium and valproate. Recent evidences support the use of olanzapine, quetiapine, and aripiprazole in long-term treatment. Long-term treatment with antidepressants is not advised in bipolar depression.

Electroconvulsive Therapy

Electroconvulsive therapy (ECT) is indicated in the following conditions:
- Acute delirious mania
- Mania not being adequately controlled by drugs

- Acute bipolar depression with suicidality
- Mania in first trimester of pregnancy
- Bipolar depression with suicidality.

Psychotherapy

Definite efficacy of psychoeducation in bipolar disorder has not yet been established. Psychological treatments such as psychoeducation promotes treatment adherence. These therapies can be initiated only when the patient is in maintenance phase of treatment. Group therapies have been conducted for patients and their families to take care of risk factors, warning signs, and coping strategies and have been found to be effective. Cognitive behavior therapy has given good results for the depressive symptoms. Individual therapies might focus on stress and conflicts of the patient and family dynamics and thus help in prevention of future episodes.

TAKE-HOME MESSAGES

- Bipolar disorders are "disorders of mood" which is also known as "affective disorders." It includes depression, mania, cyclothymia, and others. It is characterized by recurrent episodes of depression, mania, and hypomania, which generally remit spontaneously, and do not show any symptoms in the intervening period.
- The lifetime prevalence rate of bipolar disorders across the world is about 1%.
- Mania is characterized by flamboyant attitude and appearance, increased energy and activity, euphoric or irritable mood, increased volubility, pressure of speech, flight of ideas, impulsive and at times disinhibited behavior, insomnia, and lack of insight.
- Depression is characterized by generalized slowness and retardation of both speech and behavior. Mood is constantly sad with diurnal variation sometimes, and there is incapacity to experience pleasure and other emotions. Hopelessness, helplessness, worthlessness, and other cognitive emotions dominate the thinking. Sleep and appetite are reduced and there may be some cognitive impairment.
- Various genetic, biochemical, psychological, and environmental factors have been theorized to contribute to the causation of bipolar disorder.
- Management includes mood stabilizers, antidepressants, antipsychotics, sedatives, ECT, and certain psychological interventions. Lithium and valproate are important mood stabilizers. Treatment has to be given for both the acute phase and also for the maintenance phase to prevent recurrence of similar episodes.

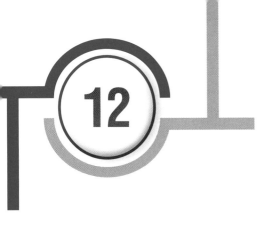

NN Raju, N Prasanna Kumar

Anxiety Disorders

INTRODUCTION

Anxiety disorders are a group of mental disorders characterized by abnormal feelings of fear and worry about current situation and future events and may be associated with physical symptoms.

Fear is a basic primary emotional state consisting of subjective apprehension and objective physiological changes. Both may be appropriate in degree and duration compared to the degree of external threat; however, at times it may be excessive and inappropriate. The physical changes, in the form of muscular, vascular, and glandular activity, prepare the organism for action which is known as flight or fight reaction. It is usually accompanied by signs of increased activity of sympathetic nervous system which include palpitation, sweating, rapid respiration, tremors, clammy and cold hands, pallor, piloerection, dilated pupil, nausea, and frequent urges to urinate and defecate. The anxiety is described as free floating when there is no conscious recognition of an external threat.

EPIDEMIOLOGY AND TYPES

Anxiety disorders with lifetime prevalence of about 29% comprise of specific phobia (10.3% annual prevalence), panic/agoraphobia (6%), social phobia (2.7%), generalized anxiety disorder (GAD—2.2%). Indian studies had reported the prevalence rate of anxiety neurosis as 10.5 per 1,000 and GAD prevalence

as 5.8% and phobias as 4.2%. Following types of anxiety disorders have been described as per International Statistical Classification of Diseases and Related Health Problems-10 (ICD-10):

- F40 Phobic anxiety disorders
- F40.0 Agoraphobia
  - .00 Without panic disorder
  - .01 With panic disorder
- F40.1 Social phobia
- F40.2 Specific (isolated) phobias
- F40.8 Other phobic anxiety disorders
- F40.9 Phobic anxiety disorder, unspecified
- F41 Other anxiety disorders
- F41.0 Panic disorder (episodic paroxysmal anxiety)
- F41.1 Generalized anxiety disorder
- F41.2 Mixed anxiety and depressive disorder
- F41.3 Other mixed anxiety disorders
- F41.8 Other specified anxiety disorders
- F41.9 Anxiety disorder, unspecified

As per Diagnostic and Statistical Manual of Mental Disorders-5 (DSM-5) anxiety disorders comprise of separation anxiety disorder, selective mutism, specific phobia, social anxiety disorder (SAD), panic disorder, agoraphobia, generalized anxiety disorder, substance/medication-induced anxiety disorder, anxiety disorder due to another medical condition, other specified anxiety disorder, and unspecified anxiety disorder.

ETIOLOGY

- *Psychodynamic theories*: The psycho-dynamic theory has explained anxiety as a conflict between the id and ego.

Aggressive, sexual, and other impulsive drives may be experienced as unacceptable resulting in repression. These repressed drives may break through repression in face of external threats or other cues and thus produce anxiety. Some examples of defense mechanism described are regression in anxiety, displacement in phobia, undoing and isolation in obsessive compulsive disorders, and conversion in somatoform disorders.

- *Learning theory*: The anxiety disorder is developed when neutral environmental cues get associated with anxiety producing events. To start with anxiety associated with naturally occurring frightful situations like accidents subsequently may produce fear to a new and different situation resulting in avoidance.
- Cognitive theory has emerged through works of Beck mainly in depression but has also been extended to various anxiety disorders in explanation and treatment. In anxiety disorders, events are interpreted by incorrect beliefs in a threatening manner. They have a tendency to overestimate the potential for danger of everything. Such beliefs (schema) result in automatic thought response to external or internal states that trigger anxiety. They tend to imagine the worst possible scenario and avoid situations they think are dangerous, such as crowds, heights, or social interaction.
- *Biological theories:* The fear and anxiety help animals in survival by leading to induction of adaptive behaviors. Current biological underpinnings point toward involvement of gamma-aminobutyric acid (GABA) receptor, benzodiazepine receptor, chloride channel complex, the noradrenergic nucleus coeruleus, and raphe nuclei and their projections.

- All anxiety disorders also seem to run in families. Familial and twin studies attribute familial aggregation to genetic etiology but no specific locus has been identified so far.
- *Areas of brain involved in anxiety:* Limbic system, locus coeruleus, and cerebral cortex are major brain components implicated in anxiety disorders. Among them hippocampus, amygdala, prefrontal cortex, and frontolimbic circuits involved in fear and anxiety. The areas implicated in potential threat include amygdala, insula, ventrolateral prefrontal cortex (VLPFC), and anterior cingulate cortex. HPA axis (hypothalamus—pituitary—adrenal axis) is reported to be associated with anxiety disorders.
- The important neurotransmitters involved in anxiety disorders include norepinephrine, serotonin, GABA, and glutamate. Several neuromodulatory systems have also been implicated in the pathogenesis of anxiety disorders. Norepinephrine is perhaps the most implicated neurotransmitter in the genesis of panic attacks. Evidence for its increased activity comes from the observation that anxiety can be provoked by activation of noradrenergic system. An increase in cerebrospinal fluid (CSF) concentration of 3-methoxy-4-hydroxyphenyglycol (MHPG) in states of anxiety has been observed. It has also been observed that yohimbine can precipitate panic symptoms, which is an alpha-2 adrenergic antagonist. Serotonin is another important neurotransmitter, which is implicated in the etiology of anxiety disorders based on the observation that benzodiazepines are effective anxiolytics by virtue of their ability to reduce the activity of serotonergic systems and also the observation that specific

serotonin reuptake inhibitors (SSRIs) may increase anxiety within first few days of its administration. A decrease in the inhibitory activity of GABA containing neuron has been hypothesized in the causation of anxiety. This is based on observation that benzodiazepines, a very effective anxiolytic agent, are known to act by enhancing GABA activity. Altered function of adenosine and cholecystokinin has also been suggested as mechanisms to cause different anxiety disorders.

SPECIFIC ANXIETY DISORDERS

Agoraphobia

Agoraphobia is a fear of being in situations from where escape might be difficult or that help may be unavailable if things go wrong. This leads to avoidance of such situations and fear of travelling alone in lifts trains, buses, or planes, crowds, public places, and entering shops.

Diagnostic Guidelines

All the following criteria should be fulfilled for a definite diagnosis:
- The psychological or autonomic symptoms must be primarily manifestations of anxiety and not secondary to other symptoms, such as delusions or obsessional thoughts;
- The anxiety must be restricted to (or occur mainly in) at least two of the following situations—crowds, public places, travelling away from home, and travelling alone; and
- Avoidance of the phobic situation must be, or have been, a prominent feature.

Panic Disorder

Panic disorder is an anxiety disorder characterized by recurrent unexpected panic attacks which are sudden periods of intense anxiety that may be associated with palpitations, sweating, shaking, shortness of breath, numbness, or feeling that one is going to be doomed. Lifetime prevalence is reported to be 7.1% in women, 4% in men. Heritability of panic disorder is 40%. Panic disorder starts in adolescence and can run chronic course with recurrent panic attacks. Stressful life events tend to precede the onset of panic disorder.

Separation anxiety disorder can predispose to panic disorder. Episodes appear suddenly with feeling of imminent danger, urge to escape, cardiac symptoms like palpitations, breathlessness, chest pain, and other symptoms include tremors, sweating, nausea dizziness, feelings of unreality (depersonalization or derealization), choking sensations, fear of dying, losing control, or going mad and also sometimes wake up from sleep at night due to panic attack. Discrete periods of intense fear with continuous concern of having another attack and worrying about the consequence of attack. Fear for consequences of attack or another attack is important in panic disorder. Panic disorder is sometimes associated with agoraphobia. Episode of panic attacks occurs not only in panic disorder but also in other disorders such as social anxiety and specific phobia.

There will be false interpretations of bodily sensations in catastrophic way as dryness of mouth interpreted as choking sensation and increase intensity of these different bodily sensations may be one of the triggering factors for panic episode. The conditioned response in panic episode may be due to conditioned stimuli of internal body sensations.

Diagnostic Guidelines

For a definite diagnosis, several severe attacks of autonomic anxiety should have occurred within a period of about 1 month:
- In circumstances, where there is no objective danger;

- Without being confined to known or predictable situations; and
- With comparative freedom from anxiety symptoms between attacks (although anticipatory anxiety is common).

Social Phobia (Social Anxiety Disorder)

Social anxiety disorder, also known as social phobia, is an anxiety disorder characterized by a significant amount of fear in one or more social situations, causing considerable distress and impaired ability to function in at least some parts of daily life.

Lifetime prevalence of SAD is reported to be 5–14% and equally common in men and women. Over protectiveness and over criticism, behaviorally inhibited temperament and interpreting neutral stimuli as fearful are predisposing factors. Fear for social situations and anxiety leading to avoidance is cardinal feature. They may feel as personal issue, under report the problem, and change their professions with less social interaction and may be associated with low self-esteem and fear of criticism. There may be complaints of nausea, or urgency of micturition, flushing, and hand tremor.

Diagnostic Guidelines

All of the following criteria should be fulfilled for a definite diagnosis:

- The psychological, behavioral, or autonomic symptoms must be primarily manifestations of anxiety and not secondary to other symptoms such as delusions or obsessional thoughts.
- The anxiety must be restricted to or predominate in particular social situations.
- Avoidance of the phobic situations must be a prominent feature.

Specific Phobias

A specific phobia is a kind of anxiety disorder that presents with excessive, unreasonable and irrational fear related to exposure to specific objects or situations. As a result, the affected person tends to avoid contact with the objects or situations and, in severe cases, any mention or depiction of them.

Lifetime prevalence of specific phobia is 12% with female to male ratio being 2:1. Specific phobia begins in childhood or early adult life and can persist for decades. Specific phobia can be natural (fear for water, high), blood, insects or animals, and type of situation (enclosed spaces and loud noise).

Diagnostic Guidelines

All of the following should be fulfilled for a definite diagnosis:

- The psychological or autonomic symptoms must be primary manifestations of anxiety, and not secondary to other symptoms such as delusion or obsessional thought.
- The anxiety must be restricted to the presence of the particular phobic object or situation.
- The phobic situation is avoided whenever possible.

Generalized Anxiety Disorder

It is an *anxiety disorder* characterized by excessive, uncontrollable, and often irrational worry, that is, apprehensive expectation about events or activities. GAD is twice common in women as in men. Patient's worries are excessive, uncontrollable, and pervasive, which persist for most of the time, resulting in significant distress and impairment. Sleep disturbance, difficulty in concentration, restlessness, irritability, and fatigue are other important components of GAD. Anxiety is generalized, persistent, and predominating in any environmental circumstances.

Diagnostic Guidelines

The sufferer must have primary symptoms of anxiety in most days for at least several weeks at a time, and usually for several months. These symptoms should usually involve elements of:

- Apprehension (worries about future misfortunes, feeling "on edge", difficulty in concentrating, etc.)
- Motor tension (restless fidgeting, tension headaches, trembling, inability to relax)
- Autonomic over activity (lightheadedness, sweating, tachycardia or tachypnea, epigastric discomfort, dizziness, dry mouth, etc.).

GENERAL MANAGEMENT

Before starting any treatment, it would be prudent to remember few common psychiatric and medical conditions which mimic anxiety disorders. The psychiatric disorders to be ruled out are depressive disorders, adjustment disorders, obsessive compulsive disorders, dissociative disorders, substance related disorders, and even psychotic disorders. The medical conditions which need to be considered are myocardial infarction, hyperventilation syndrome, hypoglycemia, hyperthyroidism, and carcinoid syndrome.

Majority of the anxiety disorders are treated by either psychotherapy or pharmacotherapy or combination of both.

Pharmacotherapy

Antidepressants like SSRIs and antianxiety drugs like benzodiazepines are most commonly prescribed medication in anxiety disorders. Following are some of the drugs extensively used both by psychiatrists and other medical specialists dealing with anxiety and related disorders:

- *Benzodiazepines:* These are agents effective in reducing anxiety irrespective of the cause or comorbid illness. Due to the concern of dependence and habit formation, many physicians are cautious in using these drugs but if they are used judiciously and properly withdrawn, they remain the mainstay of treatment. Alprazolam, clonazepam, diazepam, nitrazepam, lorazepam, and oxazepam are important molecules in this group. Discontinuation syndrome (withdrawal effects) is a major disadvantage especially with short-acting benzodiazepines, if used for long periods. Drowsiness and cognitive deficits are other unwanted effects of these drugs.
- *Antidepressants*: SSRIs are preferred as first-line of choice. The different SSRIs include citalopram (10–40 mg), escitalopram (10–20 mg), paroxetine (20–60 mg), and sertraline (50–200 mg). Some may experience gastrointestinal side effects, withdrawal syndrome, insomnia, and sexual dysfunctions with SSRIS. Serotonin norepinephrine reuptake inhibitors (SNRIs) include duloxetine (60–120 mg/day), venlafaxine (75–225 mg/day) but hypertension can occur with SNRIs. The dosages of SSRIs and SNRIs are the same for acute treatment and maintenance. But some especially those with panic attacks may experience increased anxiety during the initial periods of treatment that can be minimized by adding small doses of benzodiazepines which should be withdrawn later. A note of caution while using SSRIs in children and adolescents is that agitation and suicidal ideation are reported in such population.
- *Tricyclic antidepressants*: These are very effective in combating anxiety in array of conditions, less often used though in view of their adverse effects. Anticholinergic effects such as dry mouth, constipation, and delirium in elders, cardiotoxicity,

potential lethality in high doses are some of the unwanted actions. Imipramine, amitriptyline, nortriptyline, and clomipramine are typical drugs in this class.

Other Drugs

- *Beta-blockers*—like propranolol and atenolol, act to suppress the peripheral signs like palpitation, tremors in anxiety without reducing the fear and apprehension. They are specifically useful in panic attacks and SADs. Adverse effects include hypotension, bradycardia, erectile dysfunction, and drowsiness. They are contraindicated in person suffering from bronchial asthma.
- Buspirone—effective through its serotonergic actions is useful in GAD. The disadvantage is its slow onset of action and cannot be used to replace benzodiazepines. It may cause headache and dizziness.
- Anticonvulsants like gabapentin, tiagabine, and lamotrigine are reported to be useful at least in those who are non-responsive to other classes of drugs and therapies.
- *Nonpharmacological management*: Cognitive behavioral therapy (CBT) is the most studied and widely used in anxiety disorders. The components include identifying the negative thoughts related to anxiety, evaluating the accuracy of the beliefs, and derive alternate thoughts based on information.

TAKE-HOME MESSAGES

- Anxiety disorders are a group of mental disorders characterized by abnormal feelings of fear and worry about current situation and future events and may be associated with physical symptoms such as palpitation, sweating, rapid respiration, tremors, clammy and cold hands, pallor, piloerection, dilated pupil, nausea, and frequent urges to urinate and defecate.
- Major types of anxiety disorders are agoraphobia, specific phobias, panic disorder, social phobia, GAD, etc.
- Agoraphobia is a fear of being in situations from where escape might be difficult or that help may be unavailable if things go wrong.
- Panic disorder is an anxiety disorder characterized by recurrent unexpected panic attacks which are sudden periods of intense anxiety that may be associated with palpitations, sweating, shaking, shortness of breath, numbness, or feeling that one is going to be doomed.
- Social phobia, is an anxiety disorder characterized by a significant amount of fear in one or more social situations, causing considerable distress and impaired ability to function in at least some parts of daily life.
- A specific phobia is that kind of anxiety disorder that presents with unreasonable, excessive, or irrational fear related to exposure to specific objects or situations.
- Generalized anxiety disorder presents with excessive, uncontrollable and often irrational worry and negative anticipations, on a continuous basis, about events, or activities of life.
- Management includes ruling out of possible organic causes and by rational use of SSRIs, benzodiazepines, TCAs, beta-blockers, buspirone, etc. Non-pharmacological management includes CBT and other psychotherapeutic measures.

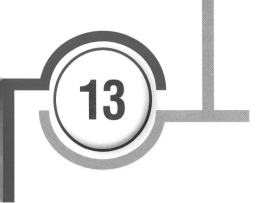

13

Obsessive-compulsive and Related Disorders

YC Janardhan Reddy, Aditi Singh

INTRODUCTION

Obsessive-compulsive and related disorders (OCRDs) include a group of disorders characterized by repetitive thoughts and/or behaviors **(Box 13.1)**. These disorders are presumed to be related to the prototype disorder, obsessive-compulsive disorder (OCD). They are grouped together because of their symptom similarity, co-occurrence, shared family-genetic risk factors and involvement of corticostriatal circuitry and often similar treatment response.

OBSESSIVE-COMPULSIVE DISORDER

Obsessive-compulsive disorder is a common mental illness with lifetime prevalence of 1–3% with almost similar prevalence rate in children and adolescents. Most adults with OCD report onset of their symptoms in childhood or adolescence. According to the World Health Organization, OCD is one among the top 20 most disabling illnesses. People suffer from OCD silently for many years before seeking treatment because of stigma, shame, embarrassment, lack of knowledge about illness, scarcity of mental health professionals and poor recognition of the illness by other health professionals.

Obsessions

Obsessive-compulsive disorder is characterized by obsessions and compulsions. Obsessions are repetitive and persistent thoughts, images or impulses/urges that are perceived as intrusive and unwanted. They are time consuming and cause marked distress and/or anxiety. Obsessions are also recognized as a product of one's own mind and not imposed from outside. This differentiates them from the delusional thoughts characteristic of schizophrenia and other psychotic illnesses.

Compulsions

Because the obsessions are intrusive, unwanted and distressing, attempts are made to ignore, suppress or neutralize them with some other action or thought (compulsions). Compulsions are repetitive behaviors or mental acts that the person feels driven to perform in response to an obsession (e.g., washing hands repeatedly in response to an obsession of being contaminated).

> **Box 13.1:** Obsessive-compulsive and related disorders.
>
> - Obsessive-compulsive disorder
> - Body dysmorphic disorder
> - Olfactory reference disorder
> - Hypochondriasis
> - Hoarding disorder
> - Body-focused repetitive behavior disorders
> - Trichotillomania (Hair-pulling disorder)
> - Excoriation (Skin-picking) disorder
> - Tourette syndrome

The compulsions are aimed at preventing or reducing distress or preventing some dreaded event from occurring (e.g., repeating same actions over and over again, praying repeatedly). Compulsions are not connected in a realistic way with what they are designed to prevent, or are clearly excessive. For example, repeating actions in a particular fashion does not in a realistic way prevent an accident from occurring.

Other Features

People who suffer from OCD often avoid cues/triggers of their obsessions (e.g., avoiding sharp instruments because of the fear of harming others) and at times make their family members perform compulsions on their behalf (proxy compulsions). Most persons who suffer from OCD have insight into the fact that their repetitive thoughts and/or behaviors are unreasonable or excessive, but a proportion of patients may have poor or absent insight. Poor or absent insight is not an indication of psychosis in the context of OCRD. Typical features of OCD are summarized in **Box 13.2**. Common obsessive-compulsive symptoms are given in **Box 13.3**.

Comorbidity

People who suffer from OCD also have other comorbid psychiatric disorders **(Box 13.4)**. Depressive and anxiety disorders are common comorbid conditions. OCD is also not uncommon in those with schizophrenia and bipolar disorders. OCRDs mentioned in **Box 13.1** can also co-occur with OCD. In children, attention-deficit hyperactivity disorder, oppositional-defiant disorder and tic disorders are other common comorbid conditions. It is important to diagnose and treat comorbid conditions as untreated comorbid conditions may negatively influence treatment outcome of OCD.

Course

Untreated OCD tends to run a chronic course with waxing and waning of symptoms. Nearly a half of those suffering from OCD remit at

---

Box 13.2: Clinical characteristics of obsessive-compulsive disorder (OCD).

- Presence of obsessions and/or compulsions:
  - Obsessions are repetitive, intrusive, unwanted thoughts (e.g., of contamination, sex, blasphemy), images (e.g., of violent scenes), or impulses/urges (e.g., to stab someone) that cause marked anxiety or distress. The obsessions are recognized by the sufferer as product of one's own mind and are not imposed from without. The individual attempts to ignore or suppress them or neutralize them by performing compulsions
  - Compulsions (or rituals) are repetitive behaviors (e.g., excessive washing in response to fear of contamination, repeated checking to prevent harm) or mental acts (e.g., praying in response to blasphemy thoughts, replacing bad thought with good thought), that are usually performed in response to an obsessional thought
- Compulsions are not connected in a realistic way with what they are designed to prevent, or are clearly excessive, but performance of compulsions result in temporary reduction of anxiety or distress
- The individuals who suffer from OCD typically recognize their behaviors as irrational, excessive, absurd or unwanted (e.g., I do not have to wash so much to keep my hands clean, but I cannot control) but some may not have good insight and consider their behaviors as reasonable and accurate [e.g., If I do not scrub my hands with Dettol every time I shake my hands with someone, I am convinced I will get acquired immunodeficiency syndrome (AIDS)]
- Individuals with OCD often avoid people, things, situations that trigger obsessions and compulsions
- The symptoms are usually time-consuming, cause marked anxiety or distress and are associated with significant impairment in day-to-day functioning

Box 13.3: Common symptoms of obsessive-compulsive disorder (OCD).

Obsessions
- Contamination related obsessions [e.g., concern or disgust with bodily secretions and waste such as stools and urine, fear of dirt or germs or infections such as fear of *catching* an illness, e.g., acquired immunodeficiency syndrome (AIDS)]
- Sexual obsessions (e.g., unwanted, forbidden sexual thoughts about family, friends, thoughts of molesting children)
- Harm/aggression-related obsessions: Fear might harm self or others, e.g., harming babies, stabbing a friend, running people over while driving), violent/horrific images of murders, fear of uttering obscenities
- Religious or blasphemy (e.g., blasphemous thoughts, fear of uttering insults to God)
- Pathological doubts about daily activities (e.g., doubts of having not locked doors, turned off gas knobs)
- Need for symmetry and exactness (e.g., concern about things being not properly aligned, symmetrical, perfect or exact)
- Miscellaneous [e.g., intrusive nonviolent images/thoughts, superstitious fears (passing a cat, cemetery), lucky or unlucky numbers, colors]

Compulsions
- Washing or cleaning in response to contamination obsessions (excessive or ritualized hand washing, showering, bathing, brushing or excessive cleaning of household items, floors, kitchen vessels, etc.)
- Checking in response to doubts (e.g., appliances, locks, stove, doors) and to prevent harm (check to make sure that you have not caused accident, examining for injuries, etc.)
- Repeating (e.g., rereading or rewriting, repeating routine activities such as going in and out of doorway)
- Counting (money, floor tiles)
- Ordering and arranging (often till you feel "just right")
- Miscellaneous (e.g., mental rituals such as praying, replacing bad thought with good thought)

Box 13.4: Comorbid disorders in obsessive-compulsive disorder (OCD).

Mood disorders
- Major depression
- Dysthymia
- Bipolar disorder

Anxiety disorders
- Panic disorder
- Generalized anxiety disorder
- Social phobia

OCD-related disorders
- Body dysmorphic disorder
- Olfactory reference disorder
- Hypochondriasis
- Trichotillomania
- Skin picking disorder
- Tic disorders

Attention-deficit hyperactivity disorder
Oppositional defiant disorder

Personality disorders
- Obsessive-compulsive personality disorder
- Anxious-avoidant personality disorder
- Borderline personality disorder
- Schizotypal personality

Other conditions
- Schizophrenia
- Autism spectrum disorders

least partially. There is some evidence that greater proportion of Indian patients remit compared to those from other parts of the world (71% vs. 48%). Early diagnosis and intensive treatment may improve long-term outcome. Early age at onset, longer duration of illness, more severe OCD and poor insight may predict poorer long-term outcome.

Etiology

Obsessive-compulsive disorder is heritable. Twin studies show higher concordance in monozygotic twins compared to dizygotic twins (75–90% vs. 10–20%). First-degree relatives of those suffering from OCD have four times greater risk of developing OCD than those of unaffected people (8% vs. 2%). Risk is even greater in relatives of those with early onset OCD. Some forms of early onset OCD may be genetically related to chronic tic disorders such as Tourette syndrome (TS). OCD is a polygenic disorder and several genes, particularly the glutamatergic, serotonergic and dopaminergic genes may play an important role in the manifestation of OCD. It is suggested that OCD manifests due to a dysregulation of genes that function in a brain network rather than single genes that simply cumulatively add risk. Environmental factors such as perinatal events, childhood trauma and stress can also contribute to manifestation of OCD.

Since clomipramine and specific serotonin reuptake inhibitors (SSRIs) are effective in treating OCD, serotonin is the most commonly implicated neurotransmitter in OCD. Other neurotransmitters such as dopamine and glutamate are also thought to be involved in OCD. This is supported by observation of efficacy of antipsychotics and glutamatergic drugs that modulate dopamine and glutamate transmission, respectively.

Neuroimaging studies have demonstrated that corticostriatal circuit that includes orbitofrontal cortex, cingulate cortex, caudate nucleus and thalamus is dysfunctional in OCD. Other brain areas such as dorsolateral prefrontal cortex and parietal cortex are also recently implicated in OCD.

Acute onset of OCD and tics is described in children following group A beta-hemolytic streptococcal infection called "pediatric acute-onset neuropsychiatric syndrome" (PANS). Autoantibodies to basal ganglia structures are postulated to be responsible for the abrupt and dramatic flare-ups of symptoms.

Some deeply held beliefs such as overestimation of danger (when things go wrong, consequences can be terrible), exaggerated sense of responsibility (even if harm is remote, I should do all that is possible to prevent it), perfectionism (things are not right if they are not perfect), intolerance of uncertainty and ambiguity (I must be absolutely certain of my decisions), importance of thoughts (having an unwanted nasty thought means I am a bad person) and perceived need to have control over thoughts (I should have complete control over my thoughts) may play a role in the manifestation of OCD.

Treatment

Pharmacological Treatment

Specific serotonin reuptake inhibitors and clomipramine are equally efficacious in treating. There is no evidence of superiority of one over the other. SSRIs are recommended first-line options since they are better tolerated with lesser side effects compared to clomipramine. Choice of SSRI depends upon the tolerability of the drug and its side effect profile. In treating OCD, higher doses of drugs are used than in conditions like depression and anxiety disorders. Doses of drugs used in treating OCD are shown in **Table 13.1**. An SSRI has to be continued at least for 1–2 years after remission. However, most patients may require indefinite continued treatment with an SSRI to prevent relapses particularly those with severe and chronic illness, past history of relapse following discontinuation and clinically significant residual symptoms. An SSRI should be continued at the same dose that resulted in improvement, unless the dose is not tolerated.

Table 13.1: Medications recommended as monotherapy in obsessive-compulsive disorder.	
Drug	*Suggested dosage*
Escitalopram	20–30 mg
Fluoxetine	60–80 mg
Fluvoxamine	200–300 mg
Paroxetine	40–60 mg
Sertraline	150–200 mg
Citalopram	40–60 mg
Clomipramine	150–225 mg
Venlafaxine	225–300 mg

Psychological Treatment

Exposure and response prevention (ERP) and cognitive behavior therapy (CBT) are effective in treating OCD. ERP involves exposing the person to triggers of obsessions that provoke anxiety/fear (exposure) and preventing compulsions (response prevention) in a graded manner. Because of repeated exposure to anxiety provoking obsessional triggers and refraining from performing compulsions, person realizes that anxiety subsides gradually on its own without having to perform compulsions and that the feared consequences do not actually occur. By this process, person gets habituated to anxiety provoking triggers and extinction of fear occurs. In CBT, along with ERP, cognitive strategies are used to correct dysfunctional beliefs such as overestimation of threat. The CBT or ERP are delivered once or twice weekly for 15–20 sessions of 90–120 minutes each spread over 8–12 weeks.

Recommended Strategy

The SSRIs and clomipramine and CBT or ERP are the first-line treatment options for OCD. They may be tried individually or in combination. In mild–to–moderate OCD, CBT or ERP may be tried as monotherapy. Severe OCD may require a combination of medications and CBT or ERP. In India, because of resource constraints, drugs are often the preferred options over CBT or ERP.

In case of a partial response to an SSRI, another medication or CBT or ERP may be added for augmentation. Commonly used augmenting medications are atypical antipsychotics like risperidone or aripiprazole. In case of nonresponse to an SSRI (i.e., no clinically significant change in symptoms with an agent after 10–12 weeks of treatment with optimum dose), another SSRI may be considered. If two SSRIs fail to produce satisfactory clinical response, clomipramine may be the next best option since some meta-analyses show that it may be somewhat superior to SSRIs. If clomipramine is not tolerated, third SSRI may be tried or CBT or ERP may be added. Venlafaxine, a serotonin-noradrenaline reuptake inhibitor, has some evidence of efficacy and may be considered if SSRIs and clomipramine are ineffective. It must be emphasized here that CBT or ERP may be considered as a potential option either as monotherapy or in combination with an SSRI or clomipramine at all stages of treatment.

Electroconvulsive therapy is not effective in treating OCD. Repetitive transcranial magnetic stimulation has been tried but there is no convincing evidence of its efficacy. Stereotactic invasive as well as noninvasive gamma knife surgery and deep brain stimulation (DBS) are indicated in chronic, severe and disabling OCD refractory to standard treatments. Common lesion-based surgeries are bilateral anterior cingulotomy and capsulotomy. DBS is a potentially reversible procedure involving high-frequency stimulation of implanted electrodes in the brain. It is hypothesized to modify dysfunctional circuits. Common sites for DBS are anterior limb of internal capsule, nucleus accumbens, subthalamic nucleus and ventral striatum. Lesion-based surgeries and DBS both seem to be somewhat equally efficacious in about 50% of patients, but in DBS, there is no permanent lesion and it is reversible. Improvement following surgery may occur over a period of 6–24 months following the procedure. Suitability for surgery should be carefully assessed considering benefits and risks. The neurosurgical procedures are not curative in nature and other standard treatments such as SSRIs and CBT or ERP may have to be continued after surgery.

BODY DYSMORPHIC DISORDER, OLFACTORY REFERENCE DISORDER AND HYPOCHONDRIASIS

Body Dysmorphic Disorder

Body dysmorphic disorder (BDD) is characterized by exaggerated concerns and marked preoccupation with a perceived physical defect **(Box 13.5)**. Lifetime prevalence of BDD in the general population is about 2%. Onset of BDD is usually during adolescence and it tends to be a chronic disorder with low rates of full remission. Those suffering from BDD consult dermatologists and cosmetic and plastic surgeons to remove their perceived defects or flaws in appearance. As a result, the underlying disorder often goes undiagnosed and untreated. Individuals with BDD often experience low self-esteem as well as feelings of disgust or embarrassment. Those suffering from BDD may become so preoccupied and distressed by their perceived defect or flaw in appearance that in severe cases, they may stop working or socializing and even become housebound. BDD is associated with high rates of suicide. Up to 80% of the patients report suicidal ideas at some point in the course of the disorder. The rates of attempted suicide range between 20 and 30%. Individuals with BDD often have poor or no insight into their beliefs concerning

---

Box 13.5: Clinical characteristics of body dysmorphic disorder (BDD), olfactory reference disorder (ORD) and hypochondriasis.

BDD
- Preoccupation with imagined defects or flaws in appearance, or ugliness in general, that is markedly excessive.
- Excessive self-consciousness about the imagined defects or flaws in appearance, often in the form of ideas or delusions of self-reference [i.e., the belief that people are noticing or talking about the perceived defect(s) or flaw(s)]
- The preoccupation about appearance is often accompanied by repetitive examination of the perceived flaws (e.g., by checking in mirrors), attempts to camouflage (e.g., wearing a cap or an oversized dark glasses to hide a perceived defect or undergoing surgery) or avoidance of social or other situations (e.g., avoiding social gatherings or meeting people)
- The preoccupation with appearance and associated behaviors are time consuming and cause marked distress or significant impairment in functioning

ORD
- Persistent preoccupation with emitting a foul or offensive body odor or breath that is either unnoticeable or only slightly noticeable to others
- Excessive self-consciousness about emitting the foul odor, often in the form of ideas or delusions of self-reference
- The preoccupation is often accompanied by repetitive checking for body odor, attempts to camouflage (e.g., using excessive perfume or deodorant, repetitive brushing, etc.), or marked avoidance of social or other situations (e.g., avoiding proximity with others, avoiding public transport, etc.)
- The preoccupation with emitting foul smell and associated behaviors are time consuming and cause marked distress or significant impairment in functioning

Hypochondriasis
- Persistent preoccupation or fear of having one or more serious illnesses
- The preoccupation is accompanied by catastrophic misinterpretation of bodily sensations, repeated behaviors such as checking of the body for proof of illness, seeking reassurance form others, undergoing multiple medical consultations or investigations that are unnecessary or avoiding medical appointments
- Hypochondriacal fears and associated behaviors are time consuming and cause marked distress or significant impairment in functioning

appearance along with ideas or delusions of self-reference. They may have delusional conviction about their appearance, yet they do not get a diagnosis of delusional disorder. BDD is typically not associated with other psychotic symptoms, such as auditory hallucinations or other delusions. In contrast to individuals with a psychotic disorder, those with BDD seem to only have delusions that center around their appearance concerns.

Olfactory Reference Disorder

Olfactory reference disorder (ORD) is characterized by persistent and exaggerated preoccupation with emitting foul or offensive body odor or breath that is either unnoticeable or slightly noticeable to others (**Box 13.5**). Clinical features of ORD are very similar to BDD. As in BDD, insight is often poor or absent often leading to a misdiagnosis of delusional disorder.

Hypochondriasis

Hypochondriasis is characterized by persistent preoccupation or fear about the possibility of having one or more serious life-threatening illnesses (**Box 13.5**). Those who suffer from hypochondriasis are often hypervigilant and have a tendency to make catastrophic misinterpretation of benign bodily signs or symptoms including normal or commonplace sensations. However, somatic symptoms can be absent or of mild intensity. Individuals with hypochondriasis have a tendency to get investigated unnecessarily and seek multiple consultations despite the assurance that they do not suffer from serious illnesses. As in OCD, those with hypochondriasis may also have poor or absent insight into their hypochondriacal fears.

Treatment

Body dysmorphic disorder and hypochondriasis often run a chronic course and are difficult to treat. SSRIs and CBT are first-line treatment options for BDD and hypochondriasis. There is scarce literature on treatment of ORD; SSRIs and CBT may be useful in treating it. Antipsychotics are not the drugs of choice in treating delusional BDD, ORD and hypochondriasis. In fact, the delusional variants of these disorders should be treated on the same lines as the nondelusional variants. Individuals with BDD should be discouraged from undergoing a surgical or cosmetic procedure for correcting their perceived defects. In most cases, the dissatisfaction and preoccupations persist even after such procedures.

BODY-FOCUSED REPETITIVE BEHAVIOR DISORDERS

Trichotillomania

Trichotillomania is characterized by hair loss due to recurrent hair-pulling (**Box 13.6**). Its 12-month prevalence is 1–2%. The onset of symptoms is usually around adolescence and a majority of individuals displays a chronic fluctuating course. The hair-pulling is usually (but not always) preceded by mounting tension and is followed by a sense of relief or gratification. The most common sites from which pulling occur is the scalp, eyebrows or eyelashes. However, hair can also be pulled from axillary, facial, pubic and other areas of the body. Hair may not be pulled at random but can be chosen based on specific characteristics (e.g., length of the hair, color, textures or placement on the hairline). Some individuals simply discard pulled hair. Others may play with the hair between their fingers, inspect the hair, bite the hair between the teeth, or ingest all or parts of the

> **Box 13.6:** Clinical characteristics of hoarding disorder, body-focused repetitive behavior disorders and tourette syndrome.
>
> *Hoarding disorder*
> - Excessive accumulation of possessions and difficulty in discarding them regardless of their actual value or utility
> - Accumulation of possessions leads to congestion and cluttering of living areas to the extent that the intended use of living spaces is compromised
> - The items are often hoarded because of their emotional value (e.g., items with a significant event or a person) or perceived usefulness (e.g., newspapers may have information that may be useful)
> - Hoarding is associated with excessive acquisition of items and distress in discarding them
> - The hoarding causes significant distress or impairment in functioning and is not attributable to other conditions such as brain injury, Prader–Willi syndrome, obsessive-compulsive disorder (OCD), schizophrenia, autism spectrum disorders or neurocognitive disorders
>
> *Trichotillomania*
> - Recurrent pulling of one's hair resulting in hair loss
> - Unsuccessful attempts to stop or decrease hair-pulling
> - Hair-pulling causes significant distress or impairment in functioning
>
> *Skin-picking disorder*
> - Recurrent picking of one's skin resulting in skin lesions
> - Unsuccessful attempts to stop or decrease skin-picking
> - Skin-picking results in significant distress or impairment in functioning
>
> *Tourette syndrome*
> - The presence of both motor tics and phonic tics that may or may not manifest concurrently or continuously during the symptomatic course
> - Motor and phonic tics are defined as sudden, rapid, nonrhythmic, and recurrent movements or vocalizations, respectively
> - Motor and phonic tics have been present for at least 1 year

hair. Ingesting hairs can result in undigested masses of hair, called "trichobezoars", which can cause gastrointestinal complications like obstruction later.

Excoriation (Skin-picking) Disorder

Excoriation (skin-picking) disorder is characterized by recurrent skin-picking leading to significant skin lesions **(Box 13.6)**. Its prevalence in the community is about 1%. The most commonly picked sites are the face, arms and hands. Individuals may pick at healthy skin, minor skin irregularities, lesions such as pimples or calluses, or at scabs from previous picking. Most people pick with their fingernails, although some use tweezers, knives, or other sharp objects. Individuals with this disorder often conceal or camouflage evidence of skin picking (e.g., using make-up or clothing). Skin-picking may be associated with rituals such as visually or tactilely examining the skin, orally manipulating, or eating the skin or scab after it has been picked. Trichotillomania, nail biting, OCD and depression are often comorbid with skin-picking disorder.

Treatment

Trichotillomania and skin-picking do not respond satisfactorily to SSRIs. Clomipramine may have some value in treating tricho-tillomania. N-acetylcysteine, the drug that modulates glutamatergic system, is found beneficial in the treatment of both trichotillomania and skin-picking. Atypical antipsychotic such as olanzapine may be useful in some people with trichotillomania. Nonpharmacological approach involves stimulus control and habit reversal training (HRT). They are effective in treating trichotillomania and skin-picking. In stimulus control, situational factors that trigger hair-pulling or skin-picking are identified and individuals are taught to eliminate or modify these factors that contribute to the behavior. For example, if hair-pulling occurs in front of mirrors, mirrors are covered or removed. If hair-pulling is triggered by feeling the hair by fingers, bandages may be applied to finger tips to prevent contact with hair. The HRT involves three components: awareness training (becoming aware of urge to pull hair), competence training (perform a task that is incompatible with hair-pulling such as making a fist), and social support.

HOARDING DISORDER

Hoarding is accumulation of possessions due to excessive acquisition or a failure to discard items of little or no value **(Box 13.6)**. It is estimated to be present in 2–5% of the general population. The individual is reluctant to part with items owing to worries about losing items that may have emotional significance, utility or some intrinsic value. Associated with the difficulty in discarding items is significant cluttering of living space, working space and sometimes even their vehicles. This might lead to substantial distress and difficulty in using these spaces appropriately as well as pose a safety hazard in very severe cases. In some individuals, hoarding could also be secondary to OCD, e.g., fear of harm to the family if possessions are discarded. The insight in hoarding is generally poorer as compared to OCD. Owing to poor insight, the individuals may not readily seek treatment. SSRIs are not found to be efficacious in treating hoarding disorder although hoarding secondary to OCD may improve. CBT involving motivational interviewing and strategies targeting hoarding specific cognitions such as beliefs pertaining to acquisition, discarding and emotional significance of possessions is found to be beneficial in treating hoarding.

TOURETTE SYNDROME

Tics are sudden, rapid, repetitive, non-rhythmic motor movements (eye blinking, nose twitching, shoulder shrugging) or vocalizations (throat clearing, snorting) which may occur multiple times in a day in bouts and wax and wane in frequency and severity. These movements may be involuntary or semi-voluntary, i.e., the person affected can suppress or postpone these for some time. Tics are usually preceded by an uncomfortable sensation or tension—the "premonitory sensation or urge". Performing a tic leads to resolution of this discomfort.

Simple tics can be motor (e.g., eye blinking, nose twitching, tongue protrusion, head jerks and shoulder shrugs, etc.) or phonic (grunting, throat clearing, coughing, sniffling, etc.). Complex motor tics involve multiple muscle groups and can be a more elaborate sequence of motor movements (e.g., tapping, circling in a pattern, hopping, jumping, touching, etc.). Complex vocal tics are repetitive, purposeless and involuntary utterances such as utterance of obscenities (coprolalia), repeating others' words (echolalia) or repeating oneself (palilalia).

Tourette syndrome is diagnosed when a person develops both vocal and motor tics, though not necessarily concurrently **(Box 13.6)**. TS affects between 0.3 and 1% of the population. TS occur predominantly in young people (before age 18 years), and it is 3–4 times more frequent in males than in females. A majority of those who had onset of TS (about 80%) before age 10 years experience a significant tic decrease during adolescence, and by age 18 years, tic intensity and frequency decreases to such an extent that the person no longer experiences any impairment from tics. Tic disorder is commonly comorbid with attention-deficit hyperactivity disorder, other disruptive behavior disorders (oppositional defiant disorder and conduct disorder), learning disability, OCD, and other mood and anxiety disorders.

For mild-to-moderate TS, α-adrenergic agonists such as clonidine (0.025–0.4 mg per day) and guanfacine (0.25–4 mg/day) are recommended. If α-adrenergic agonists are ineffective, those with moderate-to-severe TS can be treated with neuroleptics such as risperidone (0.125–4 mg/day), aripiprazole (5–15 mg/day), haloperidol (0.25–5 mg/day) and pimozide (0.5–8 mg/day). Risperidone and aripiprazole are preferred over haloperidol and pimozide because of lesser side effects. SSRIs are ineffective in treating TS. HRT is effective in treating TS and it may be considered as a first-line treatment in mild-to-moderate TS. HRT may also be used in combination with pharmacological treatment.

CONCLUSION

Obsessive-compulsive disorder and related disorders are common severe mental illnesses that can be highly disabling. They are often undiagnosed and untreated. Correct diagnosis and instituting evidenced-based treatments may improve outcome substantially. Since these disorders have a tendency to run a chronic course, with remissions and relapses, long-term treatment is needed.

TAKE-HOME MESSAGES

- OCD is a common and often disabling mental illness. Early diagnosis and treatment may improve long-term outcome. It is the prototype disorder and includes obsessions and compulsions.
- Disorders related to OCD include body dysmorphic disorder, olfactory reference disorder, hypochondriasis, hoarding disorder, trichotillomania (hair-pulling disorder), excoriation (skin-picking) disorder, hoarding disorder and Tourette Syndrome. They are often undiagnosed and untreated because of lack of sensitivity on the part of the clinicians. They need to be identified and treated aggressively as disorders such as BDD are associated with high risk of suicide.
- OCRDs are highly comorbid with each other and with other anxiety and mood disorders. Comorbid disorders need to be treated to improve outcomes.
- A combination of pharmacological and behavior therapy techniques are often used to manage these group of conditions.

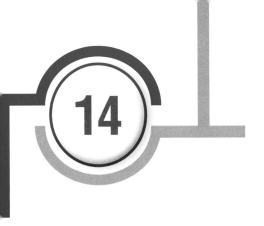

Somatoform Disorders

MS Bhatia

INTRODUCTION

Somatoform disorders (or *Somatic Symptom and Related Disorders* in DSM-5) are conditions, which present with physical symptoms that suggest a physical disorder, but for which there is evidence or a strong presumption that the symptoms are linked to psychological factors. Although the symptoms are physical, the specific pathophysiological processes involved are not demonstrable or understandable by the laboratory procedures.

The disorders discussed in this chapter are:
- Somatization disorder (somatic symptom disorder)
- Conversion disorder (functional neurological symptom disorder)
- Hypochondriasis (illness anxiety disorder)
- Factitious disorder
- Psychogenic pain disorder
- Psychological factors affecting other medical conditions.

SOMATIZATION DISORDER (SOMATIC SYMPTOM DISORDER)

It is characterized by recurrent and multiple somatic complaints, generally of several years duration, for which medical attention has been sought but which was apparently not due to any physical disorder.

Epidemiology

Symptoms usually begin in the teen years and the disorder is more commonly seen in females. Its prevalence is about 1.3–10%.

Clinical Picture

The presentation is usually vague and nonspecific, often dramatic or exaggerated. Symptoms are presented in elaborate detail but the actual chronological history and detail of treatment may be imprecise. A history of affective instability and impulsivity may be there and most patients may have consulted a number of physicians. Complaints usually involve many organ systems as given in **Box 14.1**.

In addition, there may be features related to *complications* due to unwarranted surgery, substance use disorders, depression, and interpersonal, marital, and occupational problems.

A history of somatization and antisocial personality disorders is common among family members.

Differential Diagnosis

This disorder has to be differentiated from:
- *Physical disorders* presenting with vague, multiple and nonspecific somatic symptoms [e.g., hyperparathyroidism,

Box 14.1: Symptoms of somatization disorder.

- *Gastrointestinal symptoms*:
  - Vomiting
  - Abdominal pain
  - Nausea
  - Bloating
  - Diarrhea
  - Intolerance to several foods
- *Pain symptoms*:
  - Pain in extremities
  - Back pain
  - Joint pain
  - Pain during urination
  - Other pain
- *Cardiopulmonary symptoms*:
  - Amnesia
  - Difficulty swallowing
  - Loss of voice
  - Deafness
  - Double vision
  - Blurred vision
  - Blindness
  - Fainting or unconsciousness
  - Seizure or convulsion
  - Difficulty in walking
  - Paralysis or muscle weakness
  - Urinary retention or difficulty urinating
- *Sexual symptoms*:
  - Burning sensation in sexual organs
  - Sexual indifference
  - Pain during intercourse
  - Impotence
- *Female reproductive symptoms*:
  - Painful menstruation
  - Irregular menstrual periods
  - Excessive menstrual bleeding
  - Vomiting throughout pregnancy

porphyria, multiple sclerosis, and systemic lupus erythematous (SLE)]

- *Schizophrenia with multiple somatic delusions*: It has to be differentiated from the nondelusional somatic complaints of individuals with somatization disorder.
- *Dysthymic disorder (depressive neurosis) and generalized anxiety disorder*: They are not diagnosed in individuals who have somatization disorder since mild depressive and anxiety symptoms are so ubiquitous in this disorder. On the other

hand, a superimposed major depression should be diagnosed, if there is full and persistent affective syndrome that can be clearly distinguished.

- *Panic disorder*: It can coexist with somatization disorder. In such situations, both diagnoses should be made.
- *Conversion disorder*: Usually, one or more conversion symptoms occur in the absence of full clinical picture of somatization disorder.
- *Illness anxiety disorder (hypochondriasis)*: This condition is characterized by disproportionate worry and morbid preoccupation with the idea of having a serious illness and they generally have minimal or no somatic symptoms.
- *Factitious disorder with physical symptoms*: There is strong suggestion of voluntary control of the symptoms in this disorder.

Treatment

It consists of supportive long-term care that largely focuses on containing the use of medical resources and avoiding unnecessary surgery and irrational medication use. Supportive techniques rather than intensive interpretive psychotherapy are recommended.

Psychotherapy is usually empathic, anxiety suppressing, and directed toward bolstering ego defenses. Physical symptoms should be taken seriously, but attention in individual sessions should be gradually shifted to other sources of stress such as problematic interpersonal relationships. Family therapy is useful in correcting marital and other family life crises. Comorbid psychiatric disorders (such as mood or anxiety disorders and schizophrenia) require concurrent pharmacologic management, but the use of habit-forming drugs, hospitalizations, and unnecessary diagnostic tests should be avoided.

CONVERSION DISORDER (FUNCTIONAL NEUROLOGICAL SYMPTOM DISORDER)

In this disorder, the patient is unaware about motives and there are disturbances of motor or sensory functions. The symptoms have a psychological advantage or symbolic value and they are not explained by another medical or psychiatric disorder.

Epidemiology

The exact prevalence is not known. It may be seen in any age group and is diagnosed more frequently in women.

Clinical Picture (Box 14.2)

- Symptoms correspond to the patient's own concept and understanding about illness.
- The patient usually gains some advantages ("secondary gain") from their symptoms in the form of sympathy and support from relatives and friends or being excused from various duties and responsibilities).
- The patient appears unconcerned by his symptoms *(la belle indifference)* in spite of showing exaggerated emotional reactions.

  The most frequent complications or consequences of this condition are repeated

surgical operations, drug dependence, marital separation or divorce, depression, and suicide attempts.

Etiology

Psychoanalytic Theory

It proposes that the patients suffer from the effects of emotionally charged ideas lodged in their subconsciousness at some point of time in the past. When repression of these ideas fails, possibly because of the demands of current stress, the released psychic energy manifests in the form of conversion symptoms.

Learning Theory

It holds that the symptom is a learned "adaptation" to a frustrating life situation. The patient with conversion symptoms has learned to communicate helplessness through somatic symptoms, leading to facilitation of attention and support from the environment. Hence, patient's symptoms may be reinforced by the contributory reactions of the relatives.

Genetics

There is no convincing evidence for a genetic etiology. Though it has been found to be more common in first-degree female relatives of index cases. First-degree male relatives show an increased prevalence of sociopathy and alcoholism. Conversion fits are common in epileptic patients also.

Other Theories

Some experts believe that the symptoms are derived from *corticofugal inhibition* of afferent stimulation at the level of reticular activating system. Maladaptive personality traits, history of childhood abuse and neglect, and stressful life events are the risk factors.

Box 14.2: Manifestations of conversion disorder.

- *Motor:* Paralysis, paresis, tremors, rigidity, abnormal gait, seizures, and dysphonia
- *Sensory general:* Anesthesia, paresthesia, and hyperalgesia
- *Sensory special:* Visual difficulties, blindness, deafness, and loss of taste or smell
- *Visceral:* Vomiting, retention of urine, and constipation
- Mixed symptoms

Diagnosis

The diagnosis of conversion disorder can be mistaken in three ways:

1. The symptoms are of a physical disease, which has not yet been detected (e.g., porphyria).
2. Undiscovered neurological disease may cause conversion symptoms in some unknown way (e.g., multiple sclerosis, deep or midline brain tumors, etc.).
3. Genuine physical disease may simulate elaboration of symptoms in vulnerable personalities.

To avoid mistakes, the exact form of symptoms must be established and carefully compared with those arising from known diseases. When conversion disorder is diagnosed, a mistake is less likely, if there is clear evidence of a precipitating stress and of secondary gain.

Differential Diagnosis

- *Physical disorders* presenting with vague, multiple, somatic symptoms, e.g., multiple sclerosis, SLE, acute intermittent porphyria, polyradiculopathy, cervical spondylosis, parietal or thalamic lesions, may early in their course be misdiagnosed as conversion symptoms. A diagnosis of conversion disorder is suggested, if the symptoms are inconsistent with the pattern of actual known physical disorder.
- *In undiagnosed physical disorder*, the symptoms are present, which are not explained by a known physical disorder, but there is no evidence that the symptoms serve a psychological purpose.
- *Somatization disorder* and more rarely *schizophrenia* may have conversion symptoms as integral pattern of their syndrome. In such situations, the diagnosis of conversion disorder is not made.
- *Depressive disorder*: In depression, mood disturbance is a core feature.
- *Psychogenic pain*: It can be conceptualized as a conversion symptom but because of the different course and treatment implications, all such cases are grouped as psychogenic pain disorder.
- *Hypochondriasis (illness anxiety disorder)*: Typically, there may be physical symptoms, but there is no actual loss or distortion of bodily function.
- *Factitious disorder with physical symptoms*: The symptoms are, by definition, under voluntary control.
- *Malingering*: The production of symptom is under voluntary control and is in pursuit of a goal that is obviously recognizable (this frequently involves prospect of material reward or the avoidance of unpleasant work or duty).
- *Epileptic fit*: Pseudoseizures (nonepileptic seizures) have to be differentiated from epileptic fits **(Table 14.1)**.

Management

It should begin with psychosocial assessment, in particular examining the role of precipitating life events, past history of psychological trauma, and evaluation of associated psychopathology. Direct confrontation is not useful.

If the disorder lasts more than a few weeks, the approach involves minimizing the factors, which reinforce the behavior. It is important to psychoeducate that the disability is caused by a psychological, not physical process. The use of *suggestion* is a common denominator in the treatment. *Abreaction* has been used successfully to treat acute attack. Under *hypnosis* or the effect of intravenous barbiturates, the patient is encouraged to relieve the stressful events and the accompanying emotions, which provoked conversion symptoms.

Table 14.1: Differences between pseudoseizures and true seizures.

	Pseudoseizure	True seizure
I. History		
Pattern	No neurophysiological pattern	Same pattern, which is generally stereotyped
Precipitant	Obvious emotional precipitant	May be there but less obvious
Occurrence in sleep	Not seen	May occur in sleep
Treatment	Intractable despite adequate medication	Often responds
Other features	History of sexual abuse or neglect	History of incontinence or self-injury
II. Observations		
Onset	Gradual	Abrupt
Duration	Time variable but longer (10–15 minutes or more)	Short duration up to 1–2 minutes
Consciousness	• Usually preserved • May be fluctuating but some response to pain preserved	Lost and unresponsive to pain
Aura	Aura unusual except for symptoms of hyperventilation	Aura usual
Moaning	Swoon or faint, may have moan, cry, scream, or weep	Monotonous epileptic cry
Movements	• Nonsynchronous out of phase movements (may be mild, jerky, side-to-side head movements, pelvic thrusting, limping, motionless, and unresponsive) • Opisthotonic posturing or rigidity for extended periods movements (e.g., arms in abduction)	Generalized tonic–clonic movements starting with lower amplitude progressing to larger movements
During sleep	Uncommon during physiologic sleep	May occur
Injury	Self-protection before fall, seldom self-injury	Frequent self-injury, bite tongue, hit head, hurt limb
Reflexes	No pathological reflexes	Babinski reflex and pupillary constriction after seizure
Postictal confusion	Little and patient unconcerned	Postictal confusion or transient paralysis may occur
Amnesia	Better memory for event; Nonorganic amnesia	Amnesia present
In front of significant others	Usually occurs	Independent of presence of others
Independent witness	Is usually available	May not be available

Contd...

Contd...

	Pseudoseizure	True seizure
Induction by suggestion	Readily induced or stopped	Not inducible
Induction by sleep, photic stimuli, sleep deprivation hyperventilation	Not readily precipitated	Often precipitated
Others	Avoidance behavior, arm drop, eyes may be open or closed, patient may be looking consistently towards the floor and away from the examiner, even with change in head position	Seeking help, tiredness, blank look, pupillary reflexes impaired
III. Testing		
pH immediately after fit	Normal	May change
Creatine kinase after fit	Normal	Rises (significant, if positive)
Prolactin after fit	Normal	Rises (significant, if positive)
EEG	• No epileptiform discharge, maintenance of alpha rhythm, VEEG preferred which shows only discontinuous muscle activity record during attack and absence of slowing with immediate reappearance of previous occurred alpha rhythm	• Epileptic changes in majority
	• EEG may be abnormal in 10–53% and prompt clinical and EEG recovery from a generalized convulsive episode	• Takes time to recovery

(EEG: electroencephalography; VEEG: video electroencephalography)

HYPOCHONDRIASIS (ILLNESS ANXIETY DISORDER)

Hypochondriasis is defined as an unrealistic interpretation of physical sensations as abnormal, leading to a morbid preoccupation and unrealistic fear or belief of having a serious disease. It persists despite medical reassurance and causes impairment in social or occupational functioning. RD Gillespie (1928) defined hypochondriasis as possessing the following characteristics:

- A preoccupation with a real or assumed physical or mental disorder
- The degree of preoccupation and the grounds for it are far in excess of what is justified.
- An indifference to the opinions of others about the nature of the complaints and unresponsiveness to persuasion.

This disorder is commonly seen in general medical practice with prevalence ranging from 1 to 10%. The patients with this disorder are often offended at the suggestion that their fears or beliefs are unrealistic and they frequently refuse referral for mental health clinics. The disorder frequently begins in the 30s for men and the 40s for women but it is equally common in both genders.

Transient hypochondriacal symptoms are commonly seen in response to stressful life events. If masked depression and underlying disease have been ruled out as the primary cause for the patient's symptom, the diagnosis of primary hypochondriasis should be considered. 85% of all cases of hypochondriasis are secondary (depression being the *most common* cause) and 15% are primary in nature. In secondary form, hypochondriasis represents a frequent feature of depression, anxiety disorder, schizophrenia, and early phases of dementia. It is also a common response after recuperation from any life-threatening illness.

It is a disorder of content of thought. Its severity depends on the degree of conviction and preoccupation. Clinically, the symptoms tend to be diffuse, involve multiple organ systems, and are nonlocalizing. Illness preoccupation must have been present for at least 6 months but the specific presentation may change over period of time. Headache, chest and gastrointestinal complaints, and musculoskeletal symptoms are noted more frequently. Feelings of tightness around the forehead, bloating, increased bowel sounds, constipation, chest and abdominal twinges, missed heartbeats, difficulty focusing, and lack of energy are familiar complaints. History of child abuse or serious childhood illness is important risk factor for developing this disorder in adulthood.

Hypochondriasis may be conceptualized as arising from perceptual and cognitive abnormalities of the following types:

- These patients amplify normal body sensory input,
- They incorrectly assess and misinterpret somatic symptoms of emotional arousal, and
- They are innately predisposed to thinking and perceiving in concrete rather than emotional or subjective terms.

The concept of "*sick role*" may be considered, since powerful reinforcers may exist in the family and society and the medical care system for somatic symptoms. Social and behavioral theories may explain how hypochondriacal fears are reinforced but they do not explain the obsessive internal anxiety that accompanies the disorder in its primary form.

Complications are secondary to efforts to obtain medical care. Because of the multiple physical symptoms without organic basis, true organic pathology may be missed. They may undergo exploratory surgery or become dependent on drugs. There is always impairment in social or occupational functioning.

Differential Diagnosis

Hypochondriasis has to be differentiated from:

- *True organic disease*: The early stages of neurological disorders (e.g., multiple sclerosis), endocrine disorders (e.g., thyroid or parathyroid disease), and illnesses that frequently affect multiple body systems (e.g., SLE). Transient preoccupations related to a medical disorder do not constitute hypochondriasis.
- *Psychotic disorders*—such as schizophrenia and major depression with psychotic features. In hypochondriasis,

the belief of having a disease is generally not associated with the quality of unshakeable fixity that is seen in case of a true somatic delusion.

- *Others*: Dysthymic disorder, generalized anxiety disorder, panic disorder, obsessive, compulsive, and related disorder, adjustment disorder and somatization disorder. The symptom of hypochondriacal preoccupation may appear but it is generally not the predominant disturbance. In somatization disorder, there tends to be preoccupation with symptoms rather than fear of having a specific disease.

Management

The organic pathology must be excluded. If it is thought to be secondary to some other primary psychiatric illness, such as depression, then by treating this condition, hypochondriacal symptoms generally fade away. Treatment is limited in providing support and avoidance of continuous discussion of patient's symptoms. The hospitalizations, tests, and medications with addictive potential should be avoided. The patient's social or interpersonal problems should be explored and treated.

Good outcome with psychotherapy has been associated with illness of less than 3 years duration, absence of severe personality disorder, and possibly higher social class. Poor outcome is related to the chronicity of the illness and the presence of chronic stressors.

FACTITIOUS DISORDER

It is characterized by falsification of physical or psychological symptoms or induction of injury or disease, associated with identified deception even in absence of obvious external rewards. The symptoms are not explained by another medical disorder. The symptoms can be self-induced or imposed on another (by proxy). There may be a single episode or recurrent episodes.

The various terms used for this disorder accompanied by physical symptoms are—"Munchausen's syndrome", "hospital hobos", and "hospital addicts". Ganser syndrome is also a type of factitious disorder.

Epidemiology

The exact prevalence is not known. In hospital settings, about 1% patients meet the criteria of factitious disorder.

Clinical Picture

All organ systems are potential targets, and the symptoms presented are limited only by the individual's medical knowledge and imagination. There may be uncontrollable pathological lying, in a manner intriguing to the listener about any aspect of the individual's history (*pseudologia fantasica*). The complaints of pain and requests for analgesics are common. The patients often undergo multiple invasive procedures and operations and also falsify medical tests and records. When confronted with evidence, they often deny the allegations or rapidly get themselves discharged against medical advice. In proxy form, caregivers lie about abuse injuries in dependents solely to protect themselves from liability, but their deceptive behavior is evident even in absence of obvious external rewards.

The common predisposing factors include true physical disorder during childhood or adolescence leading to extensive medical treatment and hospitalization, a grudge against medical profession, sometimes due to medical mismanagement, employment in a medical field, underlying dependent, exploitative or masochistic personality traits and an important relationship with a physician in the past.

Differential Diagnosis

It needs to be differentiated from somatization disorder, conversion disorder, malingering, and a medical or psychiatric disorder not associated with intentional symptom falsification. This disorder may be superimposed on another disorder but the objective identification of falsification of signs and symptoms confirms the diagnosis.

Management

A comprehensive and proper evaluation of family and occupational situations is required. If initial confrontation does not result in denial or flight, a plan of psychotherapy can possibly be started.

PSYCHOGENIC PAIN DISORDER (PERSISTENT SOMATOFORM PAIN DISORDER)

It is characterized by the complaint of pain in the absence of adequate physical findings but there is evidence of the etiological role of psychological factors. The disturbance is not due to any other psychiatric disorder.

The pain symptom either is inconsistent with the anatomic distribution of the nervous system or if it mimics a known disease entity (as in angina or sciatica), it cannot be adequately accounted for by organic pathology.

Epidemiology

It is common in general medical practice and is more frequently diagnosed in women. The relatives of patients have had more painful injuries and illnesses than occur in the general population. This disorder begins most frequently in adolescence or early adulthood.

Etiology

The psychological factors are etiologically involved in the pain. It may be reflected by a temporal relationship between an environmental stimulus that is apparently related to the initiation or exacerbation of the pain.

Clinical Picture

The "doctor shopping", excessive use of analgesics without relief for pain, requests for surgery, and the assumption of an invalid role are common. The individual usually refuses to consider the role of psychological factors in the pain. In some cases, the pain has symbolic significance, such as pain mimicking angina in an individual whose father died from heart attack. Dysphoria is common.

The most serious *complications* are iatrogenic, e.g., dependence on minor tranquilizers and narcotic analgesics and repeated unsuccessful surgical intervention.

Differential Diagnosis

It includes differentiation from organic pain (Table 14.2), somatization disorder, depressive disorders, schizophrenia, and malingering or pain associated with muscle contraction headaches (tension headaches).

Management

Complete disappearance of pain through suggestion, hypnosis, or narcoanalysis suggests this disorder. Temporary improvement due to suggestion has little diagnostic value since it may also occur in true physical illness. The use of narcotic analgesics or chronic use of drug should be avoided.

Table 14.2: Differences between organic and psychogenic pain.

	Organic pain	Psychogenic pain
Frequency in psychiatry clinic	Low	High
Pain	Localized, episodic	Diffuse, continuous
Waking from sleep	Often	Rarely
Pain elsewhere in the body	Unusual	Common
Associated physical disorder	Identifiable	Not-identifiable
Emotional State	Usually normal	Usually anxious, tense, depressed
Abnormalities on examination and investigations	Present	Absent
Mannkopf sign (Rise in pulse rate on pressing tender area)	Present	Absent
Response to analgesics	Present	Uncommon

PSYCHOLOGICAL FACTORS AFFECTING OTHER MEDICAL CONDITIONS

The diagnostic criteria include the presence of a medical symptom or condition, psychological or behavioral factors adversely affecting the medical condition by affecting the course, interfering with treatment (poor adherence), constituting additional well-established health risks or by influencing pathophysiology, precipitating or exacerbating symptoms, or necessitating medical attention. These psychological or behavioral factors are not due to another mental disorder (e.g., major depressive disorder, panic disorder, post-traumatic stress disorder, etc.).

Epidemiology

The exact prevalence is unknown.

Clinical Picture

Psychological and behavioral factors have been demonstrated to affect the onset, exacerbation, treatment, and course of many medical diseases. There are many cultural differences in presentation. The diagnosis should be reserved for situations in which the effect of the psychological factor on the course or outcome of the medical condition is evident. Abnormal psychological symptoms that develop in response to a medical condition are more correctly diagnosed as an adjustment disorder.

Differential Diagnosis

There is need of differentiating this category from a psychiatric disorder due to another medical condition, adjustment disorder, somatization disorder, and hypochondriasis.

Treatment

The psychological factors need to be identified and corrected. Better treatment adherence leads to better outcome of a medical condition.

TAKE-HOME MESSAGES

- Somatoform disorders are common in routine medical setting.
- They need to be correctly identified to avoid unnecessary investigations and irrational medication.
- A strong positive therapeutic relationship is essential between the physician and the patient to provide supportive care.
- Early and appropriate intervention leads to better outcome.

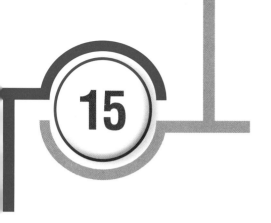

15

Adjustment and Stress-related Disorders

Nilesh Shah, Avinash De Sousa, Pragya Lodha

INTRODUCTION

The aim of the current chapter is to provide the reader an overview of stress-related and adjustment disorders, which may commonly be seen in psychiatric and general practice settings. The disorders covered under this section will be:

- Acute stress disorder (ASD)
- Post-traumatic stress disorder (PTSD)
- Adjustment disorder

Occurrence of stress and traumatic events is a common everyday reality in the life of most people. Civil unrests, riots, earthquakes, floods, tsunamis, personal tragedies, frustrations, accidents, etc., keep on happening unpredictably, leaving a huge impact on the mental health of people affected by it.

The word "stress" in ASD and PTSD does not imply the stress that we face in day-to-day lives, but refers to certain unique stressful life events that may be threatening for the life and integrity of an individual. It is important to note that both these disorders are unique because there has to be a precipitating event or prolonged exposure to repeated stressful and traumatic events, which then result in the disorder. It is important to note that trauma and stress mean different things to different people, while, one individual may bounce back rapidly from a particular stress or trauma; e.g., floods or a road accident; another individual may develop ASD or PTSD in response to this.

A plethora of emotions may be experienced after the trauma or the event, which includes depression, anxiety, guilt, anger, frustration, and the constant apprehension that the event may recur. Usually, these last for a short time, 2–3 weeks post-trauma, and when they persist, they result in the development of ASD or PTSD.

EPIDEMIOLOGY OF ACUTE STRESS DISORDER AND POST-TRAUMATIC STRESS DISORDER

There is a dearth of Indian literature when we try to review the epidemiology of these two disorders in Indian populations. The rates worldwide have been shown to lie between 15% and 35% across various nations, following various stressful events. In India, however, lower rates have been reported and may indicate that our populations are more resilient than the West.

There are a number of risk factors that may predispose an individual for developing PTSD and ASD. These include a family history of these disorders, exposure to repeated significant life events or natural calamities, living in specific regions exposed to war or natural calamities, family history of depression or anxiety, and exposure to child abuse or domestic violence.

It is important to understand that men and women may be exposed to different forms of trauma, e.g., men are more likely to be exposed to war, physical combat, and a murder attempt; while women are more likely to be exposed to trauma such as rape and domestic violence. However, certain forms of trauma may occur universally like natural calamities, child abuse, and road accidents. Certain occupations may predispose an individual to ASD or PTSD, like jobs in military, paramilitary, and police force among the firefighters. It is also common in paramedical and ambulance workers in disaster settings.

High rates of ASD or PTSD have sometimes been noted in mental health professionals and volunteers after prolonged exposure to disaster affected populations. Certain events have a greater propensity to cause PTSD or ASD, e.g., rape and child abuse, compared to road traffic accidents. It has also been reported that migrant populations, refugees, inhabitants of concentration camps and shelter homes may have more individuals with PTSD than the general population.

In India, road traffic accidents and railway accidents are commonplace and these symptoms may be seen in survivors of such calamities. It is worthwhile mentioning that sometimes ASD and PTSD may be seen in individuals who are sole survivors in such tragedies and they often tend to question their own survival (survivor guilt). Dowry-related burns and accidental burn cases causing PTSD in women are also commonly seen in India.

ACUTE STRESS DISORDER

Acute stress disorder is a disorder where there is a transient reaction to exceptional physical and mental stress where the symptoms appear either immediately after the precipitating event or within the first 2 weeks of the same. There may be an initial period of days followed by confusion and dissociative symptoms. The stressful event must be one that is a serious threat to one's personal security or physical integrity or to that of his family members. The event can also result in a sudden change in financial condition of the individual, causing him to drift down the social ladder as in natural calamities or fires that may destroy all that he owns.

The symptoms of ASD include:

- *Physical symptoms*—tachycardia, flushing, chest pain, sweating, palpitations, dizziness, breathlessness, numbness of the hands and feet, increased frequency of urination, diarrhea, acidity, hyperventilation, and fainting attacks
- *Psychological symptoms*—appearing dazed and confused, not talking to anyone, being withdrawn, refusal to eat or drink, decreased sleep and sometimes, agitation or aggression.

Factors that determine the severity of the disorder include the nature of the stress/event that has occurred, for how long it occurred, predisposing factors as discussed earlier, and presence of a psychiatric condition pre-existing in the individual.

Management

It is prudent that a combined medical and psychotherapeutic approach be used in the management of ASD. Medications like benzodiazepines may be used to reduce anxiety (Clonazepam 0.25–2 mg/day). This may be combined with drugs like selective serotonin reuptake inhibitors (SSRIs) and other antidepressants to counteract the other symptoms. Among the SSRIs, escitalopram (5–20 mg/day) is the most preferred.

Among the psychological interventions, cognitive behavior therapy (CBT) has been shown to reduce the progression of ASD to PTSD. Debriefing, which is another form of psychotherapy, has also been tried with some amount of success.

The disorder has a good prognosis and most patients show full recovery while 15–20% may progress to PTSD. Good social support, sound family functioning, and optimal premorbid functioning (functioning prior to the disorder) serve as protective factors and aid recovery.

POST-TRAUMATIC STRESS DISORDER

Post-traumatic stress disorder has been described historically in psychiatric literature right since the First World War and various terms like "shell shock", "soldier's heart", "Da costa's syndrome", "combat fatigue", and "Gulf war syndrome" have been used to describe the condition when noted in military personnel.

Post-traumatic stress disorder occurs when an individual is exposed to a stressful event/situation (short or long duration), which must be life threatening or catastrophic in nature and must have the ability to cause distress in anyone. The individual must have either, been part of the event, confronted the event or witnessed the event, thereby involving actual or perceived threat of death or serious injury.

The main symptoms of PTSD include:
- Recurrent flashbacks and memories involving the event
- Refusal to talk about the event
- Refusal to see broadcasts related to the event
- Refusal to view stimuli, which cause a flashback
- Recurrent dreams.

The patient may deny having any memory for the event that occurred. The patient may also present with anger, irritability, panic, anxiety, difficulties in concentration and attention, crying spells, emotional numbness, sleep disturbances, hypervigilance, and decreased appetite.

Important Points

The biological basis of PTSD has been studied extensively and various findings about its neurobiology have been identified.
- It has been noted that patients with PTSD show elevated serum–cortisol levels at rest and these levels rise further during stress or trauma, resulting in the PTSD-like response.
- Various brain structures like the hippocampus, the prefrontal cortex, the limbic system, and the visual cortex have been implicated in PTSD. Changes in brain metabolism and blood flow to these structures have been demonstrated via neuroimaging.
- The hypothalamic–pituitary–adrenal axis plays a role in the development of PTSD via its control on the cortisol response to stress.

Various stressors have been implicated in causing PTSD and may be classified as: natural disasters (earthquakes, tsunamis, floods, hurricanes, volcanic eruptions, etc.), transport accidents (rail and road accidents), war-related trauma (war combat, bombing, torture, and imprisonment), and domestic trauma (child physical and sexual abuse, domestic violence, rape and child neglect).

Many other psychiatric disorders may co-occur with PTSD. These include—major depression (30–50%), alcohol use disorders (15–20%), other anxiety disorders (10–15%), somatoform disorders, obsessive-compulsive disorder (OCD), and mania.

Sometimes, PTSD may occur following the death of a loved one, which is then termed as post-traumatic grief or a pathological grief reaction. This differs from normal grief that normally resolves in 2–3 weeks post the death of a loved one.

Management

It is prudent that a combined medical and psychotherapeutic approach be used in the management of PTSD.

Various psychotherapeutic treatments have been tried in the management of PTSD, these include:

- *Cognitive behavior therapy*, which involves identifying maladaptive thoughts that the patient may hold regarding the trauma and replacing these with a positive and restructured thoughts along with the use of imagery and exposure techniques to help the patient overcome any reluctance to speak about the trauma.
- *Psychodynamic psychotherapy*: This is a long-duration psychotherapy, which works by uncovering unconscious defense mechanisms and the root cause of trauma may be eliminated using this method. It is time consuming and not used widely in India.
- *Systematic desensitization and eye movement desensitization and reprocessing (EMDR)*: Here, the patient is exposed by means of images, videos, or using memory of the trauma, which is combined with relaxation techniques. In EMDR, the patient may imagine and/or relive the trauma, while he has to eye track moving fingers or lights and various exercises are provided that serve as an emotional outlet for the patient.

Medical Management

The medical management involves treatment with SSRIs to treat anxiety and depressive symptoms. All the SSRIs have been used with equal efficacy and benzodiazepines may be used to manage the panic attacks when they arise. Escitalopram (5–20 mg/day), fluoxetine (10–40 mg/day), and paroxetine (12.5–37.5 mg/day) have been used with fair success across various studies.

Family psychoeducation is paramount for relatives to understand how to manage the patient and his symptoms. It is important to remember that PTSD is a difficult disorder to treat and one must seek psychiatric expert help, if the patient does not respond to conventional treatments.

ADJUSTMENT DISORDERS

Adjustment disorder is a group of disorders, which are time limited and follow the exposure of an individual to a given stressor. It is important that the stressor be identified and then either negotiated or removed completely for the individual to recover. This is important because the disorder is nothing but a maladaptive response to the stressor.

The stressors are implicated in adjustment disorder including—life events, life changes, and continuous stressors. The most common causes seen in clinical practice include a failed love affair, divorce, marital problems, financial problems, tenant-landlord issues, exposure to riots, reactions to diagnoses like TB and cancer, death of a close near and dear ones, or mother-in-law–daughter-in-law issues.

Adjustment disorder lies on a spectrum, which can range from normal behavior to maladaptive responses to major psychiatric disorders. It is very often a diagnostic dilemma because it is poorly defined and it overlaps with multiple disorders, as it may present with many different kinds of symptoms. Many a time, it is considered as a waste-paper basket diagnosis. Its reliability and validity have been questioned in clinical circles.

The ambiguity of its diagnosis may give the clinician some strength to provide this as a temporary diagnosis before directly labeling a patient as having a major psychiatric disorder.

The disorder may also be considered as brewing pot of transient psychiatric morbidities, which may later evolve completely into a major psychiatric disorder. There is not much evidence with regard to the etiology and biology of the disorder but personal and individual vulnerability plays an important role in its genesis.

The symptoms of adjustment disorders include:

- Depressed mood
- Anxious mood
- Crying
- Fainting spells
- Dramatic behavior and violent outbursts
- Conduct disorder
- Aggression and acting out
- Somatization
- Physical symptoms such as acidity, constipation, diarrhea, chest pain, panic attacks, and sleep problems.

Sometimes, patient with adjustment disorder may take to substance use, develop medical problems related to the stress like blood pressure and diabetes, and might occasionally attempt suicide. Usually, most of these patients return to normal functioning within a few weeks.

Management

The management of adjustment disorder involves more psychological management rather than medical management. There is a need for sound psychotherapy that shall help in the following ways:

- Identify the underlying stress that is disturbing the patient
- Discuss various aspects of this stress with the patient
- Find out ways and means of eliminating and ameliorating the stress
- Solve interpersonal problems that affect relationships of the patient
- Help to make the patient psychologically stronger and resilient to the stress
- Family psychoeducation on how to handle the problem and deal with the patient.

Medications when needed for the underlying psychopathology such as depression, somatization, anxiety, and conduct issues may be used as deemed fit by the treating doctor.

CONCLUSION

Thus, stress and adjustment disorders are conditions that may not be routinely encountered in clinical practice but when encountered must be recognized and treated. It is also prudent to use both medication and psychotherapy as a combined approach while keeping in mind that in cases that are complex and involving trauma, it is better that a psychiatric evaluation and consultation are done at the earliest.

TAKE-HOME MESSAGES

- Stress-related and adjustment disorders include ASD and PTSD.
- Acute stress disorder is a disorder where there is a transient reaction to exceptional physical and mental stress where the symptoms appear either immediately after the precipitating event or shortly afterward.
- Post-traumatic stress disorder occurs when an individual is exposed to a stressful event/situation of life-threatening or catastrophic dimension, which would cause distress in anyone.
- It is prudent that a combined medical and psychotherapeutic approach be used in the management of all these conditions.
- Attention should also be paid to the management of other comorbid psychiatric and medical conditions.

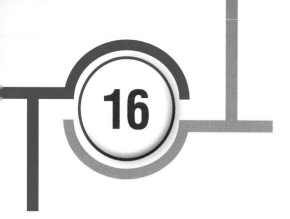

16

Normal Human Sexuality and Sexual Disorders

Shivananda Manohar, TS Sathyanarayana Rao,
Abhinav Tandon, Shreemit Maheshwari, Suhas Chandran

INTRODUCTION

According to Oxford dictionary, sex refers to being male or female based on reproductive function and biological characteristics. Gender refers to publicly lived role as male or female, more of sociocultural aspect rather than biological one. Sexuality depicts the sexual functions, activities, attitudes, and orientations of an individual. According to Levine (1989), an adult's sexuality has seven components: gender identity, orientation, intention, desire, arousal, orgasm, and emotional satisfaction. It is determined by the biological, sociocultural, and environmental factors affecting an individual. The experiences of an individual during development and relationships help in forming various aspects of the personality and sexuality of an individual.

ANATOMY AND PHYSIOLOGY

Neuroanatomy, neurophysiology, and genetic aspects of sexuality are as important as psychological and social factors.

Male

Male sexual anatomy includes external genitalia (penis, scrotum, testes, epididymis, and part of the vas deferens) and the internal components (vas deferens, ejaculatory duct, and prostate glands).

External Structures

Penis:
The word "penis" is derived from Latin that means "to hang." As per Masters and Johnson, size of the penis varies from 7 to 11 cm in the flaccid state to 14–18 cm in the erect state. Concern with the size of the penis has been found to be very common in men. Penis does not contain any muscle or bone; it is composed of three cylinders of erectile tissues that are bound together by fibrous tissue. The two uppermost cylinders lay side-by-side called corpora cavernosa and the lower cylinder is corpus spongiosum. Urethra passes through corpus spongiosum. At the tip of penis, there is a knob-like structure called Glans, which is a very sensitive structure **(Fig. 16.1).**

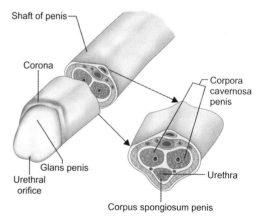

Fig. 16.1: Structure of penis.
Source: Vikramadithya Shivaram.

Female

The female sexual organs can be classified into two categories: (1) the external organs and (2) the internal organs **(Fig. 16.2)**.

The external genitals of the females consist of clitoris, the mons pubis, the outer lips, the inner lips, and the vaginal opening collectively called as the vulva. The clitoris is homologous to the glans portion of penis in males. Although not directly involved in reproductive function, it is an important structure for sexual arousal. These structures also have a rich supply of nerve endings thus making them important structures responsible for sexual stimulation and arousal.

The internal sex organs of the female consist of vagina, the uterus, a pair of ovaries, and a pair of fallopian tubes. The vagina is the organ inside which the penis is inserted during sexual intercourse and also receives the ejaculation from it. It is sometimes also referred to as the birth canal because the baby travels through it during birth. It is a tube-shaped organ that connects to the cervix of the uterus above and the introitus (vaginal opening) below. It is a very flexible organ so as to accommodate the penis during coitus. The uterus (womb) is the organ in which the fetus develops. The narrow lower third of the uterus is called the cervix which opens into the vagina. The top part is called fundus, and the main part is the body of the uterus. The main function of the uterus is to hold and nurture the fetus. The fallopian tube, two in number, extends out from the sides of the uterus. They are also called as uterine tubes. The fallopian tubes are the pathway by which the egg leaves the ovaries and the sperm reaches the egg. Fertilization of the egg occurs in fallopian tube. At the end of the fallopian tube are numerous finger-like projections called fimbriae that help in the reception of egg from the ovary. The ovaries are two organs on either side of the uterus, responsible for producing eggs (ova) and produce the female sexual hormones estrogen and progesterone. Each ovary contains many follicles which surround the egg. With the maturation of eggs, the follicles move toward the surface of ovary and release the egg in the fimbriae of the fallopian tube where it gets fertilized resulting in pregnancy.

Nerves from the autonomic nervous system (ANS) innervate the sexual organs.

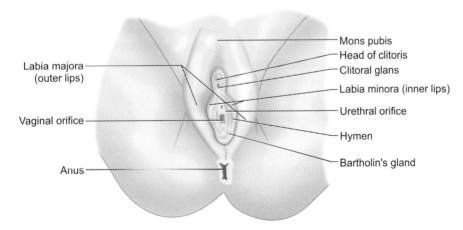

Fig. 16.2: The external genitals of a female.
Source: Vikramadithya Shivaram.

Parasympathetic nerves (S2, 3, and 4) mediate *reflex erections*. Both sympathetic and parasympathetic systems are involved in relaxing cavernosal smooth muscles which is aided by nitric oxide (NO). In females, the sympathetic system causes contraction of smooth muscles of vagina, urethra, and uterus during orgasm. The ANS is influenced by external events like stress and also by biological mediators (internal events) of sexual functioning. In males, dopamine plays an important role in erection; multiple neurotransmitters like dopamine, norepinephrine, serotonin, acetylcholine, oxytocin, GABA (gamma-aminobutyric acid), and NO are involved in ejaculation. Ejaculation is the forceful expulsion of semen and seminal fluid from the epididymis, vas deferens, seminal vesicles, and prostate into the urethra. Normal antegrade ejaculation includes three steps: (1) emission (under sympathetic control; T10–L2); (2) ejection (under parasympathetic control; S2–4); and (3) orgasm (occurs due to cerebral processing of sensory stimuli from pudendal nerve).

SEXUAL RESPONSE CYCLE

Various authors have classified sexual response cycle in different ways. Initially Master and Johnson gave the EPOR model, which included:

E = Excitation: Somatic and psychogenic stimuli lead to increasing sexual tension and subjective sense of pleasure.

P = Plateau: Intensified sexual tension and sexual pleasure.

O = Orgasm: Involuntary pleasurable climax; peaking of sexual pleasure with release of sexual tension.

R = Resolution: A sense of well-being and relaxation; men have a refractory period for subsequent orgasm whereas women can have multiple orgasms.

Through later research by Robinson and Kaplan, the above model got modified into DEOR model, here "D" stands for the "desire phase" which is influenced by sexual drive and fantasies and is the conscious desire to have sex. Sexual desire has three interactive components: (1) sexual drive—biological component; (2) sexual motivation—psychological component; and (3) sexual wish—social component. The "plateau phase" has been merged with the "excitation phase" as it is considered to be the final stage of the "excitation phase." The "desire phase" depends on the psychological makeup and is influenced by the biological characteristics of the individual. The "excitation phase" begins with psychological or physiological (or both) stimulation and leads to penile tumescence and enlargement of testes in males and vaginal lubrication, hard clitoris, formation of orgasmic platform (vagina becomes barrel-shaped with constriction in outer one-third), thickening of labia minora, increase in breast size in females, and nipple erection in both sexes. There is increase in heart rate, respiratory rate, and blood pressure. In the "orgasmic phase," sexual pleasure peaks, and there is rhythmic contraction of perineal muscles and reproductive organs; inevitable ejaculation triggers orgasm in males whereas in females there are involuntary contractions of uterus and lower third of vagina.

Resolution phase is characterized by disengorgement of blood from the genital organs; following orgasm, a general feeling of well-being and muscular relaxation occur (resolution is rapid following orgasm). However, if orgasm does not occur, resolution may take up to 6 hours and may be associated with irritability.

MASTURBATION

Masturbation is a form of stimulation which leads to sexual pleasure. Masturbation exists throughout one's lifetime, and it is a precursor of object-related sexual relationship. Though various cultures have diverse opinion about masturbation, there is no scientific evidence of masturbation causing ill health. Genital self-stimulation is often observed in toddlers at around 1.5 years of age. Masturbation acts as a method of self-stimulation and release of sexual tension in teenagers; in adults, it acts as a method of sexual satisfaction when intercourse with a partner is unsatisfactory or when the partner is unavailable. In the 1960s, Masters and Johnson described the various methods of masturbation; in women, stimulation of shaft of clitoris has been preferred. It needs professional advice and treatment only when it becomes compulsive.

SEXUAL DISORDERS

According to DSM-5 (Diagnostic and Statistical Manual of Mental Disorders), sexual dysfunction is defined as "a heterogeneous group of disorders that are typically characterized by a clinically significant disturbance in a person's ability to respond sexually or to sexual pleasure." Subtypes include lifelong versus acquired and generalized versus situational. Also (1) partner's and individual vulnerability factors; (2) relationship factors; (3) psychiatric comorbidity; (4) cultural; and (5) general medical factors need to be considered.

Epidemiology

Earlier studies done by Master and Johnson in 1970 reported that prevalence of sexual dysfunction is around 50%. Around 43% of women and 31% of men reported sexual dysfunction. In 2004, the "Committee on Epidemiology/Risk Factors for Sexual Dysfunction" with international collaboration among four countries has reported the incidence of erectile dysfunction as 25–30 cases/1,000 person years. Around 40–45% of adult women and 20–30% of adult men have at least one sexual dysfunction.

Etiology

Human sexual response involves a complex interplay of social, cultural, biological, and interpersonal factors. Sexual dysfunction may be a result of impairment of any of these factors. Sexual dysfunction can be because of partner's ill health, impairment in communication and intimacy, cultural and religious factors, or medical illness **(Table 16.1, Flowchart 16.1)**.

Table 16.1: Etiology of sexual disorders.	
Sexual disorder	*Etiology*
I. Desire disorders	• Low arousal in females is associated with thyroid problems, arthritis, irritable bowel disease • *Drugs*: Antihypertensives, psychotropics, dopamine blockers, alcohol • Androgen deficiency
II. *Arousal disorder:* Erectile disorder	• Systemic diseases, vascular insufficiency, neurological disorders, androgen deficiency, hypertension • *Drugs*: Antihypertensives, anticholinergics, psychotropics, digoxin, nicotine, estrogens
III. Disorders of orgasm	
Premature (early) ejaculation: Lifelong/acquired	Prostatic disease, increased central dopaminergic activity, increased penile sensitivity

Contd...

Contd...

Sexual disorder	Etiology
Delayed ejaculation	• Spinal cord lesions • *Drugs*: Antihypertensives, antidepressants, antipsychotics, alcohol
Female orgasmic disorder/Male orgasmic disorder	• CNS disease, Parkinson's disease • *Drugs*: SSRIs, TCAs, substance abuse
Absent ejaculation (anejaculation)	• *Neural*: Spinal cord injury, colorectal surgery, diabetes • *Drugs*: Antihypertensives, psychotropics, alcohol • Androgen deficiency
Postejaculation pain	• Psychogenic
Failure of detumescence: Priapism (primary or secondary)	• Structural penile disease, Peyronie's disease, idiopathic (primary) • *Secondary-hematological disorders*: Leukemia • *Infiltrative*: Amyloidosis • *Inflammatory*: Mumps • Neurological disorders, tumors
IV. Genito-pelvic pain/Penetration disorder	• Associated with reduced sexual desire and interest • General medical factors • Perimenopausal

(SSRI: selective serotonin reuptake inhibitors; TCA: tricyclic antidepressant; CNS: central nervous system)

Flowchart 16.1: Psychogenic causes of sexual dysfunction.

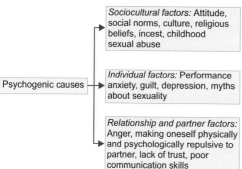

Difference between Organic and Psychogenic Sexual Dysfunction

Differences between organic and psychogenic sexual dysfunction differences are illustrated in **Table 16.2**.

CLASSIFICATION OF SEXUAL DISORDERS

Various authors have classified sexual disorders in different ways. The most recent classification is by DSM-5. But the more internationally accepted one is ICD-10 (International Statistical Classification of Diseases and Related Health Problems, 10th version) prepared by WHO, which is to be replaced by ICD-11 shortly. The difference between DSM-5 and ICD-10 in classification of sexual disorders has been depicted in **Table 16.3**.

COMMON SEXUAL DYSFUNCTIONS OR INADEQUACIES

Delayed Ejaculation

Marked delay, infrequent or absence of ejaculation on almost all or >75% occasions of sexual activity with a partner (in identified situations or, if generalized, in all situations), and without the individual desiring delay. The symptoms should be present for a minimum period of 6 months and cause significant distress.

Erectile Disorder

As per DSM-5, marked difficulty in obtaining or maintaining an erection during sexual activity

Table 16.2: Organic and psychogenic sexual dysfunction differences.

Parameters	Psychogenic	Organic
Onset of disorder	Situational	Insidious
Precipitating event	Psychogenic condition	Debilitating disease, vascular insufficiency or central nervous system abnormality, penile trauma or interfering drugs
Erectile response to other sexual stimuli	Usually present	Usually absent
Nocturnal or morning erections	Initially present and full, lost in longstanding dysfunction	Absent or reduced in frequency and intensity
Course of disorder	Episodic or transient loss of erection	Persistent and progressive erectile dysfunction
Associated ejaculatory disorder	Premature ejaculation and intermittent loss of ejaculation	Retrograde or absent ejaculation

Table 16.3: Classification of sexual disorders.

Comparison of diagnostic categories of ICD-10 and DSM-5 of sexual disorders

Disorders according to sexual cycle	ICD-10	DSM-5
Sexual desire disorders	• Lack or loss of sexual desire • Sexual aversion • Excessive sexual drive	• Male hypoactive sexual desire disorder • Female sexual interest/arousal disorder
Sexual arousal disorders	Failure of genital response	• Male erectile disorder

Orgasm disorders	• Orgasmic dysfunction
	• Lack of sexual enjoyment
	• Premature ejaculation
		• Male
		  – Premature (early) ejaculation
		  – Delayed ejaculation
		• Female
		  – Orgasmic disorder

Sexual pain disorders	• Nonorganic dyspareunia • Nonorganic vaginismus	• Female • Genito-pelvic pain/penetration disorder • Substance/Medication-induced sexual dysfunction
Other sexual disorders	• Paraphilias • Gender identity disorders • Other sexual dysfunction, not caused by organic disorder or disease • Unspecified sexual dysfunction, not caused by organic disorder or disease	• Paraphilic disorders • Gender dysphoria • Gender dysphoria in children • Gender dysphoria in adolescent and adults • Other specified gender dysphoria • Unspecified gender dysphoria

(ICD-10: International Statistical Classification of Disease and Related Health Problems 10th revision; DSM-5: Diagnostic and Statistical Manual of Mental Disorders, 5th edition)

or marked decrease in erectile rigidity on almost all or >75% occasions of sexual activity with a partner (in identified situations or, if generalized, in all situations). The symptoms should be present for a minimum period of 6 months and cause significant distress.

Male Hypoactive Sexual Desire Disorder

Persistently deficient sexual thoughts or fantasies and desire for sexual activity. The symptoms should be present for a minimum period of 6 months and cause significant distress. The judgment of deficiency or absence is made by the clinician, taking into account the factors that affect sexual functioning such as age and the context of the person's life.

Premature (Early) Ejaculation

Persistent ejaculation occurring within 1 minute of vaginal penetration and before the individual wishes on almost all or >75% occasions of sexual activity with a partner (in identified situations or, if generalized, in all situations). The symptoms should be present for a minimum period of 6 months and cause significant distress. This diagnosis may be applied in cases of nonvaginal sexual activities also.

Masters and Johnson defined a person as "premature ejaculator" if he cannot control his ejaculatory process for a sufficient length of time during intravaginal containment to satisfy his partner in at least 50% of their coital connections. Premature ejaculation has been recognized in majority of cases as psychogenic, secondary to anxiety, conditioned by early sexual experiences, guilt and hostility toward the partner.

Female Orgasmic Disorder

Marked delay, infrequent, reduced intensity or absence of orgasm on almost all or >75% occasions of sexual activity with a partner (in identified situations or, if generalized, in all situations). The symptoms should be present for a minimum period of 6 months and cause significant distress.

Female Sexual Interest/Arousal Disorder

Significantly reduced or absence of sexual interest or arousal manifested by any three of the following: (1) reduced interest; (2) absent/reduced erotic thoughts; (3) absent/reduced initiation of sexual activity or no response to partner's attempt to initiate the same; (4) absent/reduced sexual excitement; (5) absent/reduced response to erotic cues; and (6) absent/reduced genital or nongenital sensations during sexual activity. Symptoms 4 to 6 are present on almost all or >75% occasions of sexual activity with a partner (in identified situations or, if generalized, in all situations). The symptoms are present for a minimum period of 6 months and cause significant distress.

Abovementioned sexual dysfunctions can be further classified as—(1) lifelong versus acquired; (2) generalized versus situational; and (3) mild, moderate, or severe.

Genito-pelvic Pain/Penetration Disorder

As per DSM-5, persistence of any of the following symptoms: (1) difficulty in vaginal penetration; (2) significant pain during vaginal intercourse/penetration; (3) fear/anxiety related to point 2; and (4) significant contraction of pelvic floor muscles during vaginal penetration attempt. The symptoms are present for a minimum period of 6 months and cause significant distress.

Genito-pelvic pain disorder can be further classified into: (1) lifelong versus acquired; and (2) mild, moderate, or severe.

Other Sexual Dysfunctions

- Substance/medication-induced sexual dysfunction
- Other specified sexual dysfunction
- Unspecified sexual dysfunction.

For making any of the above diagnosis as per DSM-5, a nonsexual mental disorder, substance abuse/general medical cause leading to sexual dysfunction and severe relationship distress should be ruled out.

Dhat Syndrome

Dr NN Wig in 1960 coined the term "Dhat syndrome", a culture bound syndrome characterized by excessive preoccupation with loss of dhat (which is representative of semen) through urine, nocturnal emissions or masturbation. Dhat syndrome is characterized by somatic symptoms of weakness, fatigue, anxiety, decreased appetite, and guilt attributed to semen loss. This concept finds support from ancient Indian scripture Charaka Samhita which mentions that imbalance of bodily humors or excessive orgasmic ejaculations may cause damage to the dhatus. Sukra or semen is supposed to be of nutritional origin, is also believed to be all pervading in the body. According to this belief system, food is progressively transformed into blood, further to marrow, and then to semen. This syndrome is predominantly seen in Indian subcontinent; however, similar syndromes have been noted in other countries also. Dhat may be associated with depression, anxiety, sexual dysfunction, or somatic symptoms.

DIAGNOSIS OF SEXUAL DISORDERS

Adequate sexual history is the important input required for making a proper diagnosis of sexual disorders. To obtain good history of sexual functions, it is important to make patient comfortable by providing adequate privacy. Language of communication should be understandable adequately by both therapist and the patient. Differences in socioeconomic and cultural background of therapist and patient also have negative impact on adequate diagnosis of sexual disorders.

Patient's current complaint, duration, associated symptoms, mode of onset, frequency, and severity of the problem should be noted; whether the problem is generalized or situational, lifelong or acquired needs to be enquired into. Enquire regarding sexual practices, fantasies and goals, intimacy issues with partner, and relationship problems affecting the current sexual functioning. Ask regarding any other associated factors aggravating the current problem and life stressors if any. Past sexual history, mode of gaining information regarding sexual functioning, history of first sexual activity, history regarding masturbation, sexual orientation, and past history of sexual abuse need to be noted. Also note any guilt associated with sexual self-stimulation, premarital, and extramarital sexual activities, live-in relationships.

It is important to assess relationship issues among the couple, whether they are sympathetic or asympathetic toward the problem, expectations, and motivation toward treatment. High-risk sexual behavior should be assessed. In the Asian context, women are reluctant to disclose about their sexuality.

Laboratory studies should include blood tests for complete blood count, blood urea, serum creatinine, lipid profile, blood sugar, urine analysis, thyroid function, and other endocrinal and other tests as required. Rigi scan can be used for erectile dysfunction. Penile Doppler is indicated in specific conditions.

MANAGEMENT OF SEXUAL INADEQUACIES

Organicity leading to sexual dysfunction should be ruled out. However, it should be noted that associated psychosocial factors would aggravate the already existing problem.

Psychotherapeutic intervention: Sex therapy ideally involves both the partners. Therapy should emphasize that there is no use blaming one's partner or oneself, that there is no such thing as an uninvolved partner, that sex is not something a man does to a woman or woman to a man; it is something a man and woman do together. It can be a form of interpersonal communication at a highly intimate level; enhanced social communication benefits the relationship in general.

Behavioral techniques: Assessment and treatment should be tailor made to the individual client. Annon (1974) proposed a graded intervention popularly called as PLISSIT Model wherein:

P = Permission giving
LI = Limited information
SS = Specific suggestion
IT = Intensive sex therapy.

Different levels of approaches represent the different degrees and modalities of sexual problems a particular clinician encounters in his practice. The assessment and treatment need to be tailored depending upon one's setting, profession, specialty and the important of all, the type of the problem encountered in the client. The intensive therapy involves primarily sensitization and desensitization techniques.

Educating the patient is very important. Initiate discussion by giving permission to talk freely and openly about sex in a nonjudgmental way, encourage partners to see, hear, and understand each other's perception and teach communication skills and allow the couple to recognize and take responsibility for much of their treatment **(Flowchart 16.2).**

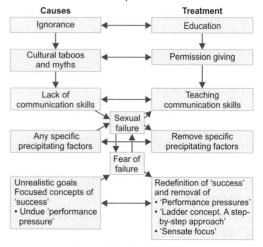

Flowchart 16.2: Causes and management of sexual problems.

Source: Elizabeth Stanley.

Sensate focus exercises: Master and Johnson pioneered the sensate focus exercise. During sensate focus exercise coitus and orgasm is prohibited. These exercises are designed to foster nonverbal and verbal communication between the partners and to establish what feels good and what does not feel good. Sensate focus exercise emphasizes mutual enhancement of erotic pleasure without orgasm. Stress of sexual performance is eliminated. After several days of exercise couple shifts to female on top position with or without intercourse. When the couple has learnt the concept of sensate focus, intercourse is allowed.

Systematic sensitization and desensitization: Squeeze technique is one of the major techniques used by therapist to treat premature ejaculation. Originally it was named "stop–start" method and was developed by Semans in 1956. The manoeuvre of squeezing the penis is used to stop the imminent ejaculation and start refers to restarting stimulation of penis in various prescribed ways. Repetition of this cycle of stop and start several times over a period helps man develop better control over his ejaculation process. Master and Johnson refined this technique further in 1970.

Pharmacotherapy for Sexual Dysfunction

Phosphodiesterase-5 inhibitors are effective drugs for erectile dysfunction. Sildenafil, vardenafil, and tadalafil are commonly used drugs of this class. Their comparative chart is given in **Table 16.4**.

Comparative chart of other drugs used for premature ejaculation is given in **Table 16.5**.

Other Treatment Methods for Sexual Disorders

- Testosterone is definitely effective only in case of hypogonadism. It can increase

Table 16.4: Comparison of phosphodiesterase-5 inhibitors.			
	Sildenafil	*Vardenafil*	*Tadalafil*
Time to maximum plasma concentration (T max) in minutes	30–120 (median 60)	30–120 (median 60)	30–360 (median 120)
Half-life in hours	2.6–3.7	3.9	17.5
Plasma protein binding	96%	94%	94%
Bioavailability	41%	15%	Not known
Onset of action in minutes	15–60	25	16–45
Duration of action	4	4	36
Absorption	Fatty meals cause a mean delay in Cmax of 60 minutes	Fatty meals cause a reduction in Cmax	Not affected by food
Dose adjustments required	• Patients >65 years old • Hepatic and renal impairment • Renal impairment • Concomitant use of potent cytochrome P450 3A4 • Inhibitors and inducers	• Patients >65 years old • Hepatic and renal impairment • Renal impairment • Concomitant use of potent cytochrome P450 3A4 • Inhibitors and inducers	• Patients >65 years old • Hepatic and renal impairment • Renal impairment • Concomitant use of potent cytochrome P450 3A4 • Inhibitors and inducers
Contraindication	• Patients receiving organic nitrates either regularly or intermittently • Hypersensitivity to any component of the tablet	• Patients receiving organic nitrates either regularly or intermittently • Hypersensitivity to any component of the tablet	• Any patient using organic nitrates either regularly or intermittently • Hypersensitivity to any component of the tablet
Side effects	• Headache • Flushing • Dyspepsia • Nasal congestion • Alteration in color vision	• Headache • Flushing • Rhinitis • Dyspepsia • Sinusitis	• Headache • Dyspepsia • Back pain • Myalgia • Nasal congestion
Recommended time between medication intake and intercourse	1 hour	1 hour	1–12 hours

Table 16.5: Other pharmacotherapeutic agents used in premature ejaculation.

Oral therapies	Recommended dose
Tricyclic antidepressant • Clomipramine	25–50 mg/day or 25 mg 4–24 hours before intercourse
Selective serotonin reuptake inhibitors • Fluoxetine • Paroxetine • Sertraline • Dapoxetine	5–20 mg/day 10–40 mg/day or 20 mg 3–4 hours preintercourse 25–200 mg/day or 50 mg 4–8 hours before intercourse 30–60 mg 1–3 hours before intercourse
Topical therapies	Dose
• Lidocaine/prilocaine cream	Lidocaine 2.5% 20–30 minutes preintercourse

the desire but has no effect on erectile functioning. It may be tried in cases of female low sex drive and anorgasmia under careful monitoring.

- Hormone replacement therapy with estrogen in case of menopausal women may help as vaginal functions, particularly lubrication improves by it.
- Hyperprolactinemia is treated by administration of dopaminergic drugs like bromocriptine.
- Smooth muscle relaxants like papaverine, phentolamine, phenoxybenzamine are used in intracavernosal injection of vasoactive drugs (ICIVAD) techniques; prostaglandin EI is a very effective agent. Various bi- and trimixes are available for use in cases of erectile dysfunction.
- Yohimbine, central alpha 2-adrenoceptor blocker, has been used for erectile dysfunction. Its effectiveness is doubtful.
- Trazodone, an antidepressant that acts by inhibiting serotonin uptake and also by influencing alpha-adrenergic and dopaminergic functions, has been tried. Results are inconsistent in erectile disorders.
- Apomorphine which acts by dopamine receptor stimulation, and L-arginine which is a NO precursor, have also been used for erectile dysfunction.

- Naltrexone, an opiate antagonist, can antagonize the inhibition of sexual functions.
- Ashwagandha, Shatavari, Korean red ginseng, and others may have beneficial effect.

Topical Pharmacotherapy

- *Nitroglycerine (2% ointment)*: A known vasodilator.
- *Minoxidil*: A vasodilator directly acting on arterial smooth muscles by opening potassium channels (2% solution).
- *Papaverine gel*: Vasodilator
- Alprostadil cream (MUSE) (prostaglandin EI) used intraurethrally.

In some selected cases when psychotherapy, behavior techniques, and drugs fail or seen to be not very effective, vacuum devices, injections, and implants, vibrators are found to be relatively effective. Ultimately, the success of sex therapy depends on a host of factors. Therapy duration ranges from 6 weeks to more than a year in occasional cases. Sexual dysfunctions respond to treatment better compared to gender identify disorders and paraphilias, which are very resistant to therapy. More than half of the cases of erectile dysfunction and almost all the cases of premature ejaculation respond to combination of therapies.

Gender Identity Disorders

Gender identity is usually set before 18 months age in a child and is irreversibly established by 3 years age. This is primarily determined by anatomical sex (biological sex) by the presence of genitals (phenotype), genetic factor (genotype), and early upbringing. Gender identity refers to the expression of gender identify toward oneself and others.

Dual role transvestism: The subject wishes to lead a double role, spending part of his time as a male and part as a female.

Gender identity disorder of childhood: Is listed in ICD-10 while DSM-5 has used the term "gender dysphoria" (instead of gender identity disorder used in DSM-IV) with different sets of criteria for children and adolescents/adults.

Intersexuality: This disorder develops as there was ambiguity about child's external genitalia at birth. Androgen sensitivity syndrome and congenital adrenal hyperplasia are the examples.

Sexual maturation disorder: Here the person suffers from uncertainty about his or her gender identity or sexual orientation which causes anxiety or depression.

Gender Dysphoria

The term gender dysphoria as a general descriptive term refers to an individual's affective/cognitive discontent with the assigned gender. According to the DSM-5, gender dysphoria is also referred to the distress that may accompany the incongruence between one's experienced or expressed gender and one's assigned gender. The incidence and prevalence of gender dysphoria is difficult to obtain due to the rarity of the condition and sensitivity of the subject. Gender identity becomes fixed in most persons by age 2 or 3 years. For natal adult males, prevalence ranges from 0.005 to 0.014%, and for natal females, from 0.002 to 0.003%. The core component for diagnosis of gender dysphoria is that individuals with gender dysphoria have a marked incongruence between the gender they have been assigned to (usually at birth, referred to as natal gender) and their experienced/expressed gender for at least of 6 months duration. There must also be evidence of distress about this incongruence. Gender dysphoria manifests itself differently in different age groups. Prepubertal girls with gender dysphoria may express the wish to be a boy, assert they are a boy, or assert they will grow up to be a man and similarly prepubertal boys may express the wish to be a girl or assert they are a girl or that they will grow up to be a woman. These children prefer cross dressing and hairstyles. Girls will display negative reactions to parental attempts to have them wear dresses and may refuse to attend social gatherings. These children may also demonstrate marked cross-gender identification in role-playing, dreams, and fantasies. Girls prefer contact sports, games traditionally for boys and have little interest in feminine toys like dolls.

Boys may role-play female figures and prefer traditionally feminine games, e.g., "playing house", etc., and avoid rough and tumble play and competitive sports. Occasionally girls refuse to urinate in a sitting position and may express a desire to have a penis or claim to have a penis or that they will grow one when older. They may also state that they do not want to develop breasts or menstruate. Similarly, boys may pretend not to have a penis and insist on sitting to urinate and rarely also express the desire or wish to have a vagina. In young adolescents with gender dysphoria, depending on the developmental level they may have clinical feature similar to children or adults with the condition. The secondary sexual characters are not fully developed but they are concerned about imminent physical changes. In adults with gender dysphoria, there is a disparity between the experienced gender and physical sexual characters. It is often, but not always, accompanied by a desire to be rid of sexual characteristics or acquire the sexual characteristics of the other gender. They may adopt the behavior, clothing, and mannerisms of the experienced gender and may feel uncomfortable with the identity of the assigned gender in the society. They may find other ways to resolve the incongruence between experienced/ expressed and assigned gender by partially living in the desired role or by adopting a gender role neither conventionally male nor conventionally female. Some adults may also seek hormone treatment (sometimes without medical prescription and supervision) and gender reassignment surgery. Management of gender dysphorias involves several phases, such as diagnostic phase, social integration phase, hormonal treatment, surgical and postsurgical phases and take several months to years. With the advancement in surgical techniques, hormonal treatment and with appropriate psychological interventions, the management of gender dysphoria is possible and should be aimed to help improve the person's social functioning, relationships, work, education, and quality of life.

Paraphilic Disorders

The term "paraphilia" is derived from the Greek words "para" which means next to and "philia" meaning love. DSM-5 describes term "paraphilia" as "any intense and persistent sexual interest other than sexual interest in genital stimulation or preparatory fondling with phenotypically normal, physically mature, consenting human partners."

DSM-5 has further described paraphilic disorders as disorders based on (1) anomalous activity preferences [further subdivided into (i) courtship disorders (voyeuristic disorder, exhibitionistic disorder, and frotteuristic disorder); and (ii) algolagnic disorders which involve pain and suffering (sexual masochism disorder and sexual sadism disorder); (2) anomalous target preferences: (i) toward humans (pedophilic disorder); and (ii) directed elsewhere (fetishistic disorder and transvestic disorder)]

These are rare and occur mostly in men. They are characterized by recurrent intense sexual urges and sexually arousing fantasies generally involving either nonhuman objects, the suffering or humiliation of oneself or one's partner or children or other nonconsenting persons. For the paraphilic patient, the imagery is persistent; the fantasies evoked are necessary for erotic arousal, for the relief from nonerotic tension, and for sexual excitement and orgasm. Many paraphilics feel no distress and represent impairment in the capacity for reciprocal affectionate sexual activity. Though increased incidence of criminality is known with extra Y chromosome, no known genetic or biological factors have been implicated in its etiology. Only upbringing, problems in mother–child relationship, etc. have been implicated. History of being sexually abused as children is common among these groups.

- *Fetishism*: Sexual arousal is produced by nonliving objects such as women's clothing.
- *Transvestism*: Must dress in women's clothes in order to become sexually aroused.
- *Frotteurism*: Sexually arousing urges to touch or rub against a nonconsenting person, usually in a crowded setting where

detection can be avoided. Common in men of 15–25 years age.

- *Pedophilia*: Sexual activity or fantasy involves prepubertal children of either sex.
- *Exhibitionism*: Recurrent and intense sexual arousal from the exposure of one's genitals to unsuspecting persons either in fantasies causing significant distress or in behavior with a nonconsenting person; seen usually in psychologically immature men.
- *Voyeurism*: Urges and fantasies about seeing unsuspecting people naked, in the act of disrobing or having sex, usually heterosexual in nature and is commonly referred as "peeping Tom." It excludes watching pornography or normal sexual play in which individuals being watched are willing. DSM-5 gives a minimum duration of 6 months for a diagnosis to be made. Voyeuristic acts are most common law-breaking sexual behaviors.
- *Masochism and sadism*: Achievement of sexual pleasure and intense sexual arousal only through physical pain or suffering of self (masochism) or others (sadism).
- *Bestiality or zoophilia*: Sex with animals in the presence of other natural sexual outlets.
- *Homosexuality*: It refers to the sexual relationship between the persons of the same sex. It is no more considered a sexual deviation. This is a disorder when it is the dominant, significant, and persistent mode of sexual relationship for that person and causes significant distress to the individual and is called ego-dystonic homosexuality. ICD-10 recognizes this as a category when sexual development and orientation are problematic to the individual. Five percent of all males and 2% of all females are reported to be homosexual. A whole spectrum of biological and social causes has been implicated in its causation.

TAKE-HOME MESSAGES

- Sex refers to being male or female based on reproductive function and biological characteristics. Gender refers to publicly lived role as male or female, suggestive more of sociocultural aspect rather than biological one.
- The concept of sexual response cycle has moved from EPOR model (excitation, plateau, orgasm, and resolution) to DEOR model (desire, excitation, orgasm, and resolution).
- Common sexual dysfunctions or inadequacies include delayed ejaculation, erectile disorder, male hypoactive sexual desire disorder, premature (early) ejaculation, female orgasmic disorder, female sexual interest/arousal disorder, genito-pelvic pain/penetration disorder.
- Dr NN Wig in 1960 had coined the term called "Dhat syndrome" to refer to a culture bound syndrome presenting with depression, anxiety, sexual dysfunction, and somatic symptoms. It is attributed to loss of semen.
- Management of sexual disorders include excluding possible organic causes and judicious use of pharmacotherapy and psychotherapy.

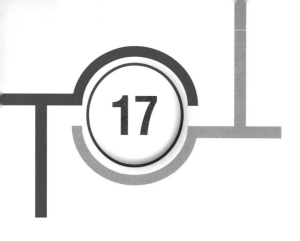

17

Sleep and Sleep Disorders

Ravi Gupta, Sandeep Grover

INTRODUCTION

Sleep is a naturally occurring, physiological, self-regulated, regularly recurrent, and reversible state of lowered consciousness, perceptual disengagement, and behavioral quiescence seen universally in nearly all organisms. During this state there is nearly no exchange of information to and fro from the environment. It is a state of reversible unconsciousness that is characterized by behavioral quiescence and brings an alteration in almost all physiological functions of the body. An adult person spends around one-third of the time in sleep, which reduces progressively with aging. Similarly, an adult spends lesser time in sleep compared to an infant. Thus, sleep duration progressively reduces as we age. Not only the duration, but also the sleep architecture changes with age, and it is depicted as reduction in the proportion of deep sleep.

SLEEP PHYSIOLOGY

Two major physiological processes regulate duration and timing of sleep: (1) the homeostatic process and (2) circadian process **(Fig. 17.1)**. Homeostatic process works on the principle that a specific amount of sleep is required for every person. If a person, for any reason, becomes sleep-deprived, pressure of sleep increases making a person somnolent. For this reason, after period of prolonged

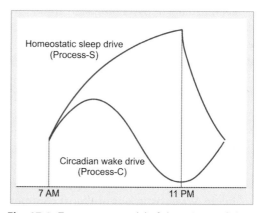

Fig. 17.1: *Two process model of sleep:* State of sleep and wakefulness depends upon two process model: Process C and Process S. Propensity to fall asleep is highest when both sleep pressure (Process S) and melatonin secretion (Process C) are at their zenith.

waking (say 18–20 hours or longer at a stretch, known as acute sleep deprivation) or when they curtail a small portion from their habitual sleep time for prolonged duration (say 30 minutes every night for 15 days; termed as chronic partial sleep deprivation) people fall asleep even when it is not required or in the situations where it is not acceptable. This is one reason people who follow regular sleep–wake schedule and feel sleepy at a given chronological time. Wakefulness is maintained by reticular activating system (RAS) that includes many nuclei which supply to almost whole of the cortex. RAS includes monoaminergic nuclei, e.g., locus ceruleus (noradrenaline), raphe nuclei (serotonin), pedunculopontine and lateral dorsal tegmental nuclei (acetylcholine), tuberomammillary nucleus (histamine), and ventral tegmental nucleus (dopamine). Several other neurotransmitters and neuropeptides colocalize with these primary neurotransmitters and modulate the functioning of brain. In addition, cerebral cortex is also rich in two other neurotransmitters: (1) Glutamate and (2) Gamma aminobutyric acid (GABA). Among these, GABA is inhibitory and promotes sleep while other transmitters (glutamate and monoaminergic neurotransmitters) promote wakefulness. Ventrolateral preoptic (VLPO) area of hypothalamus sends GABAergic signals to other excitatory nuclei to induce sleep **(Fig. 17.2)**. A third group of neurons is important for modulating the activity of sleep-promoting as well as wake-promoting areas. These are known as orexin/hypocretin neurons which are present in the posterior hypothalamus and by modulating the activity of both the areas, they try to maintain the sleep–wake status.

Circadian process decides the time of falling asleep in context of environmental lighting and thus, provides diurnal or nocturnal character to the living beings. Diurnal species like humans have predominant activity during day and fall asleep as the night

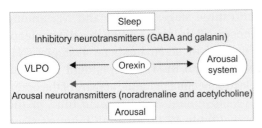

Fig. 17.2: Sleep and wake promoting areas of brain: Ventrolateral preoptic (VLPO) area of hypothalamus secretes GABA to deactivate wake promoting nuclei of reticular activating system. VLPO is connected to suprachiasmatic nuclei (SCN), the master circadian clock that regulates its activity.

approaches. Opposite is seen among nocturnal species that are most active and awake at night, e.g., preying animals. Information regarding the environmental lighting reaches the brain through retinohypothalamic tract which is then conveyed to master circadian clock located in the hypothalamus—the supra-chiasmatic nucleus (SCN) **(Fig. 17.3)**. From SCN the information is conveyed to various areas of brain to regulate other physiological processes, e.g., appetite, cardiac activity, endocrine secretion, and activity of various other physiological processes. This information also reaches to the pineal gland where it increases the secretion of melatonin that in turn induces the sleep. Among humans, secretion of melatonin is dependent upon the darkness and bright light inhibits its secretion. In the evening, natural environmental light reduces, stimulating the melatonin secretion and thus helps in inducing the sleep. However, bright light falling on the retina (whether artificial or natural) reduces secretion of melatonin, leading to increment of alertness and wakefulness.

However, it is important to understand that emotional status of a person also influences the sleep–wake cycle **(Fig. 17.4:** Regulation of sleep). Areas that regulate emotions (limbic cortex) have connections with the areas that regulate circadian and homeostatic process. This is the reason that people are not able to sleep well when they are stressed or when they are anxious. Anxiety or stress initiates the sympathetic arousal, and it increases the alertness. Hence, it is important to understand that besides two process model, multiple other factors like emotions, social situation, availability of food, environmental lighting also influence sleep–wake cycle. This understanding also has important implication in management of various sleep disorders.

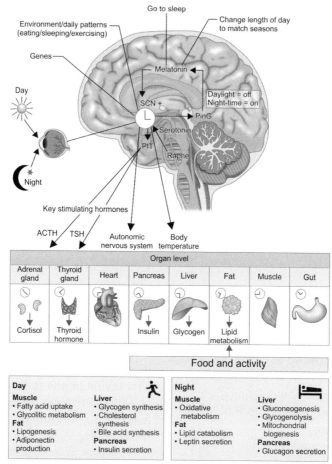

Fig. 17.3: *Master circadian clock:* Connections of suprachiasmatic nucleus.
('Master clock' SCN: suprachiasmatic nucleus (in the hypothalamus–sets the time); PIT: pituitary gland;
PinG: pineal gland; ACTH: adrenocorticotropic hormone; TSH: thyroid-stimulating hormone)

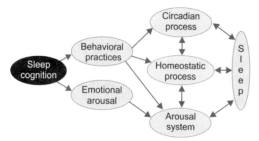

Fig. 17.4: Physiological, psychological, and
behavior model.

SLEEP CYCLE

Architecturally, sleep comprises of two
different states: (1) nonrapid eye movement

(NREM) sleep and (2) rapid eye movement
(REM) sleep. NREM sleep is further divided
into three stages N1, N2, and N3; among
these, N3 is also known as deep sleep.
Division of sleep in these 4 stages (N1,
N2, N3, and REM) is dependent upon the
electroencephalographic activity of the brain,
eye movements, and muscle tone in the
body **(Table 17.1)**. An adult initiate's sleep
with NREM sleep and from the wakefulness
drifts into N1. From N1, person passes into
N2 and then N3 sleep, unless any external
or internal stimulus wakes him up. From
N3, person comes back to N2 sleep. From

Table 17.1: Physiological characteristics of different sleep stages.

	Awake	NREM			REM sleep
		N1	N2	N3	
Brain activity as measured by EEG	Low-voltage mixed frequency activity. Posterior dominant rhythm alpha during quiet wakefulness	Low-voltage mixed frequency activity with vertex waves	Low-voltage mixed frequency activity with appearance of theta, sleep spindles and K complexes	Delta waves (0.5–2 Hz with peak to peak amplitude of at least 75 microV) present and occupies at least 20% of the epoch	Low-voltage mixed frequency activity. Saw tooth waves are characteristics of REM sleep
Eye movements	Rapid scanning eye movements	Slow eye movement	Usually absent	Usually absent	Rapid darting eye movements seen
Muscle tone	Variable	Lower than wakefulness			Lowest among all stages
Respiration	Variable in rate and rhythm	Regular rate and rhythm			Variable in rate and rhythm
Cardiac activity	Variable in rate and rhythm	Regular rate and rhythm			Variable in rate and rhythm
Blood pressure	Variable	Stable and lower than wakefulness			Variable
Brain metabolism	High	Stable and lower than wakefulness			High
Endocrine activity	None	None	None	Secretion of growth hormone	None
Thermo-regulation	Intact	Intact			Poor, prone to hypothermia

(NREM: nonrapid eye movement; REM: rapid eye movement; EEG: electroencephalogram)

the initiation of sleep, it takes around 90–120 minutes to develop REM sleep. First episode of REM is brief and is terminated by either of the following—an arousal, N1, or N2 sleep. Combination of one NREM and one REM episode is known as one sleep cycle and each cycle lasts for 90–120 minutes. In a given night person may have 3–5 such sleep cycles.

SLEEP DISORDERS

As we have seen, sleep is a neurobiological phenomenon, and it brings changes in the body physiology. Being regulated by neurotransmitters and pathways, like other psychiatric disorders, it is also liable to get disrupted. This disruption can be seen in many ways, giving rise to various sleep disorders.

Sleep disorders are among the most common clinical problems encountered in general medicine and psychiatry practice. Poor quality of sleep is associated with impairment in quality of life, accidents, job dysfunction, and increased risk of disorders like anxiety, depression, cardiovascular diseases, metabolic syndrome, diabetes mellitus, stroke, cardiac arrhythmias to name a few.

Broadly, sleep disorders can be categorized into primary sleep disorders, sleep problems secondary to psychiatric disorders, sleep problems arising due to medication or substance use, and sleep problems secondary to medical illnesses. International Classification of Sleep Disorder, 3rd Edition (ICSD-3) and Diagnostic and Statistical Manual, 5th Edition (DSM-5) divides primary sleep disorders into various categories, depending upon their clinical presentation **(Table 17.2)**. For primary sleep disorders, the etiology often remains obscure, but the pathophysiology is known. On the other hand, secondary sleep disorders, though have same pathophysiology, but are thought to be result of another disorder, medication or substance. In this chapter, common sleep disorders that are important are discussed along with their management.

Table 17.2: Classification of primary sleep disorders.	
International Classification of Sleep Disorder, 3rd Edition	*Diagnostic and Statistical Manual, 5th Edition*
• Insomnia • Sleep-related breathing disorders • Central disorders of hypersomnolence • Circadian rhythm sleep–wake disorders • Parasomnias • Sleep-related movement disorders	• Insomnia disorder • Hypersomnolence disorder • Narcolepsy • Breathing-related sleep disorders • Circadian rhythm sleep–wake disorders • NREM sleep arousal disorders • Nightmare disorders • REM sleep behavior disorder • Restless leg syndrome • Substance/medication-induced sleep disorder

(NREM: nonrapid eye movement; REM: rapid eye movement)

Insomnia

Insomnia is defined as inability or difficulty in any of the following: falling asleep, staying asleep, or waking up in the morning earlier than the usual wake time. Quantitatively, if a person takes >30 minutes to fall asleep, spends at least 30 minutes awake after catching the sleep for at least once or wakes up at least 30 minutes earlier than the usual wake time for at least 3 nights a week, diagnosis of insomnia may be considered. However, it is important to note that these difficulties must be present when the person has adequate sleep opportunity and associated daytime dysfunction. To complete the clinical picture, daytime symptoms/consequences of insomnia, e.g., headache, lethargy, daytime somnolence, poor attention and concentration, memory or mood changes, etc., must be present. In absence of daytime symptoms of insomnia, diagnosis of insomnia cannot be made and in such cases, other sleep disorders must be ruled out. If the symptoms are present for <3 months, diagnosis of short-term insomnia should be made. On the other hand, persistent symptoms for >3 months indicate diagnosis of chronic insomnia.

Diagnosis of insomnia is largely clinical. Objectively it may be diagnosed using sleep diary or actigraphy. Overnight polysomnography may show prolonged sleep onset latency (time to fall asleep), multiple nocturnal awakenings, or early morning awakenings. It affects 10–20% of the population; it is more common among females and among older adults. Other risk factors for insomnia include stressful life events, poor sleep habits, irregular sleep schedule, fear of not sleeping, anxiety or worry prone personality or faulty thinking styles, environmental factors (like noise, light, uncomfortable low or high temperature), genetic predisposition, and physiological factors like advancing age.

Pathophysiologically, insomnia is characterized by a state of neuronal hyperarousability and these patients' show signs of sympathetic arousal near bedtime, e.g., increased heart rate, increased activity of hypothalamo–pituitary axis as depicted by elevated levels of corticotrophin-releasing factor and cortisol. Electroencephalographic recordings show high-frequency waves during NREM sleep.

Insomnia must be differentiated from environmental factors causing sleep disruption, use of substances with stimulant property, circadian rhythm sleep disorders, insufficient sleep syndrome, sleep-related movement disorders, sleep-related epilepsy, obstructive sleep apnea (OSA), and restless legs syndrome (RLS).

Management of insomnia is multidimensional and includes sleep hygiene, pharmacological agents, and nonpharmacological agents. Sleep hygiene measures **(Box 17.1)** must be advised to all patients and in some patients these may be sufficient to manage insomnia. For the management of short-term insomnia, hypnotic medications should be used. These include various benzodiazepines **(Table 17.3)** and nonbenzodiazepine Z drugs **(Table 17.4)**. A particular molecule may be chosen based upon the patient's age, comorbid medical conditions, drug interaction, duration of action, and adverse effects. Pharmacological intervention is individualized, and no one molecule may fit all. Short- and long-acting benzodiazepines can have their advantages and disadvantages **(Table 17.5)**. In general, long-acting molecules should be avoided as they may lead to daytime sleepiness; they should be avoided among elderly as they may induce imbalance and increase the chances of fall. Certain antidepressants (trazodone, mirtazapine, and amitriptyline) and antipsychotics (quetiapine, olanzapine) also have sedating properties. However, it is important to note that these are usually not recommended for management of primary insomnia. These may be useful in managing secondary insomnia associated with other psychiatric disorders.

Box 17.1: Sleep hygiene instructions.

- Follow a regular sleep schedule
- *Adjust the bedroom environment*:
  - Maintain the temperature and lighting of your bedroom to a level that is comfortable for you
  - Make sure that your bedding is comfortable for you
- A regular exercise program in the morning or afternoon may help to promote sleep
- Avoid going to bed empty stomach or too full
- Avoid bright light exposure (including screens—smartphones, laptops, etc.) before bed time
- Avoid alcohol intake, nicotine intake especially in the evening
- Avoid caffeine-containing drinks especially in the late afternoon or evening

Table 17.3: Benzodiazepines.

Drug	Dose in mg	Absorption	Active metabolite	Primary metabolism route	Half life
Chlordiazepoxide	5–10	Intermediate	Yes	Hepatic	2–4 days
Diazepam	2–10	Fast	Yes	Hepatic	2–4 days
Flurazepam	7.5–30	Inter-fast	Yes	Hepatic	2–4 days
Clonazepam	0.5–1	Intermediate	Yes	Hepatic	2–3 days
Lorazepam	0.5–4	Intermediate	No	Hepatic	10–20 hours
Nitrazepam	2.5–10	Intermediate	Yes	Hepatic	24–30 hours

Table 17.4: Z-category drugs used for management of insomnia.

Drug	Dose in mg	Absorption	Active metabolite	Primary elimination route	Half life
Zaleplon	5–20	Fast	No	Hepatic	1 hours
Zolpidem	5–10	Fast	No	Hepatic	1.4–3.8 hours
Zolpidem SR	6.25–12.5	Fast	No	Hepatic	2.8 hours
Zopiclone	7.5–15	Fast	Yes	Hepatic	4–6.5 hours
Eszopiclone	1–3	Fast	Yes	Hepatic	6 hours

Table 17.5: Comparison of short- and long-acting benzodiazepines.

Measures	Short half life	Long half life
Sedative hangover effects	+	++++
Accumulation with consecutive nightly use	0	+++
Tolerance	+++	+
Withdrawal insomnia	+++	+
Anxiolytic effect next day	0	+++
Amnesia	+++	++
Rebound insomnia	++++	0
Full benefit on the first night	+++	++

For chronic insomnia, cognitive behavior therapy for insomnia (CBT-I) must be instituted that is aimed at improving the sleep-promoting behaviors and reducing sleep-defeating practices. CBT-I has various components that include improving sleep hygiene, relaxation training, sleep restriction therapy, and stimulus control therapy to name a few. Based upon the individual case, these components are instituted in various combinations.

Hypersomnia

Contrary to insomnia, which is characterized by inability to sleep, hypersomnia is characterized by an increase in duration of sleep or napping under odd circumstances. Hypersomnia may have multiple presentations. One of these is idiopathic hypersomnia (IH), which is characterized by excessive long sleep duration, usually 12–14 hours, increased efforts to wake up in the morning and short sleep latency (<8 min on multiple sleep latency testing). These patients have multiple lapses of sleep during the day; however, these naps are nonrefreshing. Symptoms must be present for at least 3 months to qualify for the diagnosis. Pathophysiology of IH is not known. Another important disorder in this category is narcolepsy. Patients with narcolepsy have irresistible urge to fall asleep during the daytime resulting in multiple naps. However, unlike naps of IH, naps in narcolepsy are refreshing. Narcolepsy can essentially be understood as a disorder of instability of sleep and wakefulness due to damage of orexin neurons that act as modulator of sleep and wake-promoting areas. Hence, sleep intrudes the wakefulness during the daytime and at night-time these patients have poor maintenance of sleep. These patients have short sleep latency (<8 min along with two or more sleep onset REM periods on multiple sleep latency testing) and or cerebrospinal fluid hypocretin level <110 pg/mL. Type I narcolepsy also has cataplexy which is characterized by sudden loss of muscle tone in response to any emotional stimuli. Pathophysiologically, cataplexy occurs due to intrusion of REM atonia during wakefulness. Cataplexy is absent in type II narcolepsy. Other associated features of narcolepsy are: sleep paralysis (persistence of REM atonia even after waking up from sleep), hypnagogic or hypnopompic hallucinations (due to intrusion of dreaming at the junction of wakefulness to sleep or sleep to wakefulness, respectively).

Diagnosis is based upon history and clinical examination. Other causes of hypersomnolence like atypical depression, medication, addictive substances, and other medical disorders like hypothalamic lesions, paraneoplastic syndrome must be ruled out. Differential diagnosis for narcolepsy includes other hypersomnias, sleep deprivation or insufficient nocturnal sleep, sleep apnea syndrome, depression, schizophrenia, dissociation/dissociative disorder, attention deficit hyperkinetic disorder, seizure disorders, chorea, and other movement disorders.

Objectively, hypersomnolence may be measured by actigraphy and polysomnography. Polysomnography also helps to conduct multiple sleep latency test that can differentiate between two conditions.

Stimulants (e.g., modafinil, methylphenidate) are used for reduction of total sleep time. Selective serotonin reuptake inhibitors may be used to control cataplexy among narcolepsy patients. Gamma hydroxy butyrate, also known as sodium oxybate, has been reported to improve all symptoms of narcolepsy. Scheduled naps may also alleviate daytime somnolence in narcolepsy.

Sleep-related Breathing Disorders

Obstructive sleep apnea (OSA) is the most common type of sleep-related breathing disorder. OSA is characterized by snoring, snorting, choking at night, pauses in breath witnessed by bed partner, nocturia, sleep-talking, nonrefreshing sleep, daytime fatigue, excessive daytime sleepiness, poor memory, and loss of libido to name a few. All symptoms are not seen in every patient and history from the bed partner is often most reliable. OSA develops owing to temporary and recurrent collapse of upper airway (pharynx) during sleep in presence of continued respiratory efforts from chest and abdomen. Pharynx is a tube-like muscular structure that does not have any bony or cartilaginous support around it to maintain its caliber. Its caliber is maintained by muscle tone during wakefulness that reduces during sleep. In addition, increased amount of parapharyngeal fat (which is proportionate to the body weight) among obese persons also push the pharyngeal airway inside and reduce the caliber of upper airway. This is why OSA is more common among obese persons. Other anatomical deformities that reduce the cross-sectional area of upper airway, e.g., macroglossia, retrognathia, retrusion of maxilla also contribute to development of OSA. In these cases, OSA may be seen despite normal body mass index. OSA is more common among males and is a disorder of middle age. Among children, it is most commonly due to adenotonsillar enlargement. Other risk factors for OSA include family history of OSA, genetic syndromes associated with anatomical deformities (Down-syndrome, Treacher Collin's syndrome), and endocrinopathies like acromegaly.

Differential diagnosis of OSA includes primary snoring and other sleep disorders, insomnias, panic attacks, and substance medication-induced insomnia/hypersomnia.

Obstructive sleep apnea can be diagnosed using overnight diagnostic polysomnography. To be clinically significant, at least five obstructive respiratory events must be present in an hour during polysomnography examination. The obstructive respiratory events may be either of the three; (1) apnea: complete cessation of breathing, (2) hypopnea: reduction in amplitude of breathing leading to significant desaturation or arousal, (3) respiratory event-related arousal: progressively increased respiratory effort culminating in an arousal.

Untreated disease may lead to cardiac arrhythmias, sudden cardiac death, systemic and pulmonary hypertension, coronary artery disease, diabetes mellitus, stroke, depression, somatic symptoms disorder, cognitive dysfunction, and congestive heart failure.

Treatment includes weight reduction and use of positive airway pressure (PAP) therapy after manual titration of PAP device. In cases with anatomical deformities, surgical correction (adenotonsillectomy, glossectomy, uvulopharyngopalatoplasty, maxillary or mandibular advancement) is recommended.

Sleep-related Movement Disorders

Willis Ekbom Disease/restless legs syndrome (WED/RLS) is perhaps the most common sleep-related movement disorder. This is characterized by an urge to move legs which is usually associated with dysesthesias in leg muscles. Symptoms usually worsen by rest and improve with moving the lower limbs; the symptoms show circadian variation as they appear only in the evening or night. Symptoms do not allow patients to fall asleep and they may present as a case of insomnia. WED/RLS has a bimodal age of onset—first during late adolescence and second during middle age and show a female preponderance. Certain conditions can precipitate the WED/RLS, e.g., iron deficiency, rheumatoid arthritis, chronic kidney disease, opioid withdrawal, pregnancy, and psychotropic medications are few of them. This disorder should be differentiated from leg edema, habitual leg movement, myalgia, arthralgia, positional discomfort, and akathisia. Management involves prescription of dopamine agonists (l-dopa, ropinirole, pramipexole) or drugs acting on alpha-2-delta ligands (gabapentin, pregabalin).

Parasomnias

Parasomnias are abnormal movements that appear during the sleep. Depending upon their appearance, they may be divided into two categories: (1) NREM sleep parasomnias and (2) REM sleep parasomnias. During NREM parasomnia, patient has incomplete awakening from sleep, does not respond to the interventions to wake him up, has amnesia for the episode, and often do not report any association of the behavior with the dreams. NREM sleep parasomnias are basically the disorders of arousal where certain areas of the brain remain in sleep while others become active. Because of the activation of certain areas the patient may perform even the complex movements and can show limited response to the environmental stimuli; however, because other areas that are still sleeping, he remains oblivious of his activities and cannot recall his act afterwards. NREM-parasomnia includes three conditions: (1) *sleepwalking*, (2) *sleep terror*, and (3) *confusional arousal*. Patients with sleepwalking get out of their bed while asleep; behaviorally, their eyes are open and they easily navigate their environment without hitting any object. They may perform movements across a wide range, starting from simple movements like walking to complex movements like cycling and driving. If anyone attempts to wake them up forcefully, they may show aggression; hence, they should be carefully handled at that time. Sleep terrors are most prevalent during childhood, and their prevalence reduces as the age increases.

Child usually wakes up from sleep screaming, he is inconsolable at that time and keeps crying, and shows signs of sympathetic arousal. Episode lasts for few minutes and then settles down. Child is not able to recall any dream that led to frightening. During confusional arousal, child wakes up for a brief period, looks around in confused manner, and again falls asleep. During childhood, these complaints are common and their prevalence reduces as the child grows. Thus, NREM parasomnias may represent a phenomenon of developing brain. Certain other factors may precipitate NREM parasomnias, e.g., fever, stress, psychotropic medications, sleeping in unfamiliar environment, and other sleep disorders like WED/RLS and OSA.

Diagnosis depends upon the clinical history. Overnight polysomnography with extended EEG montage may be done to rule out sleep-related epilepsy and other sleep disorder. When symptoms are infrequent and not threatening, reassurance may be given. The patients and their family members should be educated regarding precipitating behavior. If clinically required, screening for comorbid sleep disorders must be done. When symptoms are severe, child may be prescribed long-acting benzodiazepines. If comorbid sleep disorder is present, it should be treated.

Rapid eye movement sleep parasomnias occur during REM; and hence, these are more common during second half of night **(Fig. 17.5)**. These include nightmares and REM sleep behavior disorder (RBD). Nightmare disorder presents with episodes of awakenings, usually in response to life-threatening dreams that can be recalled. Unlike night terrors, patient achieves alertness immediately after awakening. These episodes must cause significant distress in social, personal, and occupational functioning. These are common during childhood and after major stress. They are also part of posttraumatic stress disorder.

Rapid eye movement RBD is often seen during old age and neurodegenerative conditions predispose development of RBD. These patients are often brought by their bed partners who bear the brunt of disorder. Affected individuals act on their dreams (which are often violent) and in this process may harm themselves or their bed partners. Pathophysiologically, these patients do not develop the REM atonia during their sleep. Diagnosis is based on history and polysomnography evidence of REM atonia. This can be treated by prescription of clonazepam.

Circadian Rhythm Sleep Disorders

These disorders are characterized by persistent or recurrent pattern of sleep disruption, as a result of alteration of the circadian

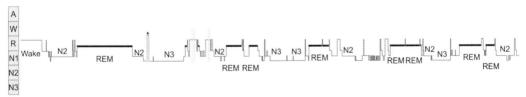

Fig. 17.5: *Hypnogram showing progress of sleep cycle in a given night:* This figure clearly shows that as the night progresses, duration of successive REM episodes lengthens while that of N3 sleep reduces. This is one reason why NREM parasomnias are predominantly seen in first half of night while REM parasomnias in second half of night. (NREM: nonrapid eye movement; REM: rapid eye movement)
Source: Sleep Laboratory, AIIMS, Rishikesh.

system or due to a misalignment between the circadian rhythm and environmental timing. Thus, the affected person's sleep–wake schedule loses the synchrony with the environmental time or sleep–wake schedule required by the profession. Diagnosis requires presence of clinically significant distress or impairment in the social, occupation, and other areas of functioning.

The circadian rhythm sleep disorders are further categorized as delayed sleep wake phase disorder, advanced sleep–wake phase disorder, irregular sleep–wake type, non-24 hour sleep–wake type, shift worker type, and unspecified type.

Delayed sleep–wake type is characterized by a significant delay in timing of falling asleep and wake timing, masquerading symptoms of initial insomnia and hypersomnia, respectively. In contrast, advanced sleep–wake type is characterized by a significant advancement in time to fall asleep and wake timing, masquerading symptoms of hypersomnia and terminal insomnia, respectively. When patients of both advance and delayed type are allowed to set their own time, they have no difficulty in quality of sleep and duration of sleep. Delayed sleep–wake type is more common than the advanced sleep–wake type.

Patients with irregular sleep–wake rhythm disorder present with history of insomnia in the night and excessive sleepiness during the day. Further history reveals that they lack a discernible sleep–wake circadian rhythm and sleep is usually fragmented in at least three periods in a day.

Shift work disorder is seen among those who work outside the normal working hours of 8.00 AM to 6.00 PM and is characterized by excessive sleep at work and impaired sleep at home, on a persistent basis. Reverting to a day work leads to disappearance of symptoms.

Many patients with circadian rhythm sleep disorders have comorbid depression and other sleep disorders. Management of all the circadian rhythm sleep disorders involves sleep hygiene and having a regular sleep schedule.

Management of delayed sleep–wake type involves either advancing or delaying the internal clock. Advancing the internal clock involves shifting the bedtime a bit earlier (about 15 minutes) on every consecutive day till the desired bedtime is reached. Delaying the internal clock involves moving the bedtime by 1-3 hours on successive nights till the desired bedtime is achieved. Management of advance sleep–wake type involves use of bright light during the early evening hours.

CONCLUSION

Sleep problems are among the most common clinical problems encountered in medicine and psychiatry. Primary sleep disorders are quite prevalent in general population. Diagnosis of sleep disorders requires proper history taking and if required carrying out various sleep-specific investigations. Untreated sleep disorders pose a threat to a healthy life and have multiple adverse health consequences. Optimal management options are available for these disorders.

TAKE-HOME MESSAGES

- Sleep is a naturally occurring, physio-logical, self-regulated, regularly recurrent, and reversible state of lowered conscious-ness, perceptual disengagement, and behavioral quiescence seen universally in nearly all organisms.

- The duration and timing of sleep is regulated by two major physiological processes; they are (1) homeostatic process and (2) circadian process.
- Sleep architecture comprises of two different states: (1) NREM sleep and (2) REM sleep. NREM sleep is further divided into three stages: N1, N2, and N3. N3 is also known as deep sleep. REM sleep is characterized by dream experience.
- Sleep disorders are among the most common clinical problems encountered in general medicine and psychiatry practice.
- Common sleep disorders are insomnia, hypersomnia, sleep-related breathing disorders, central disorders of hypersomnolence, circadian rhythm sleep–wake disorders, parasomnias, and sleep-related movement disorders.
- Sleep hygiene includes a regular sleep schedule, adjusting bedroom environment, regular exercise program in the morning, not going to bed empty stomach or too full, avoiding bright light exposure and alcohol, nicotine or caffeine intake before sleep.

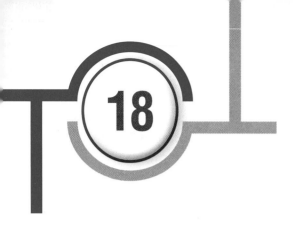

18

Eating Disorders

Rajesh Kumar, Niska Sinha

"I will feed myself and fight this illness, not feed this illness and fight myself."
(*National Eating Disorders Association*)

INTRODUCTION

It has lately been observed that the incidence and prevalence of the eating disorders, although generally considered to be rare, is on the rise. It is perceived that greater value placed by the modern society on the esthetic appeal of being slim and thin has led to rise in these disorders. Earlier it was seen mostly in industrialized and western countries, but now it has also permeated to less developed countries because of the cultural transformations, rapid industrialization, effects of media, migration, etc.

Eating disorders are actually a brain disorder which is characterized by abnormal behaviors related to food. It has significant *physical*, *psychological*, and *social* complications. They are mostly chronic and recurrent conditions with acute and chronic effects on the physical health, relationships, employment, fertility, and family life of affected individuals. They have intricate and complex issues related to negative body image, weight, and shape. These include problematic eating and various compensatory behaviors including starvation; binging; vomiting; compulsive exercise; and abuse of diuretics, purgatives, and laxatives. Eating disorders have significant physical and psychosocial morbidities including high rates of mortality, if untreated. These disorders arouse great interest among public, the media, and the scientific community. They are at times difficult to diagnose and treat because of inherent clinical and psychosocial factors. This chapter is intended to provide clear and lucid information regarding these disorders so that the readers may be able to understand, detect, manage, and refer the cases to the specialists for further assessment and management.

HISTORY

Eating disorders have a long history, and it is very difficult to trace, though cases of self-starvation have occurred from the days of biblical antiquity to middle ages. Famous case of *Martha Taylor* is presumed to be the first authentic description of a case of anorexia nervosa (AN) in 1667, which caught the attention of English physicians and England Royal Society. *Richard Morton* in 1689 first provided the medical account of AN, who described it as a nervous consumption caused by sadness and anxious care. During the nineteenth century, *Dr Charles Lasègue* wrote two articles on hysterical anorexia similar to present day AN. *Sir William W Gull* published his work on anorexia nervosa and these publications led to the term anorexia nervosa. First description of bulimia nervosa (BN) as a variant of AN was given by *Gerald Russell* in 1979.

TYPES OF EATING DISORDERS

Eating disorders are characterized by clinical presentation primarily focused on eating behavior. Its different types are given in **Box 18.1**. In International Classification of Diseases *(ICD-10)*, eating disorders have been placed under *behavioral syndromes associated with psychological disturbances and physiological factors*. In Diagnostic and Statistical Manual of Mental Disorders *(DSM-5)*, they are categorized under *feeding and eating disorders*. DSM-5 includes several changes to better represent the symptoms and behaviors of patients dealing with these conditions throughout the life span. Among the major changes are recognition of binge eating disorders (BEDs); revisions to diagnostic criterion for AN and BN; and inclusion of pica, rumination, and avoidant/ restrictive food intake disorder. Current approaches to eating disorder classification are entirely on distinctions among individuals with respect to eating and weight control behaviors and associated features. The primary goal of classification is that more people experiencing eating disorders have a diagnostic system which accurately describes their symptoms and behaviors. This chapter intends to provide brief account of the following eating disorders. *AN, BN,* and *BED*.

EPIDEMIOLOGY

The eating disorders are rare clinical syndromes. The lifetime prevalence of AN is *0.9%* in women and *0.3%* in men; BN is *1.5%* in women and *0.5%* in men; and BED is *3.5%* in women and *2%* in men. Eating disorders cause significant distress, medical morbidity, and increased mortality. These disorders usually have onset in early to mid-adolescence to young adulthood. These disorders were considered primarily a western illness having a developmental gradient across cultures with predominance in industrialized and developed countries indicating its presence primarily in affluent societies. There are acculturation pressures or rapid sociocultural changes that describe AN and BN as illnesses of modern era. The current culture of slenderness is perhaps linked to increasing occurrence of eating disorders in females. It is difficult to conclude whether cultural influences alone cause serious eating disorders. Social, individual,

---

Box 18.1: Types of eating disorders.

Anorexia nervosa:
- Resistance to maintaining body weight at or above a minimally normal weight for age and height
- Intense fear of weight gain or being "fat," even though underweight
- Disturbance in the experience of body weight or shape, undue influence of weight or shape on self-evaluation, or denial of the seriousness of low bodyweight
- Loss of menstrual periods in girls and women postpuberty

Bulimia nervosa:
- Regular intake of large amounts of food accompanied by a sense of loss of control
- Regular use of inappropriate compensatory behaviors such as self-induced vomiting, laxative or diuretic abuse, fasting, and/or obsessive or compulsive exercise
- Extreme concern with body weight and shape

Binge eating disorder:
- Frequent episodes of eating large quantities of food in short periods of time
- Feeling out of control over eating behavior
- Feeling ashamed or disgusted by the behavior
- There are also several behavioral indicators of BED including eating when not hungry and eating in secret
- No use of compensatory measure to counter the binge eating

Source: National Eating Disorders Association.

and family characteristics may be either predisposing or protective for any particular disease **(Figs. 18.1 and 18.2)**. People with AN are by definition in starvation state. Over 40% of patients with BED are obese with high rates of psychiatric comorbidities, particularly anxiety and depressive disorders. With treatment, around 40% of patients with AN will make a good 5 year recovery, 40% remain symptomatic but with limited disability, and 20% of patients suffer chronic disability. Outcomes are supposed to be better in early illness course and in children and adolescents with BN and AN. Only 50% of those with BN

go on to have a full recovery. Treatment needs to address *medical, social,* and *psychological* dimensions.

ANOREXIA NERVOSA

INTRODUCTION

The term "anorexia nervosa" was first introduced into the medical literature by *Sir William Gull* in 1874. It is a syndrome characterized by three essential criteria:

- *Self-induced starvation to a significant degree*
- *Relentless drive for thinness or of morbid fear of fatness*
- *Presence of medical signs and symptoms resulting from starvation.*

The affected individual is significantly underweight for age and height. It primarily affects adolescent girls and young women, is characterized by distorted body image and excessive dieting that leads to severe weight loss with a pathological fear of becoming fat. The DSM-IV criteria "D" requiring *amenorrhea* or the absence of three menstrual cycles have been deleted as this criterion could not be applied to *males, premenarche females, females taking oral contraceptive pills,* and *postmenopausal females.* There are two types of AN: (1) *restricting* and (2) *binge/ purge* type. The core theme of all subtypes is the highly disproportionate emphasis placed on thinness and sometime of self-esteem with weight and shape. Despite being of an abnormally low body weight, individuals with AN are intensely fearful of gaining weight and becoming fat and remarkably this fear typically intensifies as the weight falls. In the absence of an expressed fear of weight gain, this fear can be inferred by the clinicians via collateral history or observational data that indicate persistent behavior interfering with achieving or maintaining normal weight.

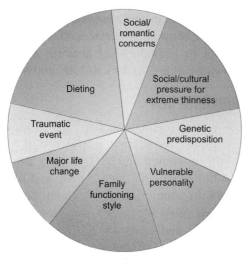

Fig. 18.1: Various etiological factors.

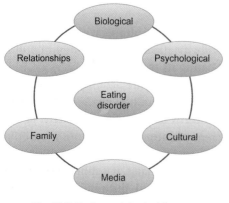

Fig. 18.2: Various etiological factors.

EPIDEMIOLOGY

It is a relatively rare illness, the average prevalence rate is *0.29%* with higher prevalence of subthreshold AN. The overall incidence rates have remained stable, but there appears to have been an increase in high risk groups of 15–19-year-old girls during the current century. This may be a reflection of earlier onset of illness, improved diagnostics, and increased utilization of health care systems. The male to female ratio is *1:10*. Some occupations such as *ballet dancing*, *fashion modeling*, and *sports activities* appear to confer particularly high risk for the development of AN.

Physiological disturbances: Multiple physical disturbances have been documented in AN. Most of these physical disturbances appear to be secondary consequences of starvation. The list of these disturbances is given in **Box 18.2**.

> **Box 18.2:** Complications of anorexia nervosa.
>
> - *Skin:* Lanugo, sunken cheeks, dull, thinning scalp hair, pitting edema of extremities
> - *Cardiovascular system:* Hypotension, bradycardia, arrhythmias, cardiac murmur (one-third with mitral valve prolapse)
> - *Hematopoietic system:* Normochronic, normocytic anemia, leukopenia, diminished polymorphonuclear leukocytes
> - *Fluid and electrolyte balance:* Elevated blood urea nitrogen and creatinine concentrations, hypokalemia, hyponatremia, hypochloremia, alkalosis
> - *Hypothermia*
> - *Gastrointestinal system:* Elevated serum concentration of liver enzymes, delayed gastric emptying, constipation
> - *Endocrine system:* Diminished thyroxine level with normal thyroid-stimulating hormone level, elevated plasma cortisol level, diminished secretion of luteinizing hormone, follicle-stimulating hormone, estrogen or testosterone, atrophic breasts, atrophic vaginitis
> - *Bone:* Osteoporosis

COMORBIDITIES

There is high prevalence of comorbid psychiatric disorders. Individuals with eating disorders are more likely to have comorbid mood or anxiety disorders. The lifetime prevalence of comorbid anxiety disorders ranges from 23 to 75% and mood disorders ranges from 24 to 90%.

ETIOLOGY

At present, the exact etiology of AN is unknown. However, it is possible to identify the risk factors which can increase the likelihood of AN. The etiology is complex with overlapping and distinct risk factors which may range from *biological, psychosocial*, to *sociocultural* factors. At present it is considered to be combination of biological, psychosocial, and sociocultural factors in the onset of the disorder.

Biological factors (genetic): AN occurs more frequently in biological relatives of patients with the disorder. Data suggest that first degree relatives of individuals with AN are 11 times more likely to have the illness in their lifetime than relatives of unaffected healthy individuals. Some evidence for a genetic component also comes from twin studies which report substantially higher concordance rates for monozygotic than for dizygotic twin pairs.

Developmental factors: As AN typically begins during adolescence, developmental factors are thought to play important etiological role. Critical challenges at this time of life include the need to establish *independence, personal identity, satisfying relationships*, etc. Family conflicts regarding *sexuality* and *pressure regarding increased heterosexual contacts* are also common. There is substantial emphasis on the self-image of adolescent boys and girls as there is significant relationship between self-esteem and satisfaction with physical appearance.

Psychological functioning: There are various theories ranging from deficit in development of object relations, deficits in self-structure, failures in early attachment, attempts to cope with underlying feelings of ineffectiveness and inadequacy, and an inability to meet the demands of adolescence and young adulthood.

Personality traits: Certain personality traits have been observed among women with AN including *obsessive compulsiveness, neuroticism, negative emotionality, low cooperativeness*, and *avoidant* personality disorder traits. The most consistent and enduring personality traits found in AN are perfectionism and harm avoidance.

Social/environmental factors: There is increased prevalence of AN in Western society as there is undue emphasis on unrealistic thin appearance of women. There is also evidence that a desire to be slim and thin is common among middle and upper class white women, and this has increased significantly in the last few decades.

ASSESSMENT

In assessment, it is important to obtain a weight history including the highest and lowest weights and the weight at which they would like to be. For women, it is useful to know the weight at which menstruation last occurred because it provides an indication of what weight is normal for that individual. The use of self-induced vomiting, purgatives, laxatives, diuretics, enemas, diet pills, and syrup of ipecac to induce vomiting should also be queried.

The greatest problem in assessment is their denial of the illness and their reluctance to participate in an evaluation. A straightforward but supportive and nonconfrontational approach is probably most useful.

As eating behaviors, body image and weight are personal and sensitive issues so it is desirable and critical that therapist provide an *accepting, nonconfrontational*, and *nonjudgmental* approach. Proper assessment is required to rule out organic causes for weight loss or menstrual abnormalities. All adolescents with such symptoms should be evaluated using certain parameters like current weight, perception about body image, weight control measures, physical activities, coexisting psychological morbidities, family, peer relationship, level of readiness to change behaviors, signs of nutritional deficiencies, and medical complications. There are some validated tools for screening and assessing eating disorders, e.g., *Eating Disorder Examination; Eating Disorder Screen for Primary Care, Eating Disorder Examination Questionnaire*, etc. Early diagnosis and aggressive management is associated with most favorable long-term outcomes.

MANAGEMENT

It requires multidisciplinary approach because people with eating disorders often have comorbid medical and psychological complications and often do not recognize the need for treatment or at times strongly resists the treatment. AN is often chronic, recurring, relapsing disorder, and requires long-term treatment. The core management goals are:

- *To engage the patient and their family members in treatment as patients usually minimize or deny their symptoms*

- *To assess and address acute medical problems such as electrolyte imbalance, cardiac arrhythmias, etc.*
- *To attain and maintain a healthy body state*
- *Normalization of all eating behaviors such as refusal/restriction of food items including compulsive exercises*
- *Dismantling the core overvalued beliefs and unhealthy cognitive schemas regarding body weight and body image*
- *Treating the comorbid psychiatric and medical issues*
- *Planning for relapse prevention for nearly 5 years after acute improvement.*

The methods of treatment include medical, nutritional, educational, psychotherapeutic, behavioral, and pharmacological components. Treatment planning depends on intensity and severity of illness.

Outpatient care: Most adolescents can be managed in an outpatient eating disorder program that provides culturally and developmentally appropriate interdisciplinary care. Essential components include medical monitoring and intervention, nutritional therapy, and individual and family therapy. Treatment is complex, long term, and may involve relapses.

Significant emphasis should be given to nonpharmacological treatment approaches like *counseling, family therapy*, and *psychotherapy.* Psychotherapies are treatment of choice for AN and other eating disorders. The best evidence for psychotherapy is cognitive behavioral therapy (CBT) in adults with BN and family-based treatment in children and adolescents with AN.

Pharmacotherapy: Pharmacotherapy is not recommended as first-line treatment. There is role of antidepressants preferably selective serotonin reuptake inhibitors for cases with comorbid depression/anxiety disorder.

BULIMIA NERVOSA

INTRODUCTION

In the late 1970s and early 1980s cases were reported for having symptoms related to AN but characterized behaviorally by *persistent binge eating and purging.* An article published in 1979 by Russell clearly described the syndrome of BN and in 1980 bulimia was first formally recognized as a disorder in DSM-III (APA, 1980). BN is characterized by frequent episodes of binge eating followed by inappropriate compensatory behaviors such as self-induced vomiting to avoid weight gain. Since 1980, there have been no major changes in its conceptualization but in the most recent iteration of DSM (DSM-5), the only modification in the criteria was an adjustment in the minimum threshold of the frequency of behavioral disturbances (compensatory behaviors) *from twice a week to once a week for 3 months*. During the episodes of binge eating the individual consumes an amount of food that is unusually large pertaining to the circumstances under which it was eaten.

Episodes of binge eating are associated with a *sense of loss of control*, once the eating has begun the individual feels unable to stop until an excessive amount has been consumed. This loss of control is mostly *subjective* as many of the individuals with bulimia will abruptly stop eating in the middle of a binge episode, if interrupted. After overeating, individuals engage in some forms of inappropriate behavior in an attempt to avoid weight gain. Most patients report self-induced vomiting or the abuse of laxatives. Other methods include misusing diuretics, fasting for long periods, and exercise extensively after eating binges.

The DSM-5 criterion requires that the binge eating episodes and the compensatory behaviors both occur at least once per week for 3 months to qualify for a diagnosis of BN along with over concern with body shape and weight. The diagnosis of BN should not be given to individuals with AN who recurrently engage in binge eating or purging behavior.

ASSESSMENT

It is very similar to AN. Patients should be asked to describe a typical day's food intake and typical binge. The therapist should explicitly enquire about self-induced vomiting including the use of laxatives, diuretics, diet pills, and enemas. A weight history should be obtained to rule out the obesity. The therapist should also enquire about history of mood and anxiety disorders and substance abuse.

Physiological disturbances/complications: In small percentage of individuals it is associated with the development of fluid, electrolyte imbalance that result from self-induced vomiting as a result of abuse of laxatives and diuretics. The most common electrolyte disturbances are *hypochloremia*, *hyponatremia*, and *hypokalemia* including alkalosis and acidosis because of excessive vomiting and abuse of laxatives, respectively. There is increased frequency of menstrual disturbances such as *oligomenorrhea* because of disturbances in hypothalamic, pituitary, and gonadal axes. Patients also develop dental erosions of upper front teeth because of persistent vomiting for many years. They also develop callous on knuckles because of self-induced vomiting which is called *Russell's sign*. This disorder is also associated with enlarged gastric capacity and delayed gastric emptying.

Comorbidities: There is increased frequency of anxiety and mood disorders, especially major depressive disorder, dysthymia, alcohol abuse, and personality disorders.

ETIOLOGY

The etiology of BN is uncertain. Several factors play role in development of BN. A personal or family history of obesity or mood disturbances also appears to increase the risk factor. Many of the psychosocial factors related to development of AN are also applicable to BN, including the influence of cultural ideals of thinness and physical fitness. BN primarily affects women; the ratio of *men to women is 1:10*. It also occurs more frequently in occupations like *modeling*, *wrestling*, and *running*. Twin studies have suggested that inherited factors are also important risk factors.

Psychological factors: There is excessive concern regarding weight and shape. They worry about the effect of the binge eating and try to restrict their food intake when they are not indulging in binge eating. The psychological and physiological restrain makes them vulnerable for additional binge eating episodes. There is significant distress about their inability to control their eating which lowers their self-esteem that contributes to disturbances of mood. They have rigid rules regarding food and eating, and the distorted and dysfunctional thoughts about body shape and weight are very similar to AN. Childhood sexual abuse has also been seen as a specific risk factor for the development of BN.

Neurobiological factors: BN is accompanied by *disturbances in the satiety* during a meal and therefore increase the likelihood of binge eating. There is also reduction in the release of *cholecystokinin*, a peptide hormone secreted by the small intestine which plays a role in terminating eating behavior. All these abnormalities may predispose the individual to overeat and therefore to perpetuate the cycle of binge eating.

Social/environmental factors: There is important role of sociocultural influences in the development of BN. The prevalence is very low in nonwestern societies but has increased substantially in last 50 years. The Western society and culture consider thinness as an ideal which is also reinforced by the media, thereby promoting concern about the perfect body weight and body shape.

MANAGEMENT

The main aim of treatment of BN is to control binge eating and inappropriate compensatory behavior. The patients should also be educated to base their self-esteem on factors other than shape and weight. There is not much conflict between therapist and patient regarding the goals of treatment unlike AN because the crucial behavioral disturbances, binge eating, and purging are less ego-syntonic and more distressing to the patients in BN.

Somatic treatment: The most common psychotropic used is antidepressant medication because of the high risk of depression among patients with BN. Fluoxetine at a dose of 60 mg per day has been found to be effective and better tolerated among other alternatives.

Psychosocial treatment: The most common psychotherapy that has been used is *cognitive behavior therapy for BN*. CBT for BN concentrates on the distorted ideas about weight and shape, on the rigid rules regarding food consumption and the pressure to diet on the events that trigger episodes of binge

eating. The therapy is very focused and highly structured and is usually conducted in 3–6 months. Approximately 25–50% patients of BN achieve abstinence from binge eating and purging.

BINGE EATING DISORDER

INTRODUCTION

Binge eating disorder is a DSM-5 diagnostic category related to, but distinct from, BN. Individuals with BED, like individuals with BN repeatedly engage in episodes of binge eating, but they do not regularly utilize inappropriate compensatory behavior like self-induced vomiting or purging. The phenomenon of binge eating among the obese was clearly described by *Stun Kard* in 1959, 20 years before BN was recognized. Yet BED has been the focus of sustained attention only recently having being identified as a formal diagnosis in DSM-5 in 2013 following 20 years of research as a putative diagnosis proposed in the appendix of DSM-IV-TR.

DEFINITION

Diagnostic criteria for BED require repetitive episodes of binge eating similar to BN. The major difference from BN is that individuals with BED do not regularly use inappropriate compensatory behaviors. Individuals with BED report a sense of loss of control over eating during binge eating episodes. The eating becomes more rapid than usual and patient eats large amount of food in absence of physiological hunger. The *eating behavior must be distressing to the individual with BED to meet diagnostic criterion, and must occur for once per week for 3 months on average.* Patients with BED do not have much concern regarding body weight and shape as is required for BN.

ASSESSMENT

It is very similar to BN. It is important to obtain a clear understanding of daily food intake and what the individual considers a binge. The therapist also needs to enquire about purging and other inappropriate weight control measures. The therapist should also enquire about weight history including symptoms of mood and anxiety disorders.

EPIDEMIOLOGY

The prevalence of BED is much greater than that of AN and BN. It is estimated to affect *3%* of adults. Among obese individuals prevalence rates estimates around *2–5%* in community samples, and as high as 30% among individuals seeking bariatric surgery or alternative weight loss treatment. In contrast to AN and BN, individuals with BED are more likely to be males (female to male ratio 1.75:1 roughly) as compared to 10:1 ratio for AN and BN.

COMORBIDITY

Mood and anxiety disorders are associated with BED and are dependent on the severity of illness and not on weight status.

COURSE

Rates of remission are higher for BED than for AN or BN. However, the illness course can be persistent similar to that seen in BN.

DIFFERENTIAL DIAGNOSIS

Binge eating is recognized on the basis of self-report of frequent consumption of large amount of food in a discrete period of time, which disturbs the individual due to inability to control. At times what precisely constitutes large amount of food, it becomes difficult to appreciate more so in an obese individual and so is the case in determining about discreet period of time as many people have habit of eating large amount of food continuously.

ETIOLOGY AND PATHOPHYSIOLOGY

The etiology remains elusive but its association with obesity is seen frequently. Childhood obesity, adverse family factors (discords within family, parental mood, and substance use disorders) are identified as risk factors. Some individuals report emotional binge eating episodes as a result of mood dysregulation. Others describe it as a result of deprivation experienced due to restrictive food intake during excessive dieting to lose weight.

TREATMENT

Treatment of BED has three goals:
- Behavioral control to cease binge eating
- Treat comorbid anxiety and depression
- Weight loss in obese.

Pharmacological and psychosocial treatments: Both psychological (cognitive behavior therapy, behavioral weight loss regimes employing caloric restrictions, interpersonal psychotherapy), and pharmacotherapy (selective serotonin reuptake inhibitors) which also takes care of comorbid mood and anxiety symptoms have been seen to be helpful. Also, weight loss agents such as *topiramate* and *orlistat* are used in obese individuals.

TAKE-HOME MESSAGES

- These are a group of brain disorders having abnormal behaviors related to food.
- Although rare clinical entities, but their incidence and prevalence have

been on the rise because of the cultural transformations, rapid industrialization, effects of media, and migration.

- The common types are AN, BN, and BED.
- These disorders are mostly found in females particularly adolescents girls and young adult women.
- The etiology is very complex and exact cause is unknown, genetic factors play an important role.
- Course of illness is usually chronic and recurrent with poor prognosis and high mortality because of comorbid medical and psychiatric complications.
- There is high prevalence of psychiatric comorbidity particularly depressive and anxiety disorders.
- The assessment and management should be done by a multidisciplinary clinical team comprising psychiatrists, psychologists, endocrinologists, and general physicians.
- There is high risk of relapse/recurrence in patients with these disorders in spite of adequate treatment.
- A comprehensive approach comprising psychological, behavioral, and pharmacological treatment is required for complete recovery.

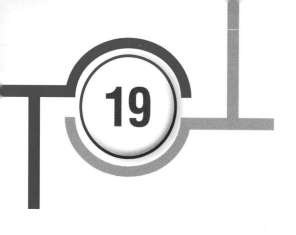

Personality Disorders

Shubhangi R Parkar

INTRODUCTION

Whenever we talk about personality of people around us, we essentially refer to the persistent impact of their behavior on our emotions and responses. The people commonly want to know regarding how and why people act as they do in common or in particular situation. Why are they different, why are some responsible, and why are some not? Why are some introverts, and why are some extroverts? Though there can be individual character, habits, thinking styles, and individualized aspect of each person in this world, they do show some pattern and clusters. Using operational view of personality that can apply to everyone is a sensible approach to discover persistent and enduring features that make any individual a unique person. Personality refers to the sum-totality of an individual.

WHAT IS PERSONALITY?

The word personality itself came from the Latin word *persona*, referring to a melodramatic or theatrical mask worn by actors in order to portray diverse roles or camouflage their identities. Personality as a concept is a common expression encountered in everyday conversation by scientist and lay people alike. However, there are many expressions, intangible perceptions, and operational definitions of personality evolved in scientific research. Personality is a distinctive and long-term pattern of inner experience and outward behavior. It tends to be consistent and regular in terms of thinking, feeling, and behavior, thereby making a person distinctive in comparison to others. The theoretical understanding of personality should be distinguished from other common expressions like temperament, traits, and character. The concept temperament recognizes features that are apparent since childhood and mainly of biological origin while character is evolved as a result of interactive process between temperament and environment. Personality "traits," represent long-term patterns of perceiving, relating to, and thinking about a variety of aspects of relationship between individual and society. Personality anticipates how a person will behave in a given situation, at the same time, it also provides flexibility of allowing people to learn and adapt to new environments. Alport's definition of personality focused on "dynamic organization" within the individuals that determines their unique adjustments to their environment. According to Alport, "dynamic organization" (unitas multiplex) is always evolving and altering, as an intrapsychic process "within the individual." Consequently, it is not inevitably a judgmental comparison of one person with another. Basic function of normal personality is to feel, think, perceive, and incorporate these aspects into purposeful behavior, during the normal course of development. The common aspects of normal personality such as belief system, attitude, and values are stable over the lifespan in spite of changing situations, emerging crisis, and related stress. These aspects of normal personality are well-known to key relatives and friends. Although, personality disorder (PD) is deeply ingrained maladaptive pattern of behavior and continues through most of the adulthood, at time it becomes less evident in old age. Nonetheless, for those with PDs, this flexibility to adapt to external as well as internal world is usually missing and leads to major disturbances in personal, occupational, and social life.

WHAT IS PERSONALITY DISORDER?

Identifying PD is a complex clinical exercise. It is acknowledged as an enduring pattern of inner experience and behavior that deviates strikingly from the expectations of the individual's culture. Though the dogma of pathological personality historically is very old, the recent impression of PD is seen in Pinel's concept of *"manie sans delire"* indicating madness without confusion of the mind. The commencement of this pathological pattern of personality can be seen during adolescence or early adulthood and is stable over lifetime. It is also inflexible and pervasive across a broad range of personal and social circumstances. It simply means the maladaptive behavior is neither situation nor event specific nor restricted to particular individual. Invariably, it leads to clinically significant subjective distress for an individual or leads to impairment in social, occupational, and other important areas of functioning in life. Some PDs may not even have subjective distress, e.g., patient having antisocial PD will not experience distress over

his reproachful and unsociable behavior. The patients with PDs demonstrate maladaptive behavior pattern of responding to their environmental stressors and inner conflicts, contributing to the chronic and invasive impairments in their capacity to adjust with others. Many of these patients have difficulty in the area of dependency pattern, aggression control, adjustment problems, and low self-esteem. The patients with PDs have major adjustment problems in personal and social relationships as they also have difficulty in the way they understand other people, social contexts, and events. Mainly, these difficulties are apparent in the area of empathizing with others, patients in fact have tendency to blame others, and suspect intentions of others. Their usual approach of blaming environment and people for their personal and social problems is clearly part of their pathological personality. Generally, these patients provoke strong emotional reactions in others but they do not have insights into their own behavior and flawed thinking styles and attitudes. As a result, their behavioral symptoms are egosyntonic. Therefore, they are not willing to change their flawed way of thinking and behavior, instead they insist on changing their environment. Hence, for detail understanding of PDs, analytical outlook of their basic psychological and social dynamics is essential. Individuals with PDs use a considerable share of mental health services. Prevalence of personality is seen in 10–20% of general population and about 50% of all psychiatric patients have a PD.

GENERAL CLINICAL PROFILE OF PERSONALITY DISORDERS

It is not easy to diagnose PDs with simple diagnostic guidelines as seen in diagnosis of major psychopathology. Very often, there are diagnostic overlaps or existence of features of two or more PDs in one individual. Quite often, this overlap is very extensive; hence, clinicians and researchers prefer to choose dimensional view of personality. At present, the *Diagnostic and Statistical Manual of Mental Disorders (DSM-5)* of APA and *International Statistical Classification of Diseases and Related Health Problems (ICD-10)* Classification of Mental and Behavioral Disorders by WHO are popular two major systems of classification with vivid description and classification of PDs. Nevertheless, consistency in personality traits and maladaptive patterns of behavior as identified by key relatives, are important clinical guiding principles to categorize PDs. Notably, PDs are neither directly attributable to gross brain damage or disease, particular situation or context nor to any other psychiatric disorder.

In general, some common features should be acknowledged while considering PDs. The patients diagnosed as PDs exhibit markedly disharmonious attitudes and behavior, involving usually several areas of functioning such as affectivity, arousal, impulse control, ways of perceiving, and thinking. The abnormal behavior pattern is durable, long standing, and not limited to episodes of mental illness. The abnormal behavior pattern is pervasive and clearly maladaptive toward a broad range of personal and social situations. The behavioral manifestations always appear during childhood or adolescence and continue during adulthood. The disorder leads to substantial personal distress but this may only become apparent later in life. As per general understanding, PDs are reported to the clinics during early and middle adulthood. They are often reported with major psychiatric disorders including addictive behaviors and suicidal behaviors. If age is below 18 years, features of personality changes must have been present for at least a year. Antisocial PD cannot be diagnosed below 18 years. Some PDs may aggravate following a significant catastrophic stressor.

ISSUES RELATED TO ASSESSMENT OF PERSONALITY DISORDERS

Assessment of PDs remains a complex clinical exercise in comparison to assessment of various other psychiatric disorders. A comprehensive history, detailed, and skilled clinical interview remain the primary dependable basis of diagnosing PDs. As per DSM-5, the pattern of PD is manifested in two or more of the following areas of— (1) Cognition; (2) Affectivity; (3) Interpersonal functioning; and (4) Impulse control. Various methods and instruments like International Personality Disorders Examination (IPDE), Structured Clinical Interview for DSM-IV Axis II personality disorders (SCID-II), Personality Diagnostic Questionnaire-4 (PDQ-4), and Millon Clinical Multiaxial Inventory (MCMI) are mostly popular in clinical practice as well as in research methods. However, clinicians need to use their clinical experience, skills, and judgment as well as psychodynamic approach for understanding PDs. Is it just trait or a psychiatric diagnosis? How much pervasiveness of these traits is required to call somebody as PD? How much psychosocial impairment or distress is attributable to PD? Very often patients or their relatives are not aware of or not ready to admit the personality traits as defective attribute or pathological feature. Due to their attitude of blaming others as a part of PDs itself, patients are unwilling to accept the relational, occupational, and social problem as a central aspect of their PD.

In presence of psychiatric disorders, the assessment of PD can be even more difficult. A number of symptoms like low energy and social disinterest in major depression or grandiosity and hypersexuality in hypomanic person may appear like features of PDs (such as avoidant PD or narcissistic PD). In cases of comorbid psychiatric disorders, it is also important to judge that personality features are persistent and not related to specific situation or triggered by particular life events or person especially in intimate relationship. By and large, gender bias is not expected theoretically with current clinical understanding of PDs. However, clinically gender prejudice should be sensitively avoided in various diagnoses of PDs such as antisocial, borderline, and histrionic personality. Clinical evaluation is even more intricate when the patients are reacting to major life event or critical life circumstances. Sometimes some medical illnesses like epilepsy or head injury are associated with impulse control problems and aggressive episodes. This needs to be evaluated with careful medical evaluation and detailed investigations.

ETIOLOGY OF PERSONALITY DISORDERS

Both genetic influences and environmental aspects are considered equally important in etiologies of PDs. Inheritance is recognized in antisocial, paranoid, schizotypal, schizoid, and borderline PD to some extent. Genes connected to serotonergic and dopaminergic neurotransmitter pathways are acknowledged as probable etiological factors. An array of early childhood harsh conditions has been associated with the origin of PD. Especially, social stressors, childhood abuse, and disharmonious families are key account of experiences in earlier period of pathological personalities. Early childhood experience of turbulent social and relational stressors is identified as critical factor in development of antisocial and borderline PDs. Breakdown

in traditional rubric of society, reduction of secure and healthy attachment, dysfunctional families, and parental psychopathology are significant aspects leading to irresponsible behavior, ethical tribulations, and impulse control problems in PDs. More than physical abuse, sexual abuse in childhood has been often identified with development of cluster B class of PDs.

COMMON CONSIDERATION OF TREATMENT OF PERSONALITY DISORDERS

There is generally prevalent view, though unfortunate, that PDs are not treatable. PDs are so ingrained that they are difficult to treat in comparison to other major psychiatric disorders but are treatable. Treatment of PDs is an important emphasis point in clinical psychiatry so as to improve prognostic outcome of comorbid disorders as well as productivity and meaningful lifestyle of patients with PDs. Many patients with PDs are not willing to take treatment as they do not have insight and motivation. Besides, majority of them also have comorbid psychiatric disorders complicating their judgment. There are no precise treatment strategies for PDs. However, treatment of PDs is based on two aspects, i.e., (1) pharmacotherapy and (2) broad range of psychosocial interventions. Based on severity and associated psychiatric comorbidity, the therapeutic intervention has to be planned carefully. Also, there are no medications exclusively to treat PDs per say. However, a variety of drugs can be used either for distressing symptom control of PDs or for associated comorbid psychiatric disorders. Most of pharmacological drugs reduce acute distressing symptoms, prevent suicidal behavior, improve social and inter-personal relationships, and reduce incidence of maladaptive behaviors. The focus of pharmacological treatment is primarily to reduce aggression, affective symptoms, and anxiety symptoms. Antidepressant drugs like SSRI (selective serotonin reuptake inhibitor) will help in increasing serotonin levels that may reduce depression, impulsiveness, rumination and may enhance a sense of well-being. Low-dose antipsychotics either typical or atypical and mood stabilizers like lithium may be effective in improving affective volatility, aggression, and reduce psychotic symptoms. Identification and management of substance use disorders is critical issue as patients with PDs tend to show bad prognosis in both. Role of various psychotherapies is acknowledged as mainstay intervention in terms of improving relationships and attending to maladaptive behavior pattern by developing insight. Psychodynamic therapy, cognitive behavior therapy, dialectical behavior therapy, motivational interviews, and problem-solving skills are identified as appreciably effective psychotherapies. Developing therapeutic alliance, setting, and securing boundaries in therapy is clinically vital. Patient and family education will go a long way to their understanding of PDs, their choice of treatment, motivation, and adherence to treatment.

CLASSIFICATION OF PERSONALITY DISORDERS

The DSM-5 and ICD-10 have operationally classified commonly seen PDs. DSM-5 identifies 10 types of specific PDs which are grouped in three clusters. While ICD-10 describes three major categories, e.g., (1) specific personality disorders, (2) mixed and other personality disorders, and (3) enduring personality changes, not attributable to brain damage and disease. There are few more PDs under evaluation. It is assumed that a person who suffers from a PD is not markedly troubled by personality traits outside of that disorder. However, these assumptions get frequently contradicted in clinical practice. In fact, the symptoms of the PDs very often than not are overlapping with each other and difficult to distinguish one from another. In addition, clinicians at times feel that particular individuals have more than one PD. This lack of agreement has raised concerns about the accuracy and reliability of these categories. Diverse cultures have different social norms, rules, and obligations about individual's acceptable and unacceptable behavior and even associated gender-specific behavior.

The DSM-5 classification of PD mentions three major clusters depending on most important, frequent, and consistent behavior pattern. The three clusters are—(1) Cluster A consisting of odd or eccentric behavior pattern of paranoid, schizoid, and schizotypal PDs; (2) Cluster B consisting of erratic, impulsive (dramatic-emotional) behavior pattern of antisocial, borderline, histrionic, and narcissistic PDs; and (3) Cluster C consisting of anxious or fearful behavior pattern of anxious, avoidant, dependent, obsessive-compulsive PDs, and other specified consisting of depressive and passive aggressive.

Some accounts of frequently identified PDs are described as below.

Paranoid Personality Disorder

Clinical Questions

Is this person primarily suspicious? Misconstrue the events and ideas of others as threatening? Finds difficulty in trusting other people? Always resentful?

Clinical Features

- Thinks that people want to harm, betray, or exploit though there is no adequate evidence for that.

- Worried by fears about the loyalty or trustworthiness of relatives and friends.
- Misconstrue common comments as threatening or disgraceful.
- Keep grudges, does not pardon insults, injuries.
- Has unfounded doubts about the faithfulness of spouse?

Differential Diagnosis

- Delusional disorder
- Paranoid schizophrenia
- Borderline PD
- Antisocial PD.

Treatment

Generally, these PDs stay away from treatment. Antianxiety and low-dose antipsychotic medication can be given symptomatically to control agitation and anxiety. Individual or group psychotherapy is helpful to work over issues of suspiciousness and mistrust.

Schizoid Personality Disorder

Clinical Questions

Is this person a loner? Aloof and disconnected? Unfriendly or cold person?

Clinical Features

- Unable to enjoy close relationships and do not have close friends or confidants
- Unable to experience pleasure in many activities
- Normally seeks private activities
- Unresponsive to praise or disapproval
- Excessive preoccupation with fantasy and introspection
- Emotionally cold, detached, or affectively flattened.

Differential Diagnosis

- Schizophrenia
- Delusional disorder

- Affective disorder with psychotic features
- Avoidant PD.

Treatment

These patients have perceptible anxiety over interpersonal relationship; hence, low-dose antipsychotics, antidepressants, and benzodiazepines will be helpful to control anxiety symptoms. Individual psychotherapy is helpful to work over issues of introspection and prospect to express thinking and emotions. Group therapy can be useful if they tolerate.

Schizotypal Personality Disorder

Clinical Questions

Is this person odd eccentric? Has difficulty in secure relationship? Has strong belief in superstition and telepathy?

Clinical Features

- Eccentricities of behavior, odd thinking
- Persistent pattern of social and interpersonal deficits
- Acute discomfort and decrease capacity for secure relationships
- Odd unusual beliefs and magical thinking that is conflicting with cultural norms
- Paranoid ideation and inappropriate affect
- Superstition, clairvoyance, telepathy, sixth sense.

Differential Diagnosis

- Schizoid and avoidant PD
- Schizophrenia
- Some patients meet criteria for both schizotypal and borderline PD.

Treatment

Antipsychotics are indicated for ideas of reference, odd psychotic thinking, and other deficit symptoms. Antidepressants are useful in the presence of depressive component. Individual therapy can be useful with sensitive and nonjudgmental therapist.

Antisocial (Dyssocial) Personality Disorder

Clinical Questions

Is this person impulsive and has difficulty controlling rage? Consistently irresponsible? Lacks remorse about wrong deeds? Unable to accept social norms?

Clinical Features

- Impulsivity and failure to plan
- Irritability, rage, resentment underneath the mask of sanity
- Inability to maintain relationship
- Disordered life functioning
- Irresponsible and has lack of regret
- Reckless with regard to the safety of self and assaults
- Shows composed, charming, and ingratiating traits.

Differential Diagnosis

- Schizophrenia
- Manic episode
- Criminal behavior not due to PD
- Substance use disorder
- Antisocial behavior secondary to substance.

Treatment

Antipsychotics are useful to control anxiety, rage, and depression. Mood stabilizer like lithium, carbamazepine, or valproate is of use in control of aggression and impulsivity. Specific treatment is necessary in presence of substance use disorder. Individual psychotherapy especially cognitive behavioral therapy (CBT) and dynamic psychotherapy can be used for controlling self-destructive behavior.

Borderline Personality Disorder (Emotionally Unstable Personality Disorder)

Clinical Questions

Does this person suffer from boredom and unstable mood? Make worried efforts to avoid rejection? Have multiple suicidal attempts?

Clinical Features

- Constant feelings of emptiness and boredom
- Unstable interpersonal relationships
- Identity disturbances
- Unstable sense of self or self-image
- Impulsivity in many areas of life such as spending, substance abuse, reckless driving, sexual activity
- Multiple attempts of self-harm and gesture
- Affective instability.

Differential Diagnosis

- Schizophrenia
- Depressive and bipolar disorders
- Paranoid and schizotypal PDs
- Identity disorder.

Treatment

Low-dose antipsychotic, antidepressant, and mood stabilizers like carbamazepine are useful to control affective instability and attempts of self-harm. Psychodynamic psychotherapies and dialectical behavior therapy are used effectively.

Histrionic Personality Disorder

Clinical Questions

Is this person dramatic and emotionally manipulative? Demanding? Wants to be the center of attention?

Clinical Features

- Dramatic expression of emotion is displayed in a theatrical, exaggerated, or self-dramatic manner
- Experiences discomfort when not the center of attention
- Interacts in a confrontational or sexually seductive manner
- Expressions of emotions are superficial and change swiftly
- Uses physical gestures to draw attention to self
- Suggestible
- Disturbances in relationships.

Differential Diagnosis

- Somatization disorder
- Borderline PD
- Brief psychotic disorder
- Dissociative disorder.

Treatment

Mainly psychodynamic and insight-oriented therapy is helpful to explore problems in their current and earlier relationships. In case of intense mood reactivity antidepressant will be effective.

Narcissistic Personality Disorder

Clinical Questions

Is this person grandiose and has undue sense of self-importance? Communicate fantasies of unlimited success? Vulnerable to threats to their self-esteem.

Clinical Features

- Preoccupation with fantasies of unlimited success, power, brilliance, beauty, ideal love
- In need for unwarranted "long overdue" admiration

- Interpersonally exploitative with lack of empathy
- Resentful of others or belief vice versa
- Egotistical, conceited, snobbish, scornful attitudes
- Prominent sense of power
- Wants to be known as superior without corresponding achievements.

Differential Diagnosis

- Borderline, histrionic, and antisocial PD
- Mania or hypomania.

Treatment

Psychoanalytical psychotherapy leading to development of insight into dynamics of PD and interpersonal problems will be the treatment of choice.

Avoidant (Anxious) Personality Disorder

Clinical Questions

Is this person not ready to become involved with people except being sure about being liked? Thinks as inferior compared with others? Have fear of being ridiculed?

Clinical Features

- Avoids social or occupational activities that involve interpersonal contact to avoid disapproval, condemnation
- Avoids relationships unless sure that they will be liked
- Reserved within intimate relationships because of fear of being shamed
- Concerned with being criticized or rejected socially
- Inhibited in new social situations due to feeling of inadequacy
- Perceives self as incompetent, unattractive, and mediocre to others
- Unenthusiastic to connect in new activities that may lead to embarrassment.

Differential Diagnosis

- Social anxiety disorders and social phobia
- Schizoid and paranoid PD
- Dependent PD.

Treatment

The patients with avoidant PD have difficulty in committing to any kind of therapy. However, they are comfortable in supportive psychotherapy to begin with. Assertiveness training and social skills training are effective in coping up with relational problems. Antidepressant and antianxiety drugs are also helpful in dealing with associated depression and anxiety symptoms.

Passive Aggressive Personality Disorder

Clinical Questions

Is this person—(1) a habitual procrastinator? (2) Stubborn to change? (3) Inefficient in social and professional life for long time?

Clinical Features

- Resistance to demands for adequate performance
- Ineffective in social and occupational life
- Indirect resistance in the form of being stubborn.

Dependent Personality Disorder

Clinical Questions

Is this person incapable of taking most necessary decisions? Has difficulty in communicating disagreement due to fear of rejection? Has difficulty in initiating new projects due to lack of confidence?

Clinical Features

- Preoccupied with fears of rejection
- Indecisive without excessive advice and encouragement

- Wants others to take on major responsibility of his/her life
- Apprehensive about expressing disagreement with others due to fear of disapproval
- Difficulty in initiating projects, because of lack of confidence
- Fears of being unable to care for self.

Differential Diagnosis

- Agoraphobia
- Histrionic and borderline PDs (traits of dependence present)
- Depressive disorder.

Treatment

These patients respond to insight-oriented therapy, family therapy, and assertiveness training. For various anxiety symptoms, antianxiety drugs will be useful.

Compulsive (Anankastic) Personality Disorder

Clinical Questions

Is this person preoccupied with minute details and set of laws? Persists that others must do things in his way? Is extremely meticulous and perfectionist?

Clinical Features

- Preoccupied with details, rules, schedules, etc., so that the primary purpose of activity is lost
- Perfectionism interferes with the completion of tasks
- Extreme involvement on work and productivity to the exclusion of friendships and leisure
- Exceedingly conscientious, meticulous
- Miserly spending approach to both self and others
- Hoards objects even though they lack sentimental value
- Rigid and stubborn.

Differential Diagnosis

- Obsessive-compulsive disorder
- Overlap with type "A" personality
- Hoarding disorder
- Narcissistic, antisocial, schizoid PDs.

Treatment

Antidepressant like clomipramine and fluoxetine in presence of depression is effective. Psychodynamic psychotherapy, behavior therapy, and social skill strategies are useful in the long run.

Persons with PDs are the largest group of patients which one comes across in psychiatric practice. Moreover, psychiatrist has to attend to these patients with commitment, as the impact of PDs is disruptive on lifestyle of the patients and contributes to the negative prognosis of associated comorbid disorders. PDs are difficult to treat because of their pervasive and durable nature of their symptoms manifesting in their thinking and behavior. Diagnosing PDs brings in a lot of stigma and social antagonism to patients; therefore, positive details of their life should be assessed and enhanced with care.

CONCLUSION

Personality disorders are a common but generally overlooked condition. Very often there are associated psychiatric comorbidities which make the management of both the conditions very difficult. Even otherwise the diagnosis and management of PDs are very difficult. PDs have grave adverse impact on the quality of life of individuals. Both genetic and environmental factors contribute to the causation of PDs. They need to be managed by judicious use of both drugs and psychotherapy.

TAKE-HOME MESSAGES

- Personality is a distinctive and long-term pattern of inner experience and outward behavior. It tends to be consistent and regular in terms of thinking, feeling, and behavior, thereby making a person distinctive in comparison to others. Personality refers to the sum-totality of an individual.
- Personality disorder is acknowledged as an enduring pattern of inner experience and behavior that deviates strikingly from the expectations of the individual's culture and generally leads to maladjustment and suffering for the individual.
- It is difficult to diagnose PDs because of their nature of symptoms, very high comorbidity, and also substantial overlap between various subtypes of PDs.
- Both genetic influences and environmental aspects are considered equally important in etiologies of PDs. Genes connected to serotonergic and dopaminergic neurotransmitter pathways as well as social stressors, childhood abuse, and disharmonious family are important contributors to its genesis.
- Treatment of PDs is based on a combination of pharmacotherapy and broad range of psycho social interventions. Psychodynamic therapy, cognitive behavior therapy, dialectical behavior therapy, motivational interviews, and problem-solving skills are identified as appreciably effective psychotherapies.
- Paranoid PD, schizoid PD, schizotypal PD, antisocial (dyssocial) PD, borderline PD, histrionic PD, narcissistic PD, avoidant (anxious) PD, passive aggressive PD, dependent PD, and compulsive (anankastic) PD are various specific subtypes of personality disorders.

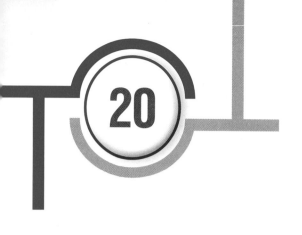

Childhood and Adolescent Disorders

Savita Malhotra, Akhilesh Sharma

INTRODUCTION

Child psychiatry is a broad discipline that deals with mental health problems during the first two decades of life, i.e., from birth to 19 years. Child at birth has 25% of the adult brain weight. There is progressive increase in brain weight after birth due to the processes of neuronal proliferation, migration, myelination, formation of synapse followed by pruning and neuronal networks. Child at birth has physiological reflexes for basic survival only, such as sucking, elimination, breathing, and sensory-motor apparatus. The journey from reflexive response patterns to adult human behavior with all its complexities and nuances of personality involves incorporation of experience and environment in development throughout childhood and adolescence and further to young adulthood, until 25 years of age. Brain development is complete by about 25 years of age with the completion of myelination of frontal lobes. This entire period of development from birth to adulthood has been categorized into infancy (up to 1 year), childhood (up to 10–11 years), adolescence (up to 19 years), and youth (up to 25 years). Development is influenced by genes as well as the environment in which the child grows to the extent that the environment is incorporated in the developing brain both structurally as well as functionally.

The environment includes parenting factors, school, family, societal factors, ecological factors, socioeconomic factors, nutrition, and so on. Unhealthy or adverse environment or genetic predispositions can steer the developmental trajectory toward maladaptation or mental ill health during childhood.

EPIDEMIOLOGY

Children and adolescents constitute 40% of the total population of the country and are considered the supreme asset for the nation. As in adults, mental health problems and disorders are also common in childhood or adolescence. About 10–15% of children or adolescents suffer from some sort of psychiatric disorder. An important thing to remember is that children and adolescents are constantly changing and evolving, their developmental needs change with age. Risk for different kinds of mental health problems and the presentation of symptoms also varies according to age.

When to suspect mental health problems in children and adolescents?

- Failure to attain age appropriate developmental milestones or delay in attainment of milestones in any of the four domains of growth: (1) gross motor, (2) fine motor, (3) social, (4) speech and language. These indicate neurodevelopmental disorders (NDDs) that manifest as the child grows.

- Child not looking into your eyes, not responding to name being called, does not show any emotional response when parents come or leave, insistence on sameness, delayed/minimal speech indicates possibility of autism spectrum disorder (ASD).
- Excessive irritability, crying, unusually quiet, self-absorbed, muttering to self, smiling to self, talking in the air, talking excessively, excessive temper tantrums, and repetitive behavior.
- Defiance, disobedience, violence, aggression, demanding behavior, over activity, fighting, quarrelling, stealing, lying, and substance use.
- Change in biological rhythms—disturbed sleep, disturbed appetite—increased or decreased.
- Avoiding familiar persons, fears, phobia, clinging behavior, excessive anxiety, and repetitive behavior.
- Complains of too many aches and pains in the body, recurrent abdominal pain, and headaches without medical cause.
- Academic difficulties, school refusal.

CLASSIFICATION

Childhood mental disorders can be broadly classified as follows:

- Neurodevelopmental disorders:
  - Intellectual disability (ID)
  - Autism spectrum disorder
  - Attention deficit hyperactivity disorder (ADHD)
  - Specific learning disorder
  - Tic disorder
- Anxiety disorders:
  - Separation anxiety disorder
  - Social anxiety disorder
  - Panic disorder
  - Phobias
  - Generalized anxiety disorder

- Mood disorders:
  - Depressive disorder
  - Bipolar affective disorder (BPAD)
  - Dysthymia
- Conduct and oppositional defiant behavior disorders
- Dissociative and somatoform disorders
- Psychotic disorders:
  - Acute and transient psychotic disorder
  - Childhood onset schizophrenia
- Obsessive compulsive disorder (OCD)
- Habit disorders:
  - Enuresis
  - Encopresis
  - Pica
  - Trichotillomania
  - Self-stimulatory behavior
  - Substance use disorders
- *Other complex mental health problems*:
  - Self-harm and suicide
  - Mental health problems arising due to or associated with physical illness
  - *Abuse and neglect*: Including sexual abuse, physical and emotional abuse and neglect.

COMMON DISORDERS PRESENTING AT DIFFERENT AGE GROUPS

0 to 3 years: This age group includes infants (<1 year) and toddlers (1–3 years). Most common mental health problems during this age are:

- *Developmental delays (fine motor, gross motor, social, speech and language) appropriate for age*: The delay in attainment of milestones can be global, i.e., all the four domains of development are affected as found in global developmental delay, or it can be isolated, i.e., in any of the four domains. Speech delay is an important predictor of later diagnosis of ASDs. Therefore, a detailed history of birth-related events, pregnancy compli-cations, birth cry, attainment of milestones should be taken while evaluating an infant or toddler.

- *Excessive crying, clinging, irritability*: Can be the presenting complaints in a number of disorders, like painful condition, constipation, lack of sleep, abuse, insecure attachment patterns, epilepsy, or a temperamental variation.
- *Failure to grow*: Infants and toddlers may be small for age in terms of weight and height norms. Referral to a higher center for evaluation should be done to look for organic conditions like neurometabolic disorders, deficiency of micronutrients and/or macronutrients, or deficient parenting.
- *Hyperactivity, temper tantrums:* Children may be reported to be overactive, angry. Temper tantrums are normal in this age group; however, parents should be cautioned to take care in the way they handle the child, or else, temper tantrums if not handled appropriately can lead to severe behavior problems later in childhood.

4-6 years of age (preschoolers): Children in this age group can present with earlier mentioned complaints and in addition, new problems, like, excessive crying while going to school (can be sign of separation anxiety), difficulty in learning new things, and coping with the academic demands (as in children with ID or soft signs of learning difficulty/disorder), bed wetting, fear of specific things, worsening of temper tantrums, defiance can occur.

6-12 years of age (school going children): Children in this age group most commonly present with complaints from school—not sitting still in class, inattentiveness, disturbing other children, poor academic performance, or being shy in class, not responding or participating in class activities, not having friends, etc. ADHD, problems due to low IQ, learning difficulty, and anxiety are common in this age group. In addition, a child presenting with these complaints should be evaluated for possibility of abuse.

12-18 years of age (preadolescents and adolescents): This is a phase of rapid physical, psychological, and cognitive growth. It is an important period of transition from childhood to adulthood with resurgence of sexuality and is usually considered a phase of stress and storm for the adolescence as well as the family. In addition to inherent problems linked with this age, it also marks the onset of many adult mental disorders like psychosis, mood disorders, depression, personality, and substance use disorders. It also marks the period when adolescents work toward forming their identity and plan future career, bringing lot of anxiety and stress with it. Rapid physical growth due to hormonal changes is another cause of anxiety; it is seen that parents come with frequent complaints of observing their children obsessed with their looks and body image. How adolescents view themselves and what opinion others carry about their looks, is important while evaluating an adolescent who comes with body image issues. All factors put together, make an adolescent at risk of having mental problems. However, if treated with care and understanding, most adolescents and families are able to sail through this phase without any trouble.

Substance use among children and adolescents is a major problem in the current times. Much of it can be attributed to the desire for experimentation, fun, peer pressure, desire to be accepted by peers, idealization of the role models who use substances.

Additional factors are easy availability of substances, exposure to media and internet, the changing lifestyle, faulty parenting, or inadequate parental control and supervision. All the adolescents do not take to drugs, but the risk is very high.

Self-harm and suicide is also witnessing an increasing trend among adolescents. Inability to cope with emotions, stresses, rejections, failure of love affairs, and examination failures are few important causes.

CAUSES OF MENTAL HEALTH PROBLEMS IN CHILDREN AND ADOLESCENTS

Mental health problems in children and adolescents arise as a result of complex interplay of genetic or intrinsic and environmental or extrinsic factors **(Fig. 20.1)**.

Genetic factors: Genetic makeup including family history of mental illness is a significant contributor to mental disorders. Risk for mental disorders is several times higher in children whose parents or close biological family members have history of major mental disorders such as schizophrenia or bipolar affective disorders. Further, children are born with intelligence which is the global capacity for understanding, thinking, and

problem solving; and temperament which is their unique style of response pattern and adaptation to environmental stimuli. Both intelligence and temperament are significantly heritable intrinsic factors that influence the development. Most of the early manifesting NDDs such as ADHD and autism have high genetic contributions and are highly heritable. But in developing countries like India still the environmental factors alone or in different combinations with genetic factors cause childhood neurodevelopmental and other psychiatric disorders.

A multitude of environmental factors arising from the social and family situations and circumstances that the child lives in, affect the mental development of children and adolescents, and contribute to occurrence of mental disorders in them.

Family factors: Family's influence on the development of the child starts even before conception in the hope, expectations, and attitude of parents toward children. Maternal stress during and after pregnancy influences how the mother cares for the newborn and this determines the bonding and attachment of infant with mother. Insecure attachment during infancy can lead to a variety of emotional and behavioral problems during infancy and later in childhood and adulthood. Apart from this, loss of parents, faulty relationship with parents, parental discord, parental substance use, parental mental illness, physical abuse, emotional abuse, and neglect are important determinants for mental health problems in childhood or even adulthood. Parental mental illness in addition to being a genetic risk factor also affects the environment in which children develop. Children may experience neglect, hostility, physical and emotional abuse at the hands of parents with mental illness. Nuclear families

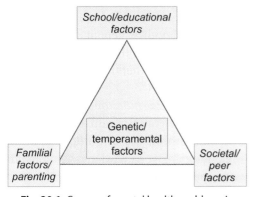

Fig. 20.1: Causes of mental health problems in children and adolescents.

and working mothers may create conditions of greater stress on infants and children for having to adapt to changing care givers, thus hampering formation of attachment. Also, at times it puts infants and children at risk of harm and abuse at the hands of care givers—making them irritable, crying excessively, clinging to parents, refusal to eat, and growth failure. Thus, a holistic family assessment is important while dealing with infants and children with behavioral problems.

Parental handling/parenting: Parenting is an art and a skill that has profound influence on child development. Parenting comprises of parental warmth and nurturance that promotes healthy growth, bonding, and trust; and parental control or discipline that imparts values of self-control and regard for the rights and needs of others. Healthy parenting requires an adequate balance which allows children to grow to their full potential with happiness, faith, trust, and secure relationships in the world on one hand; and also exercise adequate behavioral supervision and control allowing graded levels of autonomy, responsibility, and inculcation of morality and discipline. Parental overprotection and no control can make children dependent, demanding, and/or delinquent; while excessive discipline or control can make children aggressive or timid or unduly anxious in life. Deficient or faulty parenting is major contributor to mental disorders in children.

Societal factors: Poverty; substance use in neighborhood; violent, aggressive, delinquent, and antisocial subcultures make the children and adolescents living in these societies vulnerable for future substance use and delinquent or antisocial behaviors.

School and related variables: Environment at school is of utmost importance in determining whether a child likes going to school or refuses for the same. Unduly strict teachers, being bullied/teased at school, sexual and physical abuse at hands of care takers, and excessive separation anxiety from parents are important reasons for school refusal in children. Additionally, reading, writing, and learning difficulties lead to poor academic performance which can also be a reason for children to avoid going to school.

Valence of these genetic and environmental factors in the genesis of problems is different for different disorders, for different individuals suffering from the same disorder, and for same disorder expressed at different developmental period in the same child.

ASSESSMENT PROCESS

The rule of thumb is "take a good and thorough history followed by detailed physical and mental state examination." A good history remains the cornerstone of arriving at a provisional diagnosis, which can then be supported by examination findings. Enquire into:

- *Birth history*: A detailed account of mother's health during pregnancy, record of drugs taken, mode of delivery, details about birth cry, birth weight, any neonatal complications like metabolic disturbances (hypoglycemia, hypomagnesemia, etc.), neonatal jaundice, neonatal seizures, any need for neonatal ICU care, nursery care, ability to suckle mother's milk, and type of feed given.
- *Developmental milestones*: Any delay or deviance in attainment of milestones in fine motor, gross motor, social and emotional, speech, and language domains.
- Temperament of the child
- *Presenting complaints*: Onset of symptoms, duration of symptoms, evolution of illness from first complaint till the

time of examination, any exacerbating or relieving factors

- Source of referral
- Parent's understanding of illness or causation of symptoms
- Expectations from the child and response to illness
- *Family environment*: Who cares for the child predominantly, attachment pattern of child, parental discord/substance use/parental mental illness, domestic violence
- *Parental handling patterns*: Too strict or too liberal
- Enquire about socioeconomic status, decision maker in family, who has the financial control—all these have implications while formulating the management plan for the child.
- Details of past treatment taken, response to same, side effects, compliance, if noncompliance present—issues leading to noncompliance
- School report if available
- Impairment caused due to symptoms in school attendance, family relationships, relationship with peers, and social acceptability
- Expectations from treatment
- Any physical problems/illness, seizures, etc.

Physical Examination

Look for and record:

- Detailed general physical examination, including height, weight, head circumference, pulse, and respiratory rate.
- Look for neurocutaneous stigmata such as café-au-lait spots seen in neurofibromatosis, shagreen patches in tuberous sclerosis, mongoloid features in Down's syndrome, etc.
- Detailed neurological examination and systemic examination is necessary as indicated by the history.

Mental State Examination

Interview the child separately as much as possible, particularly while dealing with adolescents. Ask the child's account of issues at home, school, playground, with peers, what brings him to consult the doctor.

Examine the patient for:

- *General appearance and behavior*: Reaction to interview situation, pattern of communication with the examiner, between parents and child, response to separation from parents
- *Affect*: How the child feels or the current mood state and observation of the clinician
- *Thought content*: What does the child say about his problems, preoccupations, worries regarding anything, day-to-day fears, ideas of self-harm, or presenting complaints or symptoms
- Motivation to come for treatment and to comply with treatment.

Management Principles

General principles to be followed while dealing with children and adolescents are given below:

Based on the comprehensive understanding of the intrinsic and extrinsic factors contributing to the mental health problems in the given child, intervention should be targeted at all levels such as parents, home, school, peers, etc. Treatment is often multimodal (using several strategies) and multidisciplinary (involving several professionals like psychologists, speech therapists, occupational therapists, social workers, special educators, pediatricians, etc.).

Focus lies on symptom reduction or symptom removal, because that is what the parents and child are most concerned about, by using pharmacological and nonpharmacological approaches. None of the mental disorders in children are amenable to medication alone. Most medications are targeted at specific symptoms and none of them affect or take care of the basic underlying etiology. Medications are recommended and majorly useful in treatment of conditions such as ADHD, OCD, depressive disorders, anxiety disorders, psychotic disorders, BPAD, tic disorders, and enuresis. At times, medication is used in severe cases of aggression, violence, impulse dyscontrol, suicidality, or substance use disorders to tide over the crisis. All disorders require concomitant psychological and psychosocial interventions. Apart from symptomatic treatment, it is essential to ensure that the child is supported for growth and development through provision of adequate care, nurturance, safety, nutrition, education, and play. Efforts should be made to remove impediments that can hamper or compromise the normal growth and development trajectory. Parents need to be educated and sensitized to understand the nature of mental disorder and recommended treatment. Parental acceptance of child's illness and their cooperation in treatment is the key factor in treatment success. The child should be talked to keeping in mind his/her developmental age, and also involved in treatment. In many instances, remedial education and training to enhance developmental functions of speech, language, communication, motor development, and learning, etc., are the key intervention.

Given below is a brief overview of a few specific mental disorders, most commonly encountered in children and adolescents.

NEURODEVELOPMENTAL DISORDERS

Various categories in this broad grouping, depending on what is the central prominent atypicality in development are: (1) intellectual disability, (2) autism spectrum disorder, (3) attention deficit hyperkinetic disorder, (4) specific learning disorders (SLDs), (5) communication disorder, and (6) motor disorders including developmental coordination and tic disorders.

These children present with global or specific developmental delay especially in infancy and early childhood, which can be global delay in development as in ID, or specific delays in development of communication and language skills as in ASD, communication disorders, or in motor skills as in motor coordination disorders. In addition, there can be presence of behavioral or emotional disturbances of any kind. Some of the major risk factors of neurodevelopmental disorders are described in **Table 20.1**.

Neurodevelopmental disorders characteristically show that:

- They have an onset in infancy and/or early childhood.
- Impairment or delay in development of function is strongly related to biological maturation of CNS.
- A steady course that does not mostly involve remissions and relapses. There is mostly a natural history of improvement in varying degree but still core deficits tend to persist lifelong.
- These frequently co-occur, and generally affect males more than females.
- Nearly 15% have underlying known genetic cause. Rest do not have a single genetic etiology. It is the interaction of gene and environment which is responsible for variable degree of expression.
- There is higher incidence of epilepsy and other psychiatric disorders in their life span.
- They are more sensitive to drug side effects because of vulnerable brain.
- Behavioral manifestations seem to be more challenging and severe in childhood where brain is still growing

Table 20.1: Major risk factors of neurodevelopmental disorders.

Timing	Type	Examples
Prenatal	Chromosomal disorders	Down's syndrome, Klinefelter's syndrome, Turner's syndrome, Cri-du-chat's syndrome, Prader–Willi's syndrome, Angelman's syndrome, William's syndrome
	Single gene disorders	*Inborn errors of metabolism:* Galactosemia, phenylketonuria, MPS, Tay–sachs disease, Lesch Nyhan's syndrome, hypothyroidism
		Neurocutaneous: Tuberous sclerosis, neurofibromatosis
		Brain malformations: Autosomal recessive primary microcephaly, hydrocephalus, spina bifida
		Others: Fragile-X's syndrome, Rett's syndrome, Smith-Lemli-Opitz's syndrome
	Other conditions of uncertain genetic origin	Rubinstein Taybi's syndrome, De Lange's syndrome
	Adverse maternal/ environmental influences*	*Deficiencies:* Iodine and folate
		Severe malnutrition in pregnancy
		Substance use: Alcohol, nicotine, cocaine
		Exposure to harmful chemicals: Lead, mercury, arsenic, pollutants, abortifacients, teratogenic medications
		Maternal infections: Rubella, syphilis, toxoplasma, *cytomegalovirus*, herpes, HIV
		Others: Exposure to radiation, Rh isoimmunization
Perinatal*	• Third trimester	Eclampsia, maternal cardiac or renal disease, diabetes, placental dysfunction
	• Labor	Prematurity, low-birth weight, birth asphyxia, birth trauma
	• Neonatal	Septicemia, jaundice, hypoglycemia
Postnatal*	• Brain infections	Tuberculosis, Japanese encephalitis, bacterial meningoencephalitis
	• Head injury	
	• Chronic lead exposure	
	• Severe and prolonged malnutrition	
	• Gross under stimulation and experiential deprivation	

*Major causes in developing country like India.
(MPS: mucopolysaccharidosis)

and demands of environment are more. These tend to stabilize in adult life when a somewhat more stable equilibrium with environment is achieved.

Management: The management of NDDs focuses on three approaches:

1. To promote healthy development such as in the areas of speech and communication, motor development, and eye contact.
2. To promote learning with special education support.
3. To decrease undesirable or problematic behaviors such as rocking, over activity,

sleep problems, anger irritability, self-harming or destructive behavior, etc. as the case may be.

There is very less role of medications if there is no known specific treatable etiology or comorbid medical condition. There is no medical cure as such for most of these. Whatever may be the etiology, certain common principles of management employed are:

- Early diagnosis and early intervention are the most important first step. So, early referral to a specialist psychiatrist, pediatrician for diagnosis, and further management is recommended.
- A multidisciplinary approach with provision of special education, occupational therapy, speech and language therapy, physiotherapy, and specialized behavior therapy by clinical psychologists and special therapists on the principles of conditioning and learning after functional behavioral analysis is the key. Involvement of parents/caregivers in every step of management is crucial.
- Parental education and caregiver education. Taking care of family's emotional issues and burden/burnout.
- Possible medical comorbidies/etiologies like thyroid disorders, inborn errors of metabolism, epilepsy, etc. should be investigated and managed.
- Special medical, educational, rehabilitative, and sociolegal provision in society for removing these barriers enacted through laws based on right-based approach for disabilities.
- Once a stable equilibrium with rehabilitation is achieved then throughout lifespan many medical, psychiatric challenges also keep coming along with more broad social/financial ones as these are lifelong disabilities of varying degree in most cases but fortunately most of the persons with NDD are in mild range.

Intellectual Disability

Children with ID have delayed or arrested brain development where brain development follows the normal path but at a much slower pace and gets arrested at a lower level of attainment than what is considered normal. ID (mental retardation) is characterized by deficits in general mental abilities, such as reasoning, planning, problem solving, academic learning, judgment, and abstract thinking. The term "global developmental delay" is used for children younger than 5 years of age who are not able to achieve developmental milestones appropriate for age.

An IQ score of <70 is taken as a cut-off score for diagnosing an individual with ID; however, an assessment of adaptive functions is of *greater importance* while assessing an individual with suspected ID.

Causes of ID (mentioned above in NDD): Any pathogenic process that hampers normal brain development during prenatal, natal, or postnatal period can give rise to ID. There are more than 1,000 known genetic causes of ID; however, in 30–40% cases of ID it is still not possible to demonstrate any identifiable cause. ID occurs as a result of complex interaction of genetic and environmental (such as birth trauma/asphyxia, meningoencephalitis, epilepsy, head trauma, poisoning, etc.) factors. Severity of ID depends much on the timing (i.e., prenatal/perintal/postnatal period), intensity (i.e., severity of pathologic process), and type (i.e., genetic cause/birth asphyxia/antenatal infections, etc.) of brain insult. Brain insult in early life has far reaching negative impact on development of brain and intelligence.

Diagnosis and assessment: Use the same general principles of assessment as mentioned above. Good clinical history allows the physician to come to a close provisional diagnosis. Always try to look out for medical causes, especially reversible causes, e.g., hypothyroidism, nutritional deficiencies, hearing impairment, vision impairment, and social deprivation.

Management: General principles of management of NDDs as mentioned above apply here. *There is greater role for prevention in ID rather than cure especially in country like ours.*

Disability certification allows the individuals with ID to avail of the social welfare benefits, concession in train and bus fare, given by the Government of India to disabled persons.

Autism Spectrum Disorder

Autism spectrum disorders are NDDs characterized by deficits in social communication and social interaction across multiple contexts and restricted, repetitive patterns of behavior. ASD is different from ID in the sense that here the process of brain development is derailed or deviant and not just delayed or arrested. The child is qualitatively different in social communication from age matched typically developing children or even from those with global developmental delay whose mental age may be similar to that of the child with ASD. But in reality, there is very frequent co-occurrence of autism spectrum with intellectual subnormality, so autism spectrum is diagnostically overshadowed by intellectual subnormality. There is often excessive hyperactivity in ASD children, sensory problems of hypo- or hypersensitivity to sensory stimuli, and problems of learning.

Common presenting symptoms or signs for autism spectrum disorder are:

- Lack of eye-to-eye contact
- Delayed/absent speech development
- Speech not used for communication
- Not responding to name being called
- Avoidance or lack of response to human contact

- Absent finger pointing
- No babbling by 12 months of age
- Likes to be alone/play alone
- No meaningful play
- Absent use of conventional gestures
- Repetitive behaviors, e.g., hand flapping
- Restricted interests, e.g., fascinated by water/round objects
- Hyper- or hyporeactivity to sensory stimuli.

There is often associated history of pre- or perinatal brain insult, epilepsy, ADHD, repetitive behavior, behavioral abnormalities, and other neuropsychiatric problems.

Diagnosis and assessment: Assessment and diagnosis of ASD is specialized and skilled clinical examination and ratings. Often children with ASD are misdiagnosed as having ID.

Management: Unfortunately there is no cure for this neurodevelopmental condition. Early diagnosis followed by early intervention is the key to success. This condition is different in presentation and problem issues in comparison with ID. Treatment is multidisciplinary done at specialized centers with staff trained in handling ASD. It is a highly painstaking task with slow and small gains requiring great deal of patience and understanding on part of the therapists as well as the parents and families.

Attention Deficit Hyperactivity Disorder

Attention deficit hyperactivity disorder is one of the most common mental disorders among children and adolescents, characterized by a triad of symptoms, i.e., overactivity, inattention, and impulsivity. Approximately 5% of children under 18 years are affected by ADHD worldwide. ADHD is a familial disorder with a strong genetic component.

Attention deficit hyperactivity disorder children are highly overactive, fidgety, unstoppable, over talkative, do not wait for their turn, speak out of turn, cannot wait, intrude into conversation, impulsive, lose their things, and are disorganized. They often get into fights with others, can be rough, aggressive. There may be complaints from school or neighborhood about their behavior. They are very high risk for accidents, substance use disorders, delinquency, and scholastic under achievement.

Symptoms begin in early childhood with full manifestation occurring before 12 years. Symptoms are present in school, playground, home, and other social situations, and create problems in child's achievements. So, information from all the sources school, family, and friends is needed.

Attention deficit hyperactivity disorder is frequently comorbid with ASD, ID, specific learning disability and oppositional defiant disorder, conduct disorder, depression, substance abuse, etc. ADHD interferes with multiple areas of functioning, such as behavior at home, in social situations, school performance; treatment should seek to improve functioning in all these areas.

Assessment: Based on the general assessment principles for children and those for NDDs mentioned above, take information from school, family, and play environment.

Management of ADHD: Management comprises of medication and nonpharmacological approaches. Parental education about illness is essential.

Behavior therapy and parent management training: Behavior therapies focus on behavior modification of the child using the principles of classical and operant conditioning. Parents training is essential component of treatment where they are taught how to deal with their child's behavior by using reinforcements for desirable behaviors, setting limits, structured routine and timetable, greater supervision

for work, setting rules, and enforcing them. Liaison with school is helpful.

Pharmacotherapy: Many medications have been shown to be effective and safe for children with ADHD. Medications can be divided into stimulants and nonstimulants. *Stimulant* drugs most commonly used and effective in ADHD are methylphenidate. These drugs are very effective in controlling the symptoms of ADHD and should only be *prescribed by specialist dealing with children.* *Nonstimulant* medications are considered second-line treatments in case of intolerance, contraindications, or treatment failure.

Specific Learning Disorders

Learning disorder is the generic term to describe disorders characterized by difficulties in learning academic skills— accurate and fluent reading, writing, and arithmetic—which significantly affect academic achievement or daily functioning. These children lag in learning specific academic skills despite having adequate intelligence. Learning disorders described are dyslexia, dyscalculia, and disorder of written expression. After ruling out intellectual subnormality, functioning in various academic skills is assessed in reference to their age and grade matched performance, clinically or on psychometric tests. Children who perform two grade levels below the expected for their age on specific academic skills, on the SLD tests or on clinical examination, are diagnosed as SLD. Apart from academic difficulties, these children also have frequent comorbidity with ADHD, behavior and emotional problems, and perinatal difficulties. SLD is treated with remedial education by special educators who endeavor to teach the child using different teaching methods and aids. SLD is recognized as a disability and special relaxations are given to children with dyslexias or SLD's in Central Board of Secondary Education.

Tic Disorders

Tics are sudden, abrupt, fast movements comprising various muscle groups, with or without vocal utterances, which occur involuntarily. Tics are brief but repetitive, usually appear in short bursts or even series. They may be classified according to the degree of complexity (simple, complex) as well as their quality (motor, vocal). Tourette's syndrome is a condition that has a typical onset after 10 years of age, and presents with complex verbal and motor tics. The condition fluctuates in severity and frequency, and presents significant social disability. There is some degree of control present but then it comes in bursts. It is frequently comorbid with ADHD, OCD, depression, sleep disorders, and learning disability. Rage attacks are very common and at times Coprolalia may also be present, especially in severe forms.

- *Examples of motor tics*: Eye blinking, rolling of eyes, grimacing, shaking of head, twitching of shoulders, twitching of torso and pelvis, twitching of abdomen, movements of the hands and arms, movements of the feet and legs.
- *Vocal tics*: Throat clearing, grunting, making sounds, etc.

Genetic factors, perinatal factors, infectious agents particularly involving basal ganglia are implicated in etiology of tic disorders. Sometimes these are habit disorders where it starts as a voluntary anxiety reducing mechanism in highly anxious children becoming involuntary in due course of time. Medical tests like electroencephalogram (EEG) and detailed neurological examination are required to rule out other differential diagnosis like epilepsia partialis continua or dyskinesias.

Management: Involves education about illness that in 80% of cases it will remit on its own. For others, habit reversal therapy and/or medications like clonidine and low-dose antipsychotic (such as haloperidol, risperidone) are helpful.

Anxiety Disorder

Anxiety in children is experienced as a sense of uneasiness, unexplained fear, nausea, vomiting sensation, pain abdomen, clinging behavior, school refusal, dryness of mouth, weepiness, and sleep disturbance. Anxiety disorders can also manifest as panic attacks, social anxiety, specific phobias, separation anxiety, tics, or obsessive-compulsive symptoms. Anxiety disorders in children were thought to be relatively rare and low impact conditions. But current understanding is that most of the anxiety and depressive disorders in adults have their roots in childhood. Adult depressive disorders have childhood anxiety as their forerunners.

Various common types of anxiety disorders seen in children are given in **Table 20.2**.

There is a very frequent overlap between symptoms. It is important to understand why child is anxious. Then only ways can be designed to help them.

Sudden and atypical anxiety especially with somatic symptoms warrants detailed physical examination and necessary investigations to rule out medical conditions like epilepsy, cardiovascular, and endocrinological conditions. For younger children, it may be very difficult to verbalize their fears.

Generally understanding children as regards their triggers and allaying their fears works for most. Otherwise behavioral principles of graduated exposure in developmentally appropriate ways help in most of the cases. Specific serotonin reuptake

Table 20.2: Common anxiety disorders specific to children.

Name of anxiety disorder	Core features	Age of onset
Separation anxiety disorder	Fear or concern that something bad will happen to the child or parent/family members if they will get separated	Early to mid-childhood (around 7–8 years)
Generalized anxiety disorder	Worries about a wide range of negative possibilities that something bad will happen	Late childhood (around 10–12 years)
Social phobia	Fear and avoidance of social interactions or social performance due to a belief that others will negatively evaluate the child	Early adolescence (around 11–13 years)
Specific phobias	The core feature of specific phobias involves fear and avoidance in response to a range of specific cues, situations, or objects. There is a common belief that the object or situation will lead to personal harm	Variable depending on the type, e.g., animal phobias start in early childhood (around 6–7 years); balloon phobia or fear of darkness starts even earlier (3–4 years of age), school phobia can start any time after joining school

inhibitor group of drugs are generally indicated for severe cases and are helpful. Behavior therapy and psychotherapy either alone or in conjunction with medication are indicated. Treatment is to be generally done by specialist. Not responding or poorly responding anxiety disorders starting at this stage of development tend to last lifelong.

Depressive Disorder

Children can experience and exhibit depression in a manner similar to how it is seen in adults. While depressed children may initially present with a variety of symptoms that conceal the depression (e.g., tantrums, headaches, tiredness, and problems concentrating), a competent clinician should be able to uncover the depression. Now it is established beyond doubt through robust scientific observations and studies that depression can occur as early as infancy and is rather common in adolescence. While diagnosis is not usually difficult, depression in children and adolescents is often not detected and remains untreated. Young people tend to present initially with

behavioral or physical complaints which may obscure the typical depressive symptoms seen in adults. It is important to ascertain if the current problems represent a change from the child's or teenager's previous level of functioning or character.

Complaints which should alert clinicians to the possibility of depression include:

- Irritability or cranky mood
- Chronic boredom or loss of interest in previously enjoyed leisure activities like sports activities or dance and music lesson
- Social withdrawal or no longer wanting to "hang out" with friends
- Blaming self, ideas of worthlessness, hopelessness, or guilt
- Anxiety, fears, tearfulness, clinging behavior
- Suicidal ideas or actions
- Avoiding school
- Decline in academic performance
- Change in sleep-wake pattern (e.g., sleeping in and refusing to go to school)
- Frequent unexplained complaints of feeling sick, headaches, stomach-aches
- Development of behavioral problems (such as becoming more defiant, running away from home, bullying others)
- Abusing alcohol or other substances
- *Suicidal behavior*

Risk factors for depression are: High anxiety, physical or psychological trauma, bereavement/loss, failure, abuse, neglect, negative parenting, parent child conflict, bullying, staying in foster homes, presence of family history of depression, substance abuse in parents, female gender, puberty, chronic medical illness, and past history of depression.

Management of Depression

Many a time parents and teachers are insensitive or unaware of the child's feelings and may think that the child is deliberately behaving in that fashion. It is necessary to understand the child's feelings and thoughts and validate them. The approach has to be empathetic, reassuring, comforting, and supportive. You should try to understand the sources of stress in the child and handle them as much as possible.

Mild severity depression: Can be treated with environmental change, parental and child counseling along with social/school support.

Moderate severity: Treat with environmental change, parental, and child counseling along with social/school support. Refer to specialist if does not improve or is less than 12 years of age. The child can be given antidepressant drug such as fluoxetine 5–20 mg, under regular follow-up. Be watchful of increased agitation which can be a risk factor for suicide.

Severe depression: Those with marked agitation, marked retardation, or suicidal risk should be immediately referred to a specialist; but ask the family members to be vigilant till they reach specialist. Such a child may require hospitalization and intensive treatment with antidepressant drugs and other supportive management as required.

Suicide and Self-harming Behavior

Suicide rates in children and adolescents are rising worldwide and this trend is most sharp in India.

Suicide means the act of a person intentionally causing his or her own death. Whereas a *suicide attempt* denotes nonfatal acts or preparations intended to result in death. The suicidal act may have been abandoned, interrupted, or unsuccessful.

Suicidality refers to the cognitions and activities of persons seeking their own death, including thoughts, actions, or omissions.

Para suicide refers to, potentially life-threatening self-harming behavior which is performed without the intention to kill oneself. Because the behavior is nonsuicidal, it is termed as "deliberate self-harm" or "nonsuicidal self-injury".

Every child with depression should be assessed for suicidal risk behavior. Some parents object and even doctors hesitate to do so, thinking that leading questions about suicide should not be asked. But this is a myth, asking about suicidal ideas does not increase suicidal risk behavior, rather by not asking one can miss the opportunity to act upon saving a life. Primary care or family physician is the first point of medical help in cases of suicide, and it is at this point that the risk is to be identified and prevented. Some major risk factors for suicide among children and adolescents have been mentioned in **Box 20.1**.

Child Maltreatment and Abuse

Many children are subjected to maltreatment, physical or sexual abuse that causes serious physical injury and mental trauma which can lead to long-term harm to their development and mental health. Child abuse is an extreme form of human rights violation and a criminal

> **Box 20.1:** Major risk factors for suicide among children and adolescents.
>
> - *Presence of psychiatric illness* like major depressive disorder, bipolar disorder, conduct disorder, and substance use disorders, dysfunctional personality traits, feelings of hopelessness and worthlessness impulsive aggression, and the tendency to react to frustration or provocation with hostility or aggression
> - *Family factors*: Loss of a parent through death or divorce, family discord, family history of depression or suicide
> - *Social factors/psychological factors*: Failure, guilt, shame, rejection, low self-esteem or honor, severe trauma, stress
> - *Physical and sexual abuse*
> - *Lack of a supportive network*: Poor relationships with peers, bullying, feelings of social isolation
> - *Previous suicide attempt*
> - *Availability of lethal means*
> - *Having been exposed to suicide* (e.g., suicide or suicide attempt in family members or friends; media reporting).

offence. It occurs in about 60–70% of girls and about 50–60% of boys sometime in their life. Most cases are not reported as the victim is threatened against disclosure and society and family are unsupportive in most instances.

CHILDREN'S RIGHTS

The Convention on the Rights of the Child states that children everywhere are entitled to basic human rights which include the right to:

- Survival
- Develop to the fullest
- Protection from harmful influences, abuse, and exploitation
- Participate fully in the family, cultural, and social life.

Children who are abused appear very quiet, anxious, clingy, lack faith and trust in others. They present with unexplained somatic symptoms, dissociative symptoms, insomnia, hypervigilance, easily startled, crying, sad, hopeless, and fearful. They may deny abuse or problems as they are threatened by the abuser against disclosure.

Often the family is either unaware of the abuse or they deny any such history. Most abuse occurs within the family setup, done by a familiar person who is a family member or a family friend. The various types of child abuse are described in **Table 20.3**.

There are certain indicators that can point toward the possibility of abuse:

- Unexplained delay in seeking medical help, especially following a fracture, serious burn/scald
- Explanation offered by child or guardian is not consistent with the injury
- History of ingestion of poison, alcohol or drugs, suicidal attempts or running away
- Inappropriate response of caretaker to child's injuries such as denial that child is in pain or minimizing symptoms
- Repeated presentations with injuries, often to different doctors or health care facilities

Discovery of abuse requires high index of suspicion, careful recording of history and examination, interview of the child alone after making him/her comfortable and reassured. The family often does not accept the explanation and can threaten the doctor or the patient for having disclosed and may leave the hospital suddenly. A thorough physical and psychiatric examination is required to be carried out. Entire approach to the issue has to be sensitive and supportive from the point of view of the patient who is the victim.

Child abuse is a cognizable offence, a medicolegal issue, and doctors in emergency who may encounter such cases in the first place need to report it to police. Psychiatric intervention is needed in all cases.

CONCLUSION

Children who comprise more than 40% of our population and who represent the future of any society need special attention regarding care of their mental health. They also need special attention because they pass through rapid developmental changes during which foundations of his future and

Table 20.3: The various types of child abuse.

Physical abuse	Physical harm or injury
Neglect/negligent treatment	Failure to provide for a child's basic needs and development in all spheres such as not given food, rest, education, clothes, place to live in or sleep, play, etc.
Emotional abuse	Subjecting the child to severe criticism, derogatory comments, cursing, swearing, blaming, force, coercion, entrapment, humiliation, etc. which results in impairment of a child's emotional development or sense of self-worth
Sexual abuse	The involvement of a child in sexual activity usually by adults or children who are in a position of responsibility, have obtained children's trust, or have power over the victim. The child is either forced or lured into any form of sexual play, genital manipulation, penetrative sex, oral, or anal sex
Exploitation	The use of the child in work or other activities for the benefit of others, for financial gain, e.g., child labor

moulds of different mental faculties and value systems are being laid. Any deviation or departure at this stage may have huge impact on the future life of the individual. It also has great implications for the health of the society. Both the biological endowment and the psychosocial milieu are important in maintenance of health, causation of disorders as well as in their treatment. Because of the changing normative baseline of children during different developmental phases, it is very important to be cautious in the assessment process of disorders in children. It is very important for every psychiatrist to have a good insight into the childhood and adolescent disorders. Parents and teachers should also be sensitized to facilitate early identification of problem cases.

TAKE-HOME MESSAGES

- The importance of child psychiatry lies in the fact that it deals with mental health problems in the developmental phases of life. State of mental health in childhood has lifelong impact on health in general and mental health in particular.
- Children may suffer from a variety of NDDs, anxiety disorders, mood disorders, conduct and oppositional defiant behavior disorders, dissociative and somatoform disorders, psychotic disorders, OCD, habit disorders, substance use disorders, etc.
- Presence of a mental health problem in children should be suspected whenever there is evidence of substantial delay in developmental milestones, poor eye-contact and withdrawal, irritability, crying, defiance, disobedience, violence, aggression, smiling to self, talking excessively, excessive temper tantrum, disturbed sleep, disturbed appetite, fears, phobia, clinging behavior, excessive anxiety, headache, multiple somatic symptoms, etc.
- Mental health problems in children and adolescents arise as a result of complex interplay of genetic or intrinsic and environmental or extrinsic factors.
- Management therefore includes judicious and rational pharmacotherapy as well as, more importantly, psychosocial interventions. This would include involvement of therapists, parents, home, school, peers, etc. Treatment is often multimodal (using several strategies) and multidisciplinary (involving several professionals like psychologists, speech therapists, occupational therapists, social workers, special educators, pediatricians, etc.).

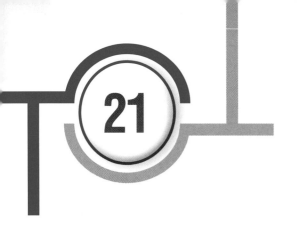

Disorder of Intellectual Development

K John Vijay Sagar, Satish C Girimaji

INTRODUCTION

Disorder of intellectual development (DID) belongs to a group of conditions called neurodevelopmental disorders (NDDs). The NDDs are characterized by impairments in various aspects of development such as cognition, general intelligence, speech, language, communication, social development, and motor functions because of aberrant neurodevelopmental processes. These developmental abnormalities may occur during neurogenesis, neural proliferation, neuronal migration, neural differentiation, axon guidance, synapse formation, synaptic pruning, and refinement.

The hallmark of DID is diminished intellectual capability with onset during developmental years. Wechsler had defined intelligence as "The aggregate or global capacity of the individual to act purposefully, to think rationally, and to deal effectively with his environment." Intellectual ability helps an individual to understand, reason, learn, imagine, remember, solve problems, adapt to and modify his environment. Intelligence is a trait that is normally distributed in the general population; in other words, it follows Gaussian or bell-shaped distribution in the community. Persons with DID are those who are in lower end of this normal distribution curve. Disorder of intellectual development causes significant life-long disability to the affected persons and generates substantial stress for the caregivers.

There are many ways to conceptualize DID; however, a comprehensive biopsychosocial perspective that takes into account the neurobiological, psychological, developmental, and the social aspects provides the best framework to understand DID in its totality.

HISTORICAL ASPECTS

The history of intellectual disability dates back to 1552 BC, when it was mentioned in the Egyptian Papyrus of Thebes. However, prior to the 18th century, there was very little scientific attention on this condition. Intellectual deficits were defined by Esquirol as conditions of incomplete mental development based on known (or unknown) biological or environmental causes. The first systematic intervention program for a person affected with DID was started in late 18th century by Jean-Marc Itard. Further progress was made when Eduard Seguin established a systematic program for "feebleminded" at Salpetrière Hospital in Paris. Intelligence assessment tests were developed in the 20th century, initially by Alfred Binet and later by others such as Wechsler.

There is a mention of DID in the ancient Indian literature. An ancient Indian Ayurvedic text on diseases of childhood titled "*Kashyapa Samhita*" makes a specific mention of children born with lesser intellectual ability ("*buddhi*"), and even offers treatments to improve the condition.

Disorder of intellectual development was earlier called by many different names such as mental deficiency and mental retardation. Another common name is intellectual disability. There has been extensive research and scientific progress in last 4–5 decades on the nature, epidemiology, causes, genetics, molecular biology, psychological evaluation, and intervention for DID. Also, there has been growing emphasis on treating these individuals with respect and dignity and recognize their rights as fellow and equal human beings.

CONCEPT AND DEFINITION

Being an NDD, DID is most often manifested in early childhood. There is usually a delay in all developmental milestones across motor, language, cognitive, and social domains. This pattern of delay is called a global developmental delay. These delays can range from being mild to severe.

Most affected individuals with DID are said to have "Static encephalopathy" which means that the some brain insult has occurred at some point in brain development and resulted in deficits, but over a period of time, there is improvement in attainment of skills and competencies. However, there is a wide variation in the quantum and rate of this improvement. A few individuals with DID have a progressive neurological disorder as an underlying cause.

Disorder of intellectual development is defined as condition characterized by significant impairment in intellectual functioning with accompanying deficits in adaptive skills, with onset in developmental period. Thus, there are three dimensions to the definition as follow:

1. Significant impairments in intellectual functioning, usually taken as an intelligence quotient (IQ) of less than 70 on a standardized test of intelligence. However, individuals with same IQ may have very different profiles of intellectual and adaptive functioning.

2. Deficits in adaptive skills, meaning diminished ability to adapt to the daily demands of the normal social environment such as self-care, communication, education, employment, and independent living skills. These adaptive skills can be classified as practical, social, and conceptual skills.

3. Developmental origin, i.e., onset before 18 years of age.

Disorder of intellectual development differs from other NDDs such as specific disorder of language development and autism spectrum disorder in the pattern of delay of developmental milestones and profile of current developmental attainments. A diagnosis of DID is considered when there is global developmental delay with marked impairments in age-appropriate current intellectual functioning such as understanding, reasoning, problem solving, learning, speed of thinking, and abstraction ability.

CLASSIFICATION

Disorder of intellectual development is classified into four categories based on level of intellectual functioning (as measured by IQ) and deficits in adaptive functioning. The four categories are mild, moderate, severe, and profound as described here.

1. *Mild DID*: Persons with mild DID acquire language with some delay but most achieve the ability to use speech as part of their daily routine, to hold conversations, and to engage in an interview with

clinicians. Most of them also achieve almost complete independence in self-help skills, mobility, transport and in simple domestic and practical skills, even if they have a slow rate of development compared to normal. The main difficulties are usually seen in academic achievement and higher order adaptive skills such as managing finances and complex social situations. Adults with mild DID are usually able to do semi-skilled work with minimum supervision. The IQ is in the range of 50–69.

2. *Moderate DID*: Persons with moderate DID are slow in developing comprehension and use of language, and their eventual achievement in this area is limited. Achievement of self-help skills and motor skills is also delayed, and some need long-term supervision. Few persons will learn the basic skills needed for reading, writing, and counting. However, the progress in academic work is limited. Adults with moderate DID are usually capable of simple practical work, especially if the work is carefully structured and skilled supervision is provided. Complete independence in activities of daily living is rarely achieved. Physical mobility and simple social activities are relatively well preserved in those with moderate DID. The IQ is in the range of 35–49.

3. *Severe DID*: Most people in this category have very limited speech and comprehension, and have some degree of motor impairment. Structural abnormalities of the brain are commonly present in this group. With training, limited self-care abilities such as eating, toilet control, and dressing will develop. The IQ is in the range of 20–34.

4. *Profound DID*: Individuals with profound ID have an IQ <20 and severe limitation in the ability to comprehend and to comply with instructions. Marked restriction of physical mobility, incontinence and presence of only limited nonverbal language skills are the hallmark of profound DID. They possess little or no ability to care for their own basic needs, and require constant help and supervision.

EPIDEMIOLOGY

The prevalence of DID across the world is around 1%. The prevalence in low and middle income countries (LAMIC) is almost two times more compared to high income countries. The highest prevalence has been reported in child and adolescent population. There is excess prevalence in males, in the ratio of 1.5:1. Prevalence also varies based on the assessment methods used for evaluation of persons with DID.

Mild DID is most common with 85% of all cases of DID followed by moderate DID about 10%, severe DID about 3%, and profound DID about 2%.

ETIOLOGICAL FACTORS

Anything that adversely affects the orderly, systematic development of the brain can lead to DID. There are hundreds of such causes, both genetic and environmental, or because of complex interplay between genetic and environmental factors. These factors can exert their adverse influence during different stages of child development. The stages are classified as prenatal, perinatal, and postnatal based on period before and after birth of the child. **Table 21.1** lists common prenatal, perinatal, and postnatal factors involved in the etiopathogenesis of DID. It is possible to identify a specific cause in about half of individuals of DID, much more so in more severe forms.

Table 21.1: Etiological factors associated with DID.

Category	Subcategory	Type	Examples
Prenatal	Embryonic	Chromosomal disorders	Down syndrome, Klinefelter syndrome, Turner syndrome, Cri-du-chat syndrome, Trisomy 18
		Microdeletions	Prader–Willi syndrome, Angelman syndrome, William syndrome, Smith–Magenis syndrome
		Single gene disorders	*Autosomal dominant:* Tuberous sclerosis, neurofibromatosis
			Autosomal recessive: Primary microcephaly, classical phenylketonuria, metachromatic leukodystrophy, Bardet–Biedl syndrome
			X-linked recessive: Hunter syndrome, Duchenne muscular dystrophy, Lesch–Nyhan syndrome
			X-linked dominant: Rett syndrome, Fragile X syndrome, Aicardi syndrome, Coffin–Lowry syndrome
		Copy number variations	17q21.31 microdeletion, 1q21.1 microdeletion
	Adverse maternal/ environmental influences	Deficiencies	Iodine deficiency, folate deficiency
		Exposure to other harmful chemicals (teratogens)	Exposure to medications such as thalidomide, phenytoin and warfarin sodium in early pregnancy, heavy metals, pollutants, abortifacients
		Maternal infections	Toxoplasmosis, rubella, cytomegalovirus, herpes (TORCH infections), syphilis, HIV, Zika
		Using substances	Alcohol (fetal alcohol syndrome), nicotine, and cocaine during early pregnancy
		Maternal diseases	Chronic renal or cardiac disease
		Others	Severe malnutrition in pregnancy, excessive exposure to radiation, Rh isoimmunization, hyperthermia
	Brain malformations of uncertain or multiple etiology		Lissencephaly, double cortex, heterotopias, polymicrogyria, schizencephaly, congenital hydrocephalus
Perinatal		Third trimester	Complications of pregnancy: Eclampsia Maternal Diseases: Cardiac, renal, diabetes Placental dysfunction/deprivation of supply
		Labor	Severe prematurity, very low birth weight, hypoxic-ischemic encephalopathy (birth asphyxia), birth trauma
		Neonatal	Septicemia, severe prolonged jaundice, hypoglycemia
Postnatal			Neuroinfections (tuberculosis, Japanese encephalitis, bacterial meningoencephalitis), head injury, chronic lead exposure, severe and prolonged malnutrition, gross under-stimulation and experiential deprivation

CLINICAL PRESENTATION

Delay in developmental milestones, difficulty to learn new things, slowness in activities of daily living, impaired speech and comprehension, partial or complete dependence on caregiver for self-help skills, poor scholastic performance and poor memory are the common presenting complaints. Few children are primarily brought for consultation due to behavior problems such as hyperactivity, poor concentration, impulsivity, self-injurious behavior, or sleep/appetite disturbances. History of recent onset change in behavior of a person already having developmental delay is another important presenting complaint, and needs careful evaluation to rule out comorbid psychiatric disorder. A child can be brought by parents for assessment of IQ which can further assist for certification to obtain disability benefits, school admission, and so on. Comorbid medical disorders like seizures lead to initial consultation and during evaluation found to have developmental delay.

Comorbid Disorders

A number of medical, behavioral, and psychiatric problems can co-occur with DID. These are described below:

- *Comorbid psychiatric disorders*: Persons with DID have a 4–5-fold higher risk of developing comorbid psychiatric disorders. These comorbid disorders are often missed during routine clinical evaluation due to mainly two factors; features of psychiatric disorders modified or "masked" by the cognitive and language limitations leading to non-specific symptoms (diagnostic masking) and the tendency to subsume the symptoms of a comorbid psychiatric disorder within the diagnosis of DID (diagnostic overshadowing). Attention deficit hyperactivity disorder (ADHD), oppositional defiant disorder (ODD), depression, anxiety disorders, stress-related disorders, psychotic disorders, and sleep disorders are the common comorbid disorders in persons with DID. History of a recent onset change in behavior, overall functioning, sleep, and appetite patterns often points toward a comorbid psychiatric disorder.

- There are certain well-known behavioral patterns associated with certain genetic syndromes. These are termed "Behavioral Phenotypes". Examples include self-injurious behavior in Lesch–Nyhan syndrome, obsessive compulsive disorder in Prader–Willi syndrome, autistic behaviors in Fragile X syndrome, and psychosis in velocardiofacial syndrome.

- *Comorbid medical disorders*: DID is commonly associated with medical disorders, both neurological and non-neurological. These are often missed during routine evaluation of persons with DID. These disorders result in significant impairment in functioning of the affected person. The list of common medical comorbidities is listed in **Table 21.2**. The prevalence of seizures in a child with DID

Table 21.2: List of common medical comorbidities.

- *Neurological disorders*:
  - Seizure disorder
  - Cerebral palsy
- *Other medical disorders*:
  - Congenital heart disease
  - Cleft lip and cleft palate
  - Hypothyroidism
  - Orthopedic conditions—congenital talipes equinovarus (CTEV), congenital dislocation of hip (CDH)
  - Nutritional, vitamin, and mineral deficiencies
  - Recurrent infections
  - Visual impairment
  - Hearing impairment

ranges from 15 to 30%. Those with severe to profound DID have a higher prevalence of seizures.

CLINICAL EVALUATION

A thorough clinical evaluation is needed to arrive at a comprehensive diagnosis and to plan the management in persons with DID. Steps in clinical evaluation include history taking, behavioral observation and interview, physical examination, psychological testing, medical investigations, and diagnostic formulation.

- *History taking*: A good clinical history is the most important aspect of clinical evaluation. History needs to be obtained from multiple informants including parents, other caregivers, teachers and the child himself/herself. A detailed review of the previous medical records needs to be done. History taking has to be done in a structured format so that all the relevant information is elicited from the informants. The history taking format must include the following sections and details:
  - *Presenting complaints and duration*
  - *Family history*: Three generation genetic diagram (pedigree chart) drawn with internationally accepted symbols, family history of any NDDs or any psychiatric disorders or neurological disorders, family background, current living arrangements, parenting and childrearing practices, caregiver stress, social support, coping and adaptation by the family.
  - *Personal history*: Birth and developmental history which includes pre-, peri-, and postnatal details, developmental milestones and developmental course or trajectory (onset of delay, dates of acquisition of key milestones, delay in all areas or not, severity of delay), schooling history, and menstrual history.
- *Medical history*: Seizures, feeding problems, recurrent gastrointestinal symptoms (constipation, diarrhea, reflux esophagitis), and recurrent infections.
- *Psychiatric history*: If there is any history of a psychiatric or behavioral disorder, the onset, course, and progression of symptoms.
- *Treatment history*: Help seeking in the past with the specific nature, duration, and response to any past medical or psychosocial intervention.
- *Current developmental attainment of the child*: Current level of attainment of milestones in motor, cognitive, language and social domains, and parents' estimation of mental age of the child.

- *Behavioral observation and mental status evaluation*: Child's behavior has to be observed right from the time he/she enters the consultation room. The consultation room should have minimum furniture and should enable the child to move around without hurting self. The child should be made comfortable in the room. Age-appropriate play and art materials are helpful in eliciting cooperation from the child. The clinician should be prepared to leave his chair and move around to effectively interact with the child. Interview with the child has to be done in a nonjudgmental manner with simple questions. Some children with marked language delay may not communicate using words. The key areas to be assessed include attention and concentration, activity level, language and communication skills, general fund of information, reasoning and abstraction abilities, speed of thinking, quality of interaction with parents/caregivers, sociability, mood, play behavior, and academic skills. The examiner needs to form an impression about the individual's current intellectual abilities in comparison to same-age peers and the degree to which it is delayed. It is also worthwhile to note the strengths of the individual.

- *Physical examination*: A thorough head-to-toe physical examination of all the organ systems has to be done for all children with DID. Physical examination gives vital clues to the etiologic factors and underlying medical conditions. It will also help the clinician to plan the necessary medical investigations. Examination needs to be done in a child-friendly manner to elicit child's cooperation. Recording of any major and minor congenital anomalies (MCAs) needs to be done as described in **Table 21.3**, four or more of these MCAs suggest possible influence of prenatal factors in the etiopathogenesis.

  Clinicians should be well-versed with features observed in common genetic syndromes associated with DID. **Table 21.4** lists some common genetic syndromes and the associated physical examination findings.

- *Psychological testing*: Psychological testing is useful for several reasons such as confirming the presence and severity of DID, formulating a baseline of skills and deficits before planning intervention, monitoring the impact of intervention, and for provision of disability benefits by government. Commonly used tests in India are Vineland Social Maturity Scale (VSMS), Binet–Kamat Test (BKT), Malin's

Intelligence Scale for Indian Children (MISIC), Vineland Adaptive Behavior Scale (VABS), Raven's Progressive Matrices, Wechsler Intelligence Scale for Children (WISC), and Bhatia Battery. An Indian adaptation of Bailey's Scale for infants is also available (Developmental Assessment Scale for Indian Infants). Checklists such as Portage checklist, BASIC-MR from National Institute for the Empowerment of Persons with Intellectual Disabilities (NIEPID), Secunderabad, are also useful for planning targeted intervention. The tests for developmental screening of infants include Trivandrum Developmental Checklist, Bayley Scale for Infant Development (BSID), and Denver Developmental Screening Test (DDST).

- *Medical investigations*: Medical investigations have to be planned after a thorough clinical evaluation. Choice of tests depends on many considerations such as need to elucidate causative factors, further exploration of associated conditions, and diagnostic yield of tests. Parents have to be involved in the discussion prior to decision making on any investigations. The role of investigation has to be clearly explained to the parents with sufficient time for clarification of any queries. Children with DID may not cooperate for invasive tests and the clinician should approach this issue sensitively. Care must be taken to initiate interventions at the earliest without waiting for the result of investigations. Audiological and ophthalmological evaluation should be done when required. Neurological investigations such as imaging and EEG are not required in all cases and have to be done when they are likely to lead to a better understanding of the problem. Tests to detect underlying cause have to be

Table 21.3: Physical examination in disorder of intellectual development.

Aspect of examination	Examples of anomalies
Facial appearance or facial gestalt	Typical facies (down, coarse, progeroid), elongated, triangular, midfacial hypoplasia
Height	Short stature, tall stature, increased arm span, gigantism
Weight	Obesity, emaciation
Head circumference	Microcephaly, macrocephaly
Shape of skull	Brachycephaly, scaphocephaly, trigonocephaly, oxycephaly, plagiocephaly
Ears	Low set, small, large, malformed, protruding, posteriorly rotated, preauricular tags, cup-shaped
Skin	Dry and coarse, café-au-lait spots, abnormal pigmentation, hemangioma, ichthyosis, eczema, absence of sweating
Nose	Depressed nasal bridge, short and stubby, beak-shaped, bulbous tip, flaring or hypoplastic nostrils
Vision	Optic atrophy, refractive error, nyctalopia
Hearing	Partial or complete loss
Neck	Short, webbed, torticollis
Eyes	Deeply set, proptosis, microphthalmia, upslanting/downslanting eyes, telecanthus, hypertelorism, epicanthal folds, strabismus, nystagmus, ptosis, bushy eyebrows, synophrys, microcornea, corneal clouding, K-F ring, cataracts, coloboma of iris, blue sclera, telangiectasia
Palate	High arched, shallow, clefting, bifid uvula
Hair	Hirsutism, light colored, double whorl on scalp, easily breakable, low anterior/posterior hairline
Other facial features	Long/absent philtrum, micrognathia, sloping forehead
Hands	Simian crease, spade-shaped, small
Fingers	Clinodactyly, camptodactyly, arachnodactyly, short little finger, syndactyly, polydactyly, broad thumb
Chest	Pectus excavatum, pectus carinatum, nipple anomalies, gynecomastia, inverted nipples, cardiac problems
Abdomen	Protuberant, umbilical hernia, hepatosplenomegaly, inguinal hernia
Spine	Kyphosis, scoliosis, spina bifida
External genitalia	Hypogenitalism, macro-orchidism, undescended testis, ambiguous genitalia, hypospadias, absent secondary sexual characteristics, shawl scrotum
Feet	Pes Planus, Pes Cavus, Valgus/Varus anomaly, broad Hallux, increased distance between first and second toe
Skeletal	Exostoses, increase carrying angle, joint hypermobility

planned on case-to-case basis and include chromosomal analysis, fluorescent in situ hybridization (FISH), molecular genetic tests, biochemical tests such as screen for inborn metabolic disorders and TORCH screen.

- *Diagnostic formulation*: Diagnosis of DID should be based on a thorough

Table 21.4: List of common genetic syndromes associated with disorder of intellectual development (DID).

Syndrome	Key features
Down syndrome	Typical facies, short stature, medial slanting of eyes, clinodactyly, simian crease, cup-shape ears, cardiac problems
Fragile X syndrome	Elongated, triangular face, protruding/prominent ears, macro-orchidism in postpubertal boys
Rett syndrome	Normal development till around 1 year of age in a girl child followed by plateauing and regression, loss of hand functions, midline hand stereotypies
Cornelia de Lange syndrome	Hirsutism, long eye-lashes, synophrys, bushy eyebrows, microcephaly, flat philtrum
Prader–Willi syndrome	Obesity, hypogenitalism, small hands and feet
Tuberous sclerosis	Sebaceous adenomas, ash-leaf spots, shagreen patches, seizures
Congenital hypothyroidism	Lethargy, growth failure, coarse and dry skin, constipation, feeding problems, protuberant abdomen, bradycardia
Mucopolysaccharidoses	Typical facies, coarse skin, skeletal anomalies, macrocephaly
Homocystinuria	Marfanoid features, behavioral changes
Phenylketonuria	Light-colored hair, abnormal smell of urine, microcephaly, seizures
Autosomal recessive microcephaly	Severe congenital microcephaly with only mild to moderate DID, no other anomalies
Rubinstein Taybi syndrome	Prominent beak-shaped nose, broad thumb and hallux

clinical evaluation. Once a diagnosis of DID is made, the clinician must ascertain the severity of DID based on clinical estimation of mental age. Estimated mental age has to be divided by chronological age and then multiplied by 100 to yield a rough estimate of IQ. The IQ needs to be confirmed by psychological testing. Care must be taken while evaluating persons with mild degree of DID, as errors in either overdiagnosis or underdiagnosis may happen. Individuals with borderline intelligence (IQ between 70 and 85) should not be labeled as having DID.

Persons with cerebral palsy, psychiatric disorders like psychosis and severe depression, visual/hearing impairment, specific language delay, autism spectrum disorder, and specific learning disability with normal intellectual functioning may be erroneously diagnosed as having DID. However, these conditions may occur as comorbidities with DID and it is important not to miss the diagnosis of comorbidities. A comprehensive diagnosis should include information about degree of DID, causative factors, comorbid medical and psychiatric problems, and relevant psychosocial factors such as parents' level of awareness, attitudes, stress in the family, and problems in parenting such as overprotection and permissive parenting.

MANAGEMENT

By its nature, DID is developmental in origin and leads to life-long impairments. There is no evidence supporting use of medications in "improving intelligence". However, a variety of interventions can help in development and well-being of individuals with DID, better adaptation within the families looking after them, and building a society that is conducive to the well-being of these individuals and their families. Ideally, a multidisciplinary team approach is needed for management. Key aspects are described below:

Key Principles in Management

These include a rights-based inclusive approach, home-based family care with parents as partners in care, and early detection and intervention.

- *Rights-based inclusive approach*: From a rights-based perspective, every person with DID has a right to live with respect and dignity and to freely exercise their choices. The society at large has a responsibility in providing such an environment conducive to the holistic development and well-being of persons with DID. Inclusive approach means that they are considered very much part of mainstream society and not excluded or discriminated or stigmatized. Every effort needs to be made to ensure that they get the same opportunities to learn, develop, participate, and work.
- *Home-based family care*: The concept of home-based family care with parents as partners is a key principle of management especially in the LAMIC where there are huge gaps in the multidisciplinary professional resources required for the effective management of DID. The clinician has to actively collaborate with the parents right from the first consultation and eventually empower them to take up the role of effective cotherapists in providing intervention.
- *Early detection and intervention*: Research studies in animal models and humans have clearly shown that early intervention

by providing adequate stimulation to the brain helps in fostering the development of children with developmental delay and those "at risk" including premature infants, those with low birth weight, neonatal hypoxic ischemic encephalopathy, neonatal septicemia, and other brain insults. Such early intervention capitalizes on neural plasticity (capacity of the brain to change and reorganize itself) and experience-dependent learning, which is maximal in early years of life.

It is often seen that parents may detect developmental delay in their children, but are not aware of the need for intervention or do not have access to professionals providing the required evaluation and intervention. In most of the LAMIC, the screening of developmental deficits in infants and toddlers is not done in a systematic manner. Except motor development, the other areas (cognitive, language, social) are largely ignored. An alert and aware clinician can detect early developmental delays and initiate early intervention and help the child to develop well.

Medical Management

These include treatment of underlying causes, management of comorbid disorders, and genetic counseling. They are briefly described below:

- *Treatment of underlying causes*: Potentially treatable conditions such as phenylketonuria, homocystinuria, and other neurometabolic disorders, and hypothyroidism, if detected, can be managed. Recently, novel treatments such as enzyme replacement therapy, gene therapy and stem cell therapy have emerged for the management of a few inherited metabolic disorders.

- *Pharmacotherapy for comorbid disorders*: Psychotropic medication like antipsychotics, antidepressants, anxiolytics, and mood stabilizers are required in the management of comorbid psychiatric disorders. Neurological disorders such as epilepsy and the other medical conditions also require management by medication. Caution must be exercised while prescribing these medications. Consent of parents has to be obtained prior to starting any medication. Medication must always be started at a low dose and subsequently increased if needed on an individual basis. Children with DID are sensitive to the adverse effects of medication. Regular follow-up while on medication needs to be ensured. Medication per se does not improve the intellectual functioning and adaptive behavior of a person with DID. Use of pharmacotherapy should always be done in combination with psychosocial intervention to obtain optimum and sustained improvement.
- *Genetic counseling*: Prospective parents, especially couples who already have a child with DID are keen to know the risk of their next child being affected. Professional advice to such parents may help them to make informed decisions about having the next child. Such genetic counseling could be as simple as telling parents who have a child with DID caused by postnatal neuroinfection that the risk for their next child is very low or it could be a very complicated process needing several expensive investigations when a genetic cause is suspected. Recently, there have been rapid advances in the field of genetics that are relevant to diagnosis, prevention, and management of genetic disorders that cause DID. A new set of molecular genetics techniques such as array CGH and exome sequencing have evolved, that are able to identify genetic deviations and help parents to take informed reproductive decisions.

Psychosocial Management

The key components of psychosocial management include psychoeducation of parents, addressing caregiver stress, early intervention, education, and skills training and behavioral modification.

- *Psychoeducation*: Psychoeducation starts from the time of initial contact with the family for history taking. The clinician should first elicit the understanding of the parents in a nonjudgmental manner. Adequate amount of time has to be provided for open discussion about the understanding of the parents. Myths and misconceptions, if any, have to be addressed. Common myths and misconceptions about DID include notions such as DID is always heritable, children with DID become completely normal when they grow up to be adults, marriage can cure DID, medications can cure DID, and persons with DID are dangerous as they do not have control over their behavior.

  Parents should be provided clear information about DID being an NDD and about the possible causative factors. Psychoeducation materials prepared in the language that parents understand are very useful. Counseling individuals with DID also needs to be done wherever necessary.
- *Addressing caregiver stress and empowering parents*: DID causes enormous caregiver stress in parents. Once a diagnosis of DID is made by the clinician and parents are educated about the same, most parents go through a difficult

phase with feelings of shock, disbelief, disappointment, anger, guilt, misery, helplessness, and worry about their child's future. A diagnosis of DID impacts several aspects of family life such as daily care demands, psychological impact on parents (such as depression, anxiety), interpersonal difficulties between parents, financial difficulties, and adverse social consequences (such as social isolation and stigmatization). Counseling would include providing psychological support, allowing parents to ventilate, giving practical tips to manage the child, and teaching them coping skills. Parents are also encouraged to become members of parent associations.

- *Early intervention*: This is the systematic teaching of skills and competencies so that the child starts acquiring developmental milestones that he or she is lagging in. It is done through a mutually enjoyable parent–child interaction. Parents are taught how to engage with child, observe the child's responses and respond/reinforce the child's responses so that child learns new activities. Children are taught how to use their sensory and motor organs (sensory-motor stimulation), learn concepts of physical characteristics of objects, time, space (cognitive stimulation), speech/language/communication, and how to take care of themselves (self-help skills)? In addition, physiotherapy and occupational therapy are useful to improve child's functioning.
- *Education:* Children with DID have a right to education and must attend schools as far as possible. This will enhance not only their academic skills but helps in social inclusion and social learning. Government of India has a special program for inclusion of children with special needs called Sarva Shiksha Abhiyan (SSA).

Depending on the availability and nature of child's problems, education can occur in inclusion settings (regular schools) or in special schools.

- *Skills training*: For older children and adolescents, the focus is usually on self-help skills, social skills, self-protection skills, skills of domestic work, mobility, transport, shopping, and prevocational skills. The nature of training inputs depends on the child's age, degree of DID, and the assets and liabilities in the child. It is important to train all family members so that each one can provide the inputs during the available time with their children. Adults require vocational training and job placement.
- *Behavior modification techniques*: Behavioral modification is an effective method to develop/inculcate new skills and to reduce the severity of behavioral problems. Behavioral modification is based on principles of learning such as conditioning and social learning. The techniques of behavioral modification for skills training include goal specification, task analysis, modeling, shaping, chaining and prompting and rewarding appropriate behaviors. Techniques used for reducing problem behavior frequency and/or intensity include disregarding, ignoring, time out, differential reinforcement of other behavior, blocking, limit setting, and gradual guidance.
- *Life-span issues*: Individuals with DID and their families face different challenges at different phases of life. For instance, emerging sexuality and behavioral issues are common issues in adolescence; whereas work, marriage, meaningful daily routine, and guardianship are common issues in adulthood. A helpful clinician can make a major difference to them in facing these challenges.

Relevant legislations: Government of India has passed Rights of Persons with Disabilities Act to ensure equal rights and opportunities for persons with DID. Another important institution is National Trust for Persons with Mental Retardation, Cerebral Palsy, Autism and Multiple Disabilities set up under National Trust Act. Many social security measures such as disability pension, job reservations, and travel/income tax concessions have been introduced.

PREVENTION OF DISORDER OF INTELLECTUAL DEVELOPMENT

It is possible to reduce the incidence and prevalence of DID and also limit its severity and the consequent disability by a series of public health and social measures. These can be conceptualized as levels of prevention proposed by World Health Organization, and is presented in **Table 21.5**.

Level	Approach	Example of steps
Primary prevention (preventing the occurrence of DID)	Health promotion	Health education, especially for adolescent girls
		Improvement of nutritional status in community
		Optimum healthcare facilities
		Optimal pre, peri and postnatal care
	Specific protection	Universal iodization of salt
		Rubella immunization for women before pregnancy
		Folic acid administration in early pregnancy
		Genetic counseling
		Prenatal screening for congenital malformations and genetic disorders
		Detection and care for high-risk pregnancies
		Preventing Rh isoimmunization
		Universal immunization for children
Secondary prevention (halting disease progression)	Early diagnosis and treatment	Neonatal screening for treatable disorders such as phenylketonuria, and congenital hypothyroidism
		Intervention with "at risk" babies
		Early detection and intervention of developmental delay
Tertiary prevention (preventing complications and maximization of functions)	Disability limitation and rehabilitation	Speech and language therapy, occupational therapy, physiotherapy, education, skills training, vocational training, treatment of comorbid disorders
		Inclusion and mainstreaming
		Support for families
		Parental self-help groups
		Social security for individuals and families

Table 21.5: Prevention of disorder of intellectual development (DID).

CONCLUSION

Disorder of intellectual development is a common NDD caused by diverse etiologies and results in significant impairment of affected person's functioning. Clinicians need to be well versed with developmental history taking, behavioral examination, mental status evaluation, and physical examination for the diagnosis and management of DID and its comorbid disorders.

TAKE-HOME MESSAGES

- Disorder of intellectual development is a neurodevelopmental disorder characterized by significant impairments in intellectual and general adaptive development, usually from early childhood.
- In terms of severity, it is categorized as mild (IQ 50–69), moderate (IQ 35–49), severe (IQ 20–34), and profound (IQ <20)
- It may be caused by a large number of both genetic and environmental factors that adversely affect brain development and maturation in pre, peri or postnatal developmental periods.
- It is often associated with other neurodevelopmental disorders, various medical disorders as well as behavioral and emotional problems.
- Management includes parental psycho-education and empowerment, early detection and intervention, treatment of underlying and associated disorders, education, skills training, prevocational and vocational training of the affected person, and social security measures.
- A clinician who is knowledgeable, skillful, and capable of instilling hope and optimism can make big difference to these individuals and families.

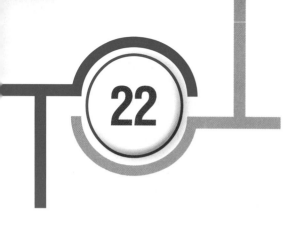

22

Geriatric Mental Health

Om Prakash, Amit Khanna

INTRODUCTION

One of the most perplexing clinical challenges that young medical graduates face is the situation when they have to deal with the elderly, especially those presenting with mental and behavioral symptoms. Elderly patients most often present with comorbid medical illnesses which color and modify the presentation of psychiatric disorder in them. To complicate the clinical situation further, a substantial proportion of this age group presenting to the hospital have history of neglect, physical abuse, and abandonment by their own family members.

Trainee doctors will find it difficult to solve this conundrum of old-age issues in the absence of specific knowledge related to the psyche of elderly, physiological changes in old-age, and the common neuropsychiatric maladies in this vulnerable population. With the increasing patient load, limited time of clinicians and "defensive" psychiatric practices of resorting to neuroimaging at the earliest, the art and skill of history taking and mental status examination especially in the elderly has suffered and needs to be revived. Young doctors need to know that there is no replacement for a good history and examination and one should not give into the pressures of modern technology. Some common difficulties encountered by young clinicians in dealing with the elderly during

Box 22.1: Common difficulties encountered by clinicians in the course of history taking of elderly persons.

- Doctors should not give in to patient's explanations of a given set of problems such as "I guess I am Old", or "People at my age become slow"
- Age-specific normal physiological changes may be perceived to be abnormal by the patient
- Difficulty in expression during old age and in understanding the advice of the clinician may fluster the doctor who rushes the interview
- Exhaustive list of problems presented by the elderly patients can often cause the clinician to lose his patience
- Forgetting past medical/psychiatric events can result in difficulty in establishing a diagnosis
- Elderly persons with a disordered personality type or dementia patients can get agitated on detailed probing by the clinician
- Difficulty in sharing sexual history and changes in sexual activity out of shame when it may be of primary importance
- Need to interview many family members can result in the clinicians exhaustion compromising the ability to isolate the problem
- Inexperience in dealing with the family and mobilizing psychosocial support systems of the elderly
- Young clinician being "written off" by the elderly patient citing age and experience can result in difficulty in rapport formation

initial stages of assessment are given in **Box 22.1**.

Almost all clinicians have experienced the above-mentioned difficulties during the course of their training. The trainee doctor should be honest in informing the patient, the specific need to elicit the information and prevent rushing the interview or turning it into a mechanical exercise. The doctor may take help of a senior colleague in dealing with difficult patients. This chapter attempts to provide general overview of geriatric mental health issues, of care, treatment and management in the elderly.

PSYCHOLOGICAL ASPECTS IN THE GERIATRIC AGE

Perhaps the most well-understood psychological theories of human development, i.e., Eric Eriksons' theory of personality development, divide human development into eight stages and the 8th stage of *Integrity versus Despair* is the hallmark of the aged population. Trainee doctor should always keep in mind that a failure to master each step can lead to difficulties later. Final stage of Erikson begins by 60 or after 65 years following retirement, death of spouse or a major life event. During this stage, old age persons would like to analyze their own life and how they have treated it and vice versa. If they get a sense of satisfaction in what they have done, it results into integration of the ego; else it can lead to a sense of utter despair.

There is enough evidence available to suggest that old persons who have made plans preretirement are better adjusted postretirement. Similarly, there is higher incidence of depression in the elderly following death of spouse. Although an arduous task, trainee doctors need to approach the elderly patients with a psychological bent of mind and attempt to resolve their conflicts for better adjustment.

The Seattle Longitudinal Study (SLS) investigated the decline in intellectual and cognitive abilities in multiple cohorts between 18 and 88 years and found that noticeable decline in the cognitive abilities of the elderly

begins to occur between 60–70 years and by 80 years is actually half that of young people. As one ages, the total body water content decreases, fat content increases, there is gross brain atrophy with ventricular enlargement and decline in cerebral blood flow. These changes must be born in mind as it may predispose the elderly to drug toxicities.

EPIDEMIOLOGY OF GERIATRIC MENTAL HEALTH DISORDERS

There is genuinely a great need of epidemiological studies in the elderly population across the globe. Multicentric studies on noninstitutionalized patients with a large sample size which may be nationally representative are far and few in the elderly population. Among psychiatric disorders in this population, anxiety disorders are commonly found in community samples followed by depression and cognitive disorders.

Hospital studies from India found the highest percentages for mood disorders (mainly depression) up to 26% followed by mild cognitive impairment (15%), substance use disorders (4.5%), and dementia (3.4%). The overall prevalence of psychiatric morbidity in the elderly in urban settings is 13–49% and in the rural areas is 27–43%. The prevalence of psychiatric morbidity is found higher in in-patient settings, both psychiatric and nonpsychiatric facilities, and still higher in old-age homes. It is noteworthy to mention that among the medically ill elderly attending hospital clinics in India, as high as 50% have hypertension, 15% osteoarthritis, 13% diabetes, and 8% constipation. In this category, roughly 18% had depression and 11% other diagnosable psychiatric disorders. Some of these common mental health issues of relevance to the medical undergraduates have been briefly described in the next section.

COMMON PSYCHIATRIC AND NEUROBEHAVIORAL SYNDROMES IN THE ELDERLY

Depression

By now most of the researches across the globe are in accord with the fact that the most common mental health issue in the geriatric age group is depression. Epidemiological studies although few in number in this age group report that 4% of the older adults above 60 years suffer from major depressive disorder, although a significant number (27%) report depressive symptoms. Various subtypes of depression that may be seen in elderly are given in **Box 22.2**.

It is often difficult for a young medical graduate to fathom depressive symptoms in the elderly mistaking it for normative behavior in the old age. Such patients may report persistent sadness of mood, loss of interest in pleasurable activities, religious activities, loss of energy and drive, cognitive impairment, loss of sleep and appetite and sexual drive which is commonly not explored by the trainee having feeling that it may be culturally inappropriate to do so, and hence ignored in the elderly. To be able to differentiate these changes from normative findings in the old age, one needs to look for functional loss in the patient. If either of these complaints has become a reason for distress, discomfort or concern for the elderly, then it needs to be addressed. Major concern in the elderly appears to be presence of suicidal

ideation. It is important to ask explicitly from these patients about death and suicidal thoughts because in contrast to depression in young adults, elderly less often report suicidal ideas but are more likely to commit suicide. It is for this reason that behavioral observation report from significant family members is essential and the slightest hint toward suicidality must not be missed. The various facets of depression in the elderly range from merely experiencing transient stress related depressive symptoms to full blown depressive disorder and bipolar disorder.

All these possibilities of a depressive spectrum must be kept in mind when doing an assessment of a depressed geriatric patient. As mentioned above, memory problems in depression can compel the young trainees to entertain a diagnosis of dementia, and hence the term "Pseudo dementia" is also used for depression in the elderly with prominent cognitive symptoms. On the contrary, 50% of dementia patients may have depressive manifestations, and hence a thorough neurological examination, including a detailed higher mental function assessment cannot be understated in the elderly.

Bipolar Disorder

The Epidemiological Catchment Area (ECA) study found low prevalence (up to 0.5%) of bipolar in those above 65 years in comparison to 1.4% in the young adults and 0.4% in the middle aged adults. In comparison to bipolar illness in young adults, the episodes are more severe and disabling with a propensity toward rapid cycling or mixed manic states. Further, there may be significant residual psychopathology, high relapse rates, and high mortality. Comorbid medical and neurological insults such as stroke can complicate the clinical presentation and make management difficult.

Box 22.2: The subtypes of depression in late life.

- Subsyndromal depression
- Bereavement
- Adjustment disorder with depressed mood
- Dysthymia
- Depressive disorder with or without psychotic symptoms
- Bipolar disorder
- Depression associated with medical illness

> **Box 22.3:** Clinical presentations of elderly bipolars.
>
> - Those diagnosed with early onset bipolar disorder and have reached old age
> - Previously experienced a depressive episode and now developed a manic episode
> - Late onset manic episode in the background of a medical/neurological disorder
> - Those diagnosed with bipolar disorder but previously misdiagnosed with another disorder
> - Late onset mania with no underlying medical/neurological cause

Some earlier studies attempted to distinguish between early onset (adolescence to young adults) bipolar disorder and late onset bipolar disorder (between 30 and 50 years). From a clinical viewpoint, the delineation has relevance in terms of clinical presentation. Most cases of bipolar disorder that a young trainee may see in the geriatric clinics are likely to fall in the five categories as mentioned in **Box 22.3**.

It is prudent to categorize elderly bipolar patients in this manner for ease in decision making for treatment and management. Research evidence suggests that mania in the elderly is characterized by presence of psychotic symptoms and cognitive symptoms more often than seen in depression in the elderly, thus making treatment of mania equally difficult in this age group.

Schizophrenia and Other Psychotic Disorders

It may be of some interest to know that Sir Issac Newton too had suffered a psychotic breakdown at the age of 51 years for the first time during which he had paranoid ideation and self-withdrawn behavior. Schizophrenia and other psychotic disorders are not so uncommon in the elderly as commonly thought and evidenced by history. Although accurate data on prevalence is unavailable because of methodological differences across studies but it is believed that about 13% of schizophrenia patients have onset of their illness in the fifth decade and about 7% have onset in the seventh decade. The most common feature of late-onset schizophrenia is persecutory delusions along with auditory hallucinations. Negative symptoms are less common in this age group and psychosis responds to lower dosages of antipsychotics. Caution needs to be exercised in this age group. Medical causes such as electrolyte disturbances, cerebrovascular insults and degenerative illnesses need to be ruled out before prematurely diagnosing the patient with schizophrenia or other psychotic disorder.

Substance Use Disorders in the Elderly

Substance use disorders in the elderly were perhaps unheard of 30–40 years ago, but with the improvement in healthcare services and longer life-spans, it is not unexpected that a substantial percentage of elderly population would have issues related to drug and alcohol use. Alcohol seems to be the most common drug of abuse (85%) in the elderly population followed by benzodiazepines and prescription drug abuse. Alcohol can have significant health impact affecting majorly the central nervous, gastrointestinal, and hepatobiliary systems. Psychiatric manifestations range from anxiety and depressive symptoms, sleep disturbances, cognitive disturbances, confusional, and hallucinatory states. For this reason, trainee must ask the pattern of use of alcohol and other substances even in the elderly population. The *CAGE* questionnaire **(Box 22.4)** is relevant for screening in the elderly as much as it is in adults. Other tools such as the Short Michigan Alcohol Screening Test (Geriatric version) have also been

Box 22.4: CAGE questionnaire.

- *Cut down*—have you ever felt the need to cut down on your drinking?
- *Annoyed*—have people annoyed you by criticizing your drinking?
- *Guilt*—have you ever felt guilty about your drinking?
- *Eye opener*—have you ever felt you needed a drink first thing in the morning to steady your nerves or to get rid of a hangover?

developed for use in the elderly population which may be useful in clinical practice.

Dementia and Other Neurocognitive Disorders

The term "Neurocognitive" refers to all such clinical conditions where the hallmark is decline in cognitive functioning which is acquired and not developmental in nature. The most common clinical syndrome in this category is dementia. Alois Alzheimer, a psychiatrist and a neuropathologist, was the first person who published in 1907 the description of a typical case of dementia, while recording his observations made on a patient named Auguste Deter at Frankfurt's State Asylum. This condition was later given the label of Alzheimer's disease by another famous psychiatrist and his colleague, Emil Kraepelin. The diagnosis of dementia is based on evidence of involvement of several areas of cognition, i.e. amnesia along with aphasia, apraxia and/or agnosia; and a thorough history and examination is therefore required in making a clinical diagnosis. According to the current estimates, more than 4.3 million people in India are living with dementia which is projected to increase to 14.3 million by 2050. Globally, 5% of the elderly above 65 years of age have dementia. More than 50% of all cases of dementia are of Alzheimer's type.

Patients with Alzheimer's dementia typically presents with progressive forgetfulness, i.e., inability to remember what they had eaten in the morning or at night, loosing himself in the neighborhood, difficulty remembering names of relatives and of objects and word substitution. On formal higher mental status testing, there is usually deficit in immediate and recent memory wherein recall of names after 5 minutes is also impaired. It is important to mention here that these deficits comprise what is called as anterograde amnesia and only in the later stages of the disease does the patient develop retrograde amnesia. It is possible that these patients may continue to remain very good at tasks involving "habitual" memory such as playing a musical instrument, driving a cycle or a car, as only declarative memory is affected and procedural memory remains unimpaired. But this should not deter one from considering a diagnosis of dementia.

Alzheimer's Dementia/Dementia of Alzheimer's Type (DAT)

Alzheimer's dementia has been clinically graded into mild, moderate and severe categories. In mild forms, early cognitive deficits are common like inability to name objects, language difficulties, etc. As the disease progresses, there is worsening of cognitive deficits with aphasia, apraxia and agnosia. Classic *"Mirror"* sign has been described in these patients who fail to recognize themselves when they look at themselves in the mirror. In the final stages of the disease, the patients become doubly incontinent and vegetative, speech may be jargon in nature and there is a higher propensity to develop delirium. Often delirium may be superimposed on dementia making the clinical picture more complex. Because of degeneration in several areas of the brain, behavioral and psychological symptoms of dementia (BPSD) **(Box 22.5)**

Box 22.5: Behavioral and psychological symptoms of dementia (BPSD).

- Affective and motivation symptoms such as irritability, apathy, depression, and anxiety
- Thought and perceptual disturbance such as delusions and hallucinations
- Disturbances of basic drives, including sleep, sexual functions, and feeding
- Socially inappropriate and disinhibited behavior

and neurological symptoms such as gait disturbance, seizures, and incontinence may also emerge. Incidentally, Alzheimer's first case, Auguste Deter presented to him with delusion of jealousy regarding her husband; hence one should be aware of the spectrum of behavioral and psychological symptoms of dementia, else there is a high chance that such findings may be missed. Alzheimer's dementia needs to be distinguished from other forms of dementia in the elderly.

Vascular Dementias

Cardiovascular morbidity is one of the most leading causes of death and disability in the elderly across the globe. Often in the evaluation of an elderly with cognitive deficits, there may be history of hypertension, diabetes, myocardial infarction and stroke. This needs to be given precedence in the assessment of dementia. Broadly for simplification for medical trainees, vascular dementias classically have a *"step-ladder"* pattern of progression. The patients remain in a stage of clinical plateau for a substantial but variable period of time and then have worsening of symptoms following another cerebrovascular event. It is largely of three types:

1. *Multi-infarct dementia* where more than one region of the brain is involved following a large cortical or subcortical bleed.
2. *Lacunar dementia* characterized by a lacunar syndrome specific to the region of the brain involved.

3. *Binswanger's disease* or "white matter disease" characterized by micro-angiopathy. In view of the involvement of white matter (subcortical areas), there is more executive function loss along with cognitive loss.

Lewy Body Dementia

This clinical subtype of dementia was first described by Okazaki in 1961. The onset of Lewy body dementia (LBD) is gradual and usually in the seventh decade. Patients either present with dementia or with Parkinsonism and in the terminal stages an admixture of the two. The hallmark of dementia of Lewy body is frequent episodes of delirium and early onset hallucinations or delusions. More than half of the patients have fluctuations in consciousness lasting for hours to days without any apparent precipitating factor. Reality distortions (delusions and hallucinations) are seen in two-thirds of all cases and tend to be visual or complex in nature. Delusions of persecution and misidentification symptoms may be present in some cases.

In the Parkinsonian variant of LBD, although the presentation is similar to Parkinson's disease with tremors, rigidity and bradykinesia but there is a symmetric onset and less tremors, in addition, myoclonus may be present in LBD, which is rare in Parkinson's disease. These patients display an abnormal "neuroleptic sensitivity" and tend to worsen with antipsychotics. REM sleep behavioral disorders are also frequently present years before the onset of LBD, and these patients tend to "enact their dreams".

Pick's Disease

The onset of Pick's disease is between 40 and 70 years of age, although younger onset is also known. Pick's disease has been known for over a century and classically presents with changes in personality. Patients with the disease are disinhibited and have motor or verbal perseveration. Memory impairment and aphasia is a late feature unlike Alzheimer's dementia. Interestingly, neuroimaging studies reveal gross frontal and temporal atrophy, often frontal more than temporal.

Frontotemporal Dementia

Historically, Pick's disease was considered a subtype of frontotemporal dementia (FTD) but subsequent researches have attempted to distinguish the two for clinical and nosological clarity. FTD accounts for majority of cases of dementia below 65 years of age. However, the age range varies from fourth to eight decade. There are three clinical variants of FTD namely, (1) FTD, personality change variant, the most common presentation; (2) semantic dementia; and (3) progressive nonfluent aphasia.

Although in clinical practice, there is usually an admixture of symptoms but it is also true that a mixture of the three variants is also seen in the terminal stages of the illness. The personality changes in FTD are of primarily two types, the frontal variant typically presents with frontal lobe syndrome, i.e., with disinhibition, lack of empathy, poor self-care, mood changes, utilization behavior also called *environmental dependency syndrome* may be seen in 80% of the cases, wherein the patients are compelled to pick up and "utilize" objects in the immediate environment as if they have lost their autonomy and are dependent on the environment.

The temporal variant of FTD is characterized by repetitive nongoal-directed activities called "stereotypies" which may manifest in the form of clapping, clicking, counting, hoarding, etc. These patients may have ritualized behaviors, mental inflexibility and follow strict patterns in diet, routes, ideas or opinions. In a small fraction, hyperphagia, hyperorality, hypersexuality, and abnormal placidity (Kluber-Bucy symptoms) may be found. However, irrespective of the variant, almost all patients have an absence of insight into their behavioral oddities.

Patients with semantic dementia may have loss for words for common objects and may often be confused with Alzheimer's dementia. In contrast to the sensory aphasia in Alzheimer's disease, patients with FTD have progressive nonfluent aphasia and find it difficult to initiate speech. Among all types of dementia, FTD is the most lethal and patients progress to death in 5–10 years' time.

MANAGEMENT OF GERIATRIC MENTAL HEALTH DISORDERS

When a geriatric patient presents to the emergency or outpatient setting, medical trainee must learn the process of approach for handling such case. It must be remembered like in most other cases, more so in the elderly age group, that the doctor must have a biopsychosocial approach to treatment and care. During the process of history taking and physical and mental status examination, it is imperative that specific issues related to the medical problems are addressed along with psychological and social issues for effective and holistic management. Necessary investigations must be sent at the earliest with a caution not to subject the elderly to undue discomfort. Adequate time and analysis must go into history taking and examination and formulation of the case.

In the era of modern science, the geriatricians and medical practitioners have a range of options to choose from depending on their suitability for the patient. However, due to physiological changes in old age, the drugs need to be chosen with great caution as the elderly are very prone to develop side effects. As a general rule, the clinician must follow the principle of starting low and going slow; hence, any medication must be administered in half the dose than that for an adult. The clinician must be familiar with drug–drug interactions as it is common to find elderly patients on medications prescribed for treatment of other medical disorders. Despite these challenges, treatment of geriatric mental health issues provides a huge relief to the caregivers in terms of reducing the burden of care.

Pharmacological Interventions

There is enough evidence to support the use of selective serotonin reuptake inhibitor (SSRI) in the elderly. Citalopram, escitalopram, and sertraline are preferred over fluoxetine and paroxetine because they are safer and well tolerated. They are used for treatment of depression, anxiety disorders, aggression, and for behavioral problems in patients of dementia. It is important to monitor electrolytes in these patients on SSRI's as they have a propensity to cause syndrome of inappropriate secretion of antidiuretic hormone (SIADH) resulting in hyponatremia and its associated complications. SSRIs also affect platelet activation, and hence increase the risk of gastrointestinal bleeding or postsurgical bleeding. It must also be given cautiously in patients receiving nonsteroidal anti-inflammatory drugs (NSAIDs) and/or aspirin.

There is an evidence to support use of venlafaxine, duloxetine, bupropion and mirtazepine but they are not the first line of treatment in the elderly for their respective indications. Particularly, venlafaxine must be avoided in the elderly with hypertension because of its propensity to cause dose-dependent escalation of blood pressure. Among the tricyclic antidepressants (TCAs), which are less often prescribed in the elderly chiefly because of their anticholinergic side effects, the safer ones are nortriptyline and desipramine. SSRIs because of their safety profile have replaced TCAs and monoamine oxidase (MAO) inhibitors in the treatment of depression and anxiety disorders. The use of psychostimulants such as methylphenidate has little support in geriatric patients and should not be used for patients reporting attention deficits, apathy, etc.

For treatment of psychotic symptoms in depression or independent psychotic states, atypical antipsychotics are preferred over typical antipsychotics primarily because of higher side effects with the latter. Geriatricians prefer quetiapine because of its sedative effect and safety profile in comparison to risperidone and olanzapine. Clozapine use in the elderly is limited by its serious side effects and requirements for monitoring and should therefore be preferably avoided. Anticholinergic side effects (such as urinary retention, cognitive dysfunction and delirium), antihistaminic (sedation), and antiadrenergic side effects (postural hypotension) of various psychotropics are particularly disabling and can lead to falls and fractures. In some cases with issues of intermittent noncompliance to medications, long acting injectables can also be used, which can help in reducing the oral dosages of the psychotropic medications. Typical antipsychotics are used with caution because of risk of development of extrapyramidal syndrome and neuroleptic malignant syndrome.

Mood stabilizers are the first line of treatment in the management of bipolar disorders. Most of the researches are available on lithium, valproate, and carbamazepine. Although, the efficacy of lithium in the elderly has been substantiated across different studies but the use in clinical practice gets limited due to its side effects. Lithium should be monitored properly by frequent measurements of morning blood sample. Valproate has been found to be safe and effective in the elderly, however some caution needs to be exerted as it can cause thrombocytopenia and hepatic enzyme derangements. Carbamazepine is less often used in this age group as it may lead to drug-induced leukopenia, agranulocytosis and ataxia which can be very problematic in the elderly. Of the newer anticonvulsants, lamotrigine has been found to be more effective than placebo in bipolar disorder-prophylaxis; however there is risk of developing severe and at times fatal rash. Gabapentin and pregabalin have not been systematically studied in the elderly.

The use of benzodiazepines should be avoided in the elderly as it causes sedation, falls, and cognitive impairment. Nonbenzodiazepines drugs such as zolpidem may be used but in low dosages.

Cognitive enhancers which include cholinesterase inhibitors (donepezil, rivastigmine and galantamine) and NMDA (N-methyl-D-aspartate) receptor antagonist (memantine) have shown modest evidence toward improving cognitions and preventing cognitive decline and are often recommended in all the clinical stages of dementia with some exceptions.

The use of electroconvulsive therapy (ECT) in old age, contrary to popular belief even among medical practitioners is rather safe and effective. ECT is the first line of treatment in severe depression with suicide risk, acute schizophrenic episode, and catatonia with inanition. Geriatric patients with comorbid Parkinson's disease can also be safely administered ECTs. However, if one is involved in the care of an elderly who has been administered ECTs, then the higher mental functions must be monitored before and after each ECT as it can cause transient anterograde and retrograde amnesia. Newer intervention techniques such as repetitive transcranial magnetic stimulation (rTMS) have not been systematically studied in the elderly population.

Nonpharmacological Interventions

The basics of psychotherapy hold true for this age group of patients as well, i.e., the therapist should have an unconditional positive regard for the patient with a noncondemning and noncritical attitude. There should be trust and confidentiality, empathy, and genuineness. The standard therapies used in adult population have been slightly modified for the elderly population. A young medical trainee may find useful, certain elements of at least two specific therapies in dealing with an elderly client namely supportive psychotherapy and cognitive behavioral therapy. In supportive therapy, the patient is allowed to ventilate his feelings and receives comfort from the therapist in terms of being heard, reassured and guided wherever necessary and goes a long way in instilling hope for the future. In other therapy called "Life Review and Reminiscence Psychotherapy", the patient is encouraged to reflect upon his life and deduce a meaning of his life. For systematic and structured psychotherapies, the patient should be referred to a clinical psychologist or psychiatrist.

Occupational therapy interventions can enhance adaptability of elderly patients to new environments, increase independence in skilled tasks, and improve the overall quality of life of such persons. The basic strategies adopted in occupational therapy include assessment of the difficulties of the person, breaking the task into easy, small and understandable steps, as in early stages attention and concentration difficulties are common. Patients are first made competent in establishing their activities of daily living such as bathing, washing, wearing clothes, eating and structuring their daily routine. In case the person has difficulty remembering, an aid such as a diary or a smart phone alarm may be used to assist the person. Attempts to understand difficulties in communication with others and problems in social engagement can be addressed by involving the person in group activities on outpatient basis. Some patients with dementia have fear of fall and occupational therapy intervention can help prevent falls in the elderly thereby preventing disability due to injuries. The goal of occupational therapy is to achieve mastery over basic and specific skills for daily living and go a long way in prevention especially in patients with mild cognitive impairment.

Diet and lifestyle modifications also have immediate and long-term health benefits even in the elderly patients and must always be emphasized in the clinics. The services of a physiotherapist would need to be taken to improve mobility, decrease pain, and improve overall quality of life.

Home-based care by family members for the elderly holds meaning and utility for both urban and far off rural areas with poor access to mental health facilities. Often elderly patients especially those with severe dementia, only require supportive care by family members which is best done in a familiar environment such as home. Changes may need to be made in the home environment for comfort and safety of the elderly such as removing heavy furniture to prevent falls, locking door at night to prevent

wandering, putting calendars and improving the ambient light conditions in the room for proper orientation. All these comprise what is called as "Nidotherapy", i.e., the planned, systematic and collaborative change within the nest or home environment for care of the mentally ill. Medical trainees must not only be aware of this but also advocate it at their level to patients and their families.

POLICIES AND PROGRAMS FOR THE ELDERLY

There has been a paradigm shift in the family systems in India. Families have become more and more nuclear, young people both men and women are engaged for longer hours at work leaving the elderly relatively neglected and alone as opposed to a couple of decades back, when the closely knit ties of the joint family systems provided for healthy aging in terms of social support, social engagement, and medical care. Further, the elderly are subjected to physical, emotional abuse and neglect by their own kith and kin as is evidenced from the rising crime rates against elderly in the recent past. Perhaps, it is for this reason that more attention is now being given to the social depravity of the elderly population than in the past. The Government of India follows a multipronged approach to safeguard the interest of the elderly population. "Maintenance and Welfare of Parents and Senior Citizens Act, 2007" has been an important legislative step toward ensuring the protection of the elderly population especially by their children. Under this act, children (sons, daughters, grandchildren but not minors) are legally bound to provide maintenance (food, shelter, clothing, medical care needs) to the elderly parents. They have also been made liable for penalty on failure to provide maintenance.

Ministry of Social Justice and Empowerment has been implementing an

Box 22.6: Objectives of National Policy on Senior Citizens 2011.

- Promote the concept of "Aging in Place" or aging in own home, housing, income security and homecare services, old age pension and access to healthcare insurance schemes and other programs and services to facilitate and sustain dignity in old age
- Mainstream senior citizens, especially older women, and bring their concerns into the national development debate with priority to implement mechanisms already set by governments and supported by civil society and senior citizens' associations
- Support promotion and establishment of senior citizens' association, especially among women
- It recognizes institutional care of senior citizens as the last resort. It recognizes that care of senior citizens has to remain vested in the family which would partner the community, government and the private sector
- Long term savings instruments and credit activities will be promoted to reach both rural and urban areas. It will be necessary for the contributors to feel assured that the payments at the end of the stipulated period are attractive enough to take care of the likely erosion in purchasing power
- Being a signatory to the Madrid Plan of Action and Barrier Free Framework, it will work toward an inclusive, barrier-free and age friendly society
- Recognize that senior citizens are a valuable resource for the country and create an environment that provides them with equal opportunities, protect their rights and enable their full participation in society
- Toward achievement of this directive, the policy visualizes that the states will extend their support for senior citizens, living below the poverty line in urban and rural areas and ensures their social security, healthcare, shelter and welfare. It will protect them from abuse and exploitation so that the quality of their lives improves
- Employment in income generating activities after superannuation will be encouraged. All States will be advised to implement the Maintenance and Welfare of Parents and Senior Citizens Act, 2007 and set up Tribunals so that elderly parents unable to maintain themselves are not abandoned and neglected
- Support and assist organizations that provide counseling, career guidance and training services
- States will set up homes with assisted living facilities for abandoned senior citizens in every district of the country and there will be adequate budgetary support

"Integrated Program for Older Persons (IPOP)" since 1992 wherein the States have been mandated to regulate the functioning of old age homes, day care centers for Alzheimer's dementia and physiotherapy clinics for the elderly, through the NGO sector. As health is of utmost priority for the elderly, the Ministry of Health and Family Welfare launched "National Program for Healthcare for the Elderly (NPHCE)" in 2010. The program envisaged and encouraged strengthening of healthcare services at primary healthcare level, district hospitals and community centers with 10 bedded facilities meant exclusively for the elderly at district hospital level. Regional medical institutions were upgraded and equipped to provide dedicated tertiary medical care facilities for the elderly including postgraduation in geriatric psychiatry which has been started in KGMC (Lucknow) and NIMHANS (Bangalore). National policy on senior citizens was also framed in 2011 **(Box 22.6)**.

Other welfare programs of importance ensuring a safe and comfortable life for the elderly include Indira Gandhi National Old Age Pension scheme (IGNOAPS) under the National Social Assistance Program (NSAP) launched in 1995 by the Ministry of Rural Development. The pension amount for elderly is revised from time to time. Although, these schemes have brought about some relief for the elderly population but change is slow to come and requires commitment and dedication at all levels.

CONCLUSION

Geriatric mental health is a challenging field with a huge body of work already available; however a lot more needs to done to meet the prevailing challenges in this field. It is imperative that we identify the basics of geriatric mental health and orient undergraduates, both in medical and paramedical fields and thereby equip them to deal with all such cases within a biopsychosocial paradigm. Given the current scenario in India, it would be utopian to imagine holistic geriatric care, being available under one roof by a multidisciplinary team adequately equipped and trained to deal with geriatric mental health issues for all such patients. We need to go on improving services for the elderly and an important step towards that is to increase awareness about geriatric mental health issues at grass root levels of medical education **(Flowchart 22.1)**.

Flowchart 22.1: Illustrative flowchart for undergraduate medical students for management and care of elderly patients.

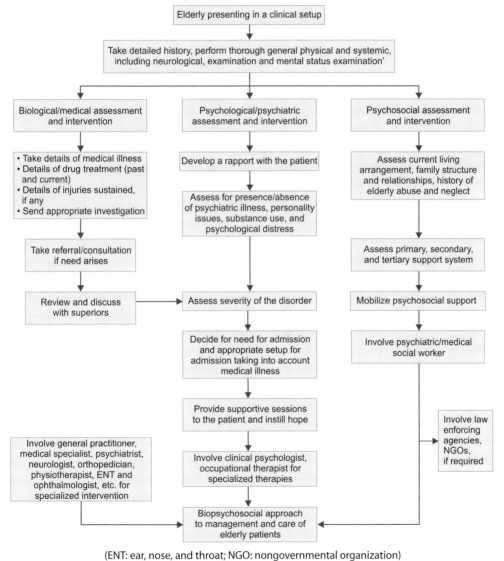

(ENT: ear, nose, and throat; NGO: nongovernmental organization)

Only when undergraduate medical trainees are imparted proper orientation and a sense of what geriatric mental health entails and know the magnitude of the problem, we can ever hope to have enough qualified professionals in our country who can work towards improving the quality of life of elderly patients and their family members.

TAKE-HOME MESSAGES

- Geriatric psychiatry is an emerging subspecialty in psychiatry, which encompasses all mental health-related issues of the elderly.
- The magnitude of geriatric mental health problems are immense and range from depression, bipolar disorder, schizophrenia, anxiety disorder, dementia, substance use disorders, sleep disorders, to mention a few. Alzheimer's disease accounts for about 50% cases of dementia.
- A biopsychosocial approach to treatment and care of geriatric patients is essential, inclusive of judicious and cautious use of indicated drugs, supportive psychotherapy, cognitive behavior therapy, occupational therapy, diet and lifestyle modification, optimization of the environment, "nidotherapy", etc.
- Treatment of elderly mentally ill persons requires multidisciplinary team approach which needs to be managed and led by a mental health expert.

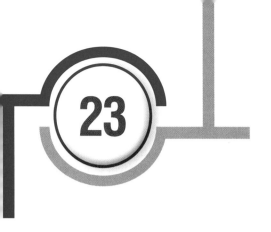

23

Consultation-Liaison Psychiatry

Swaminath G, Ajit V Bhide

INTRODUCTION

Consultation-liaison psychiatry (C-L psychiatry), or liaison psychiatry is a subspecialty of psychiatry concerned with the study, practice, and teaching of the interplay and relationship between physical and psychiatric disorders. Lipowski (1983), whose seminal work laid a foundation for this specialty, provided the definition, "Consultation-liaison psychiatry is a subspecialty of psychiatry that incorporates clinical service, teaching, and research at the borderland of psychiatry and medicine". This interface between psychiatry and other specialties usually takes place in a hospital or medical setting. Consultation occurs when the primary care team queries the psychiatric team about a patient's mental health or seeks to know how a patient's suffering is affecting his or her care in treatment. The liaison of the psychiatric team is between the patient and the medical team. Thorny issues such as fresh physical symptoms as a result of mental disorder or its treatment, conflicting problems in both physical and mental health, and capacity to consent to treatment and conflicts with the primary care team require diligent management.

PSYCHIATRY IN THE GENERAL HOSPITAL

A palpable lack of funds to establish new lunatic asylums led to a fortuitous consequence in the early 20th century in the form of initiation of the process of shifting psychiatrically ill patients to general hospitals. General hospital psychiatry units (GHPUs) were started in the West in early 1900s and in India came in 1930s, the first one being at RG Kar Medical College at Kolkata in 1933. This adaptation turned out to be quite refreshing and has continued to gain momentum; GHPUs are now a major part of the public health system that takes care of the mental health problems of majority of the population. This process has also reduced the stigma associated with psychiatric disorders, in medical professionals and establishments, as well as in members of the public.

In the beginning, medical professionals were not too keen to admit psychiatrically ill patients in general hospitals. However, the speciality was appreciated and eventually integrated owing to two factors. The understanding that emotions and psychological states played a role in the causation and maintenance of few physical diseases, drawing attention to concept of psychosomatic relationships was one factor. The other was the recognition of psychological symptoms and reactions in medical and surgical departments.

Several models have been offered for the association between psychiatric and physical illness:

- Emotional reactions to medical illnesses and surgical procedures

- Acute or chronic brain syndromes such as delirium and dementia resulting from medical disorders affecting brain function
- Medical complications of maladaptive behavior such as drug abuse, overeating or deliberate starvation
- Somatic symptoms with no organic basis like chronic pain or fatigue secondary to emotional disorders
- Physiologic concomitants of emotional states, like the classical psychophysiological medical disorders, e.g., irritable bowel syndromes
- Psychosomatic diseases such as eczema, peptic ulcer disease, hypertension and migraine
- Physical illnesses presenting as emotional or psychological problem, e.g., myxedema, thyrotoxicosis
- Psychological adverse drug reactions to drugs used for medical illnesses such as antihypertensives
- Medically ill patients being more prone to develop psychiatric disorders than healthy people.

Medically ill patients with psychiatric comorbidity seldom seek psychiatric help. The reason for this neglect is the lack of awareness among patients, the stigma of "mental" consultation, and nonavailability of psychiatric services. Psychiatric disorders in the medically ill are generally underdiagnosed and undertreated. Doctors who are not sensitive to psychological matters fail to spot psychiatric symptoms. There is often a lack of services for proper referral to a psychiatrist. Other hurdles to proper management include nonadherence to treatment recommendations, difficulty in obtaining consent for procedures and the inherent risk to patients and staff. This can have dangerous consequences on the patient's health outcome, quality of life, and medical treatment.

INTERFACE WITH MEDICAL SPECIALTIES

The considerable interface between psychiatry and other medical specialities is complex. It spans from contribution to and causation of medical illness to psychiatric symptoms secondary to medical illnesses, especially chronic or life threatening ones. During the management of medical illnesses, there can be interactions between drugs used for physical illnesses and psychopharmacological agents as well as psychiatric side effects of medications and procedures.

Some of the interfaces have developed into super specialities such as:

- Psycho-oncology—psychiatric aspects of cancer
- Psychonephrology—psychiatric aspects of renal diseases
- Psychocardiology—psychiatric aspects of heart diseases
- Psycho-ophthalmology—psychiatric aspects of eye diseases
- Psycho gynecology—psychiatric aspects of gynecological disorders
- Perinatal psychiatry—psychiatric issues pertaining to the period around childbirth
- Neuropsychiatry—psychiatric aspects of neurological diseases.

It goes without saying that psychosurgery is not psychiatric aspects of surgery, psychopathology is not psychiatric aspects of pathology and orthopsychiatry is not psychiatric aspects of orthopedics.

Medically ill patients have a high prevalence of psychiatric disorders. Indian studies have found that 38.6% of patients seen in medical OPDs seem to be suffering with a psychiatric condition, with depressive disorders (28.2%) being the most common. Psychiatrists in GHPUs are now frequently called to provide services for psychiatric emergencies arising in medical and surgical wards including intensive care units (ICUs). In ICUs, delirium and symptoms of substance intoxication or withdrawal are the most common reasons for referral. The integration of psychiatry with various medical and surgical specialities is on the rise.

CONSULTATION-LIAISON PSYCHIATRY

In C-L psychiatry, the psychiatrist renders services as a consultant, providing expert advice on the referred patient to his referring colleagues. He is an advisor to the treating doctor in issues of diagnosis and management of patients who has sought his expert opinion and advice. He does not take over the case but only advises, and his role is in assisting through advice in the acute management of the referred cases. In essence, the C-L psychiatrist has two quarters to address, the specialist seeking the consultation for a case (consultee), and the patient who is the case. The obligation to the consultee often extends to serving the interests of the healthcare facility, and of society at large. Sometimes this leads to an internal conflict, such as in situations when the perceived interest of the patient conflicts with the desires of the consultee, the needs of the hospital, and/or of society.

The consultation process could be a *referral* wherein the psychiatrist is asked to take over the psychiatric care of the patient if indicated, while in *consultation*, the psychiatrist renders an opinion or advice to the requesting physician about the patient, but does not take over the complete responsibility of the patient. Here, there is collaborative care of the patient on the request of the physician. To prevent diffusion of accountability of direct care, the consultee is in direct charge of treatment including ordering medicines as well as communication with care givers.

The consultations can be:

- *Patient oriented*: Wherein the consultation benefits the patient by provision of diagnosis, management, and rehabilitation.
- *Colleague oriented*: Wherein the consultation is provided to medical/surgical colleagues with a view to educate them about the role of the psychiatrist, concept of psychosomatic medicine, stress, and its role in medical disorders.
- *Agency related*: Here the focus is directed at the agency that has sought consultation. The psychiatrist counsels the organization which has sought help on the issues of psychological importance as in emergency settings in hospitals, schools or workplace mental health issues.

"Liaison" of C-L is an area of cooperation or relationship between psychiatry and their medical–surgical disciplines in a general hospital for patient care, education, and research. Here, the psychiatrist is part of the medical/surgical team in providing care to its patients. By being part of the treating team, the psychiatrist takes part in all activities, such as attending ward rounds, interacting with patients, carers and other members of the treating team. He makes suggestions about patient care which may not be evident to the medical/surgical team. He is a regular member of treatment teams in transplant programs, cancer centers, or dialysis units. The focus is on early recognition, early intervention and prevention of chronicity and disability. His role, however, as in the consultation model is advisory and he does not take over the care of the patient.

The liaison involves interpretation and mediation, i.e., the consultant psychiatrist mediates between patients and members of the clinical team, and between the mental health team and other health professionals, respectively. Consultation and liaison are mutually complementary. The patient, the consultee, and the therapeutic team form three interlocked foci in the consultation process. The psychiatrist having a personal contact with both the patient and caregivers is crucial for effective management.

The educational function is an important part of liaison psychiatry. An essential exercise is to pass on relevant information to patients, their family and friends, physicians, nursing staff, and others in the healthcare system. This includes teaching all of them about the psychological needs of patients, recognition of common psychiatric symptoms, identification and management issues, emergency management, use of psychotropic drugs as well as the determination of capacity to consent to procedures. Importance is given to the doctor-patient relationship as well as harmonious relationship with various members of the medical team in patient care. Psycho-education of patients and caregivers is required also to ensure treatment adherence and proper follow-up. It is important that the education be accurate yet imparted in simple language shorn of technical jargon as much as possible. Gentle repetition and getting the addressed party to verbalize the material shared are often necessary in this process.

Administrative and legal functions of the C-L psychiatrist is mandated by either the institution or the government, and governed by the local laws regarding care of persons with mental illness. Most hospitals direct evaluation of an acutely suicidal or homicidal patient by a psychiatrist, who decides on further issues such as involuntary care or referral to a psychiatric facility if required. Another example is the C-L psychiatrist

deciding on testamentary capacity in a patient with suspected dementia.

Research plays a key role in C-L psychiatry. The evidence that psychiatric intervention reduces the cost of healthcare by optimizing medical utilization is an upshot of scientific exploration. It has been shown that a collaborative care model with close interaction between the primary care physician, and a care manager (mental health worker) supervised by a C-L psychiatrist is more effective than care as usual in primary care settings. There are exceptional opportunities to study the role of epigenetic factors in organ dysfunction through the study of the gene-brain-environment interaction in the C-L setting.

In addition, the role of psychosocial factors of relevance to medical disorders and psychiatric aspects of medical disorders are two prominent areas of research. The study of attitudes of various members of the team toward psychiatric illnesses as encountered in the C-L setup would assist in delivery of humanistic and holistic treatment to patients.

Role of the C-L Psychiatrist

Consultation liaison psychiatrists are skilled clinicians as well as a psychological experts, who liaison in the general hospital setting for optimizing the treatment outcomes. They sometimes act as "med-psych detectives", and assist in complex cases as well as interact with primary teams, nursing teams, ancillary services, and patients and family members. They assess psychiatric symptoms, suggest treatment, and explore interactions between medicine and psychiatry.

Roles and Responsibilities

The role of the C-L psychiatrist and the types of referrals seen will vary by the hospital type, the population served, and the speciality mix within the hospital.

- *Direct consultation*: Requests for advice on diagnosis, prognosis, and management of psychiatric disorders.
- *Direct liaison with specialist units*: Closer relationship with specialist unit, with involvement in individual clinical cases as well as in training, staff support, and policy development.
- *Emergency department*: Assessment of patients presenting with symptoms suggestive of mental disorder, following deliberate self-harm and of patients brought in by police to a "place of safety".
- *Outpatient referrals*: From general medical, surgical, obstetric and gyneco-logical clinics and GP referrals, especially cases of somatization and "medically unexplained symptoms".
- *Teaching and training*: Formal teaching of undergraduate and postgraduate medical trainees and training of paramedical and nursing staff.
- *Research and audit*: Research into psychological aspects of medical illness and deliberate self-harm.

The domain of C-L psychiatry extends to both inpatient and outpatient services. In India, the functional aspect of C-L psychiatric services have not been highlighted. C-L services are mostly in the line with the consultation model, wherein on receiving a referral from the physician/surgeon, a psychiatrist evaluates the patient and psychiatric inputs are provided.

The wide range of psychiatric disorders and situations presented to the C-L psychiatrists for evaluation, opinion, and advice are broadly listed here:

- Patients presenting after deliberate self-harm or with suicidal thoughts or plans
- Assessment of mood or anxiety symptoms

- Issues of consent, capacity or detainability
- Assessment of confusion or cognitive impairment
- Assessment of psychotic symptoms
- Request for advice in a patient with pre-existing psychiatric problems
- Patients referred during pregnancy, labor and most commonly, the puerperium
- Medically unexplained physical symptoms
- Alcohol or substance abuse related problems
- *Assessment prior to listing for organ transplantation:* Both donor and recipient
- Psychiatric symptoms secondary to organic illness
- *Altered psychobiological functions:* Sleep, eating, elimination, and sex.

Scope of C-L Psychiatry

- Assisting in diagnosis is the most important role of the C-L psychiatrist. It involves accurately assessing the situation and in recognizing the psychological illness or significant psychological factors in the patient which have a bearing on the medical-surgical condition.
- Psychiatric symptoms caused by medical conditions have important implications, not only for diagnosis but also for evaluation, treatment, and management of both the medical and psychiatric conditions. The medically ill patient with psychiatric symptoms may first present to psychiatric settings and often delay the diagnosis of medical illness. Similarly the patient with medical illness-induced psychiatric symptoms may be dismissed as not medically ill. Any delay in comprehensive diagnosis may lead to difficulties in treatment and exacerbation of the illness. It is always prudent to review diagnosis in case of nonresponse to

treatment in search of underlying medical or psychological cause or illness.

Certain medical conditions have overt psychological symptoms:

- Endocrine: Hypo- or hyperthyroidism, hypoglycemia or hyperglycemia, Cushing disease, Addison's disease, and parathyroid disorders
- Brain neoplasms and neurodegenerative diseases, e.g., Parkinson's disease and Huntington's disease
- Seizure disorders
- HIV-AIDS and other sexually transmitted disease such as syphilis
- Trauma–both to head or generalized
- Metabolic encephalopathy
- Vitamin deficiency disorders—B_1 (Thiamine), B_{12} deficiencies
- Miscellaneous—systemic lupus erythematosus, multiple sclerosis, Wilson's disease, acute intermittent porphyria, and pheochromocytoma.

The C-L psychiatrist has a major role in assisting in the management of patients referred to him or as part of liaison services. They include organic mental conditions and psychiatric emergencies in medical wards. Conditions which interfere with proper adherence to treatment such as depression, hopelessness and anhedonia require management. Even maladaptive defensive mechanisms such as denial of illness, or nonadherence can affect outcome. Eating disorders compromise metabolic regulation especially in diabetics. Psychiatric medications with metabolic side effects warrant close collaboration with primary healthcare providers.

Patients with the following psychiatric problems land up with the C-L psychiatrist:

- Suicidal attempt or threat
- Depression
- Agitation
- Anxiety, quite often in the form of concern over a physical problem/diagnosis
- Hallucinations and psychotic illness
- Sleep disorder
- Confusion
- Noncompliance or refusal to consent to procedure
- Medically unexplained symptoms (absence of organic basis for symptoms).

The C-L psychiatrist has to advise about psychopharmacological, psychotherapeutic and behavioral management as appropriate. Maintaining continuity of care by arranging regular after care and follow up is also a vital responsibility of the C-L psychiatrist.

Management Issues

In comparison to psychiatrists working elsewhere, there are many challenges to a CL psychiatrist working in GHPUs. Most of the patients have comorbid illnesses and these raise a unique set of issues in management.

Issues in Pharmacotherapy

Special care needs to be exercised in the treatment of medically ill persons with psychopharmacological agents. The pharmacokinetic and pharmacodynamic properties of prescribed drugs and the underlying clinical and medical status of the patient are important considerations in treatment. The choice of medication and dosing regimen require careful assessment after taking into account the complex variables specific to each individual case.

In those who cannot take oral agents, the choice changes to intramuscular, intravenous or rectal routes. Buccal wafers and topical patches are other newer options. In patients who are hypovolemic or with reduced protein binding the dosage may have to be altered. Coprescription drugs such as antacids slow the distribution of drugs such as benzodiazepines. The presence of liver disease alters metabolism of psychotropic drugs, mandating lower dosage. Drug-drug interactions can raise or lower drug levels by either inhibition or induction of metabolism by cytochrome P450 enzymes. Many psychiatric medications have narrow therapeutic indices, and alteration of the blood levels due to either inhibition or induction of the isoenzyme involved in metabolism could cause problems.

Excretion via kidneys is reduced in acute and chronic renal failure and patients receiving medicines which are excreted predominantly via renal route would require lower dosing.

Pharmacodynamic issues involve the alteration of a drug's intended action by another drug or mechanism at the site of action. There needs to be a frequent review of all the medicines taken by the patient, both in the present and in the past. The review should consider the underlying medical conditions, possible drug interactions, and possible dosage adjustments. Other variables include nonadherence and polypharmacy, especially in patients being treated by several providers. There is a need to simplify medication regimens, and sometimes directly observe the process of taking the pills.

Few examples of medical complications include the serotonin syndrome which may be fatal when selective serotonin reuptake inhibitors (SSRIs) interact with certain drugs such as dextromethorphan or meperidine to produce a potentially fatal problem characterized by confusion, ataxia, hyperreflexia, nausea and hypertension. Similarly, bleeding in the gastrointestinal (GI) tract could be prolonged by SSRIs and hence prescribed in caution especially in the elderly. Confusion and decrease in bladder and bowel motility is associated with the anticholinergic effects caused by very many drugs. Sedation which is an issue in elderly is often associated with falls, and could be secondary to benzodiazepines.

All of these justify caution in prescription of drugs to elderly and those with concomitant medical illnesses.

Psychotherapy in the Medically Ill

Communication is the most crucial element of the consultation and treatment process. Clear communication by ensuring accurate, timely, and helpful interactions improves the process of consultation as well as the outcome. It also improves rapport and cooperation of the patient to interventions.

Therapies for hospitalized patients are usually brief and supportive. The type of intervention depends on patient's cognitive status, disease state, and treatments. Delirious patients require filling in of gaps of memory and replacing misperceptions with accurate information. Frightening hallucinations, especially those secondary to substances, require reassurance that they are secondary to drugs.

Cognitively intact patients could suffer from depression, feelings of hopelessness, helplessness, and suicidal thoughts. Some could have been severely upset and demoralized after witnessed the failure of revival of a roommate. Supportive psychotherapy helps eliciting these fears and emotions and initiating helpful measures. Exploration of the patient's idea of the illness, the distress and negative consequences as well as their attempts at overcoming the illness helps in planning therapy. Many patients have difficulty in discussing these with their primary physicians. Distortions of causal factors, prognosis, and treatment effects require correction, and this reduces anxiety and improves optimism. One needs to recognize and handle maladaptive strategies such as denial and refusal of care as well as to strengthen such healthy defences as the patient may have. It is important to utilize available family support in assisting the patient. Destitute patients can pose quite a challenge. Ascertaining the patients' assets (e.g., a good support system or individual, finances, faith) and liabilities (e.g., unemployment, lack of social supports) helps in planning a comprehensive management plan. It is not uncommon that a patient in a depressed state overlooks or underestimates his assets.

For the long term, in ambulatory and rehabilitation settings, cognitive and behavior therapy, interpersonal therapy, graded exercise, and most importantly psycho-education assists in comprehensive management.

Motivational Interviewing

A combination of relationship building principles with cognitive behavioral methods to target the patient's motivation to change, forms the crux of this method. This approach helps to resolve ambivalence about altering problematic behavior. This intervention has been used for alcohol and other substance related disorders as well as in lifestyle diseases (e.g., diabetes, obesity), smoking cessation, and medication adherence.

The techniques involve open-ended questioning which addresses patients' concern about change as well as encourage him to talk about change ("What would you like to see different in the current situation?," "What makes you feel it's the right time to change?"). Reflective listening validates how a patient is feeling ("I'm getting a sense that you want to change, but have concerns about becoming sober"). Normalizing the difficulties is another strategy, which helps

patient understand change is commonly difficult ("A lot of people find it difficult to become sober"). Affirmative statements to convey recognition of strength and effort to change ("It is clear you are making efforts to change"; "You are showing determination and strength to be sober"). Finally summaries to end and frame the conversation to end ambivalence is useful. Motivational interviewing techniques provide multiple approaches to empathize with patients, to meet them where they are and to elicit talk of change from patients themselves instead of forcing them through persuasion.

Clichéd as it seems, the art of listening is of great importance in any psychotherapeutic process, and this cannot be overemphasized in the context of C-L psychiatry. Also the taciturn or reluctant patient needs patient handling to try to draw out conflicts and concerns.

Consultation-liaison Psychiatry in Special Situations

There are few areas of medicine and surgery where evaluation of psychiatric symptoms and psychological issues form a dominant part in their assessment and management.

Intensive Care Units

These include cardiac, pulmonary care, trauma and critical care units, and neurological and similar units which rigorously care critically ill patients. All ICUs deal with patients who experience anxiety, depression, and delirium. Both patients and staff frequently observe cardiac arrests, deaths, and medical disasters, which leave them all autonomically aroused and psychologically defensive. Patients display hopelessness, helplessness, and apprehension and this is shared by relatives and caregivers too. A condition called ICU syndrome or ICU psychosis is well recognized, predominated by delirium and emotional and sleep disturbances. Both environmental factors such as light and noise levels, and medical factors like metabolic dysfunctions, pain, medication side effects, and missed infections can contribute to this.

Intensive care unit nurses experience high levels of stress resulting in nurse burnout, high turnover rates, and may undermine their efficiency. The C-L psychiatrist may educate and support the staff in resolving stress as well anxiety and depression.

Hemodialysis Units

Patients in this unit cope with lifelong, debilitating, and limiting illness and are totally dependent on machines. Repeated dialysis disrupts patient's personal routines. Psychological issues are usual in patients on chronic dialysis. They require to be prepared to deal with frequent, often daily, dialysis for long as well as adapting to a lifelong and sometimes life threatening illness. Patients need to be helped to develop a sense of autonomy and independence and staff of dialysis units too require psychological support. The vast experience of the C-L psychiatrist can help patients in preparing them to adapt to chronic illness, dealing with denial and unrealistic expectations. Care should also be taken to ensure that both dependence and sick role does not develop in the patient.

Surgical Units

There is now enough evidence that those patients who show clear depression and anxiety, but deny it, have higher risk for morbidity and mortality than those who are given similar depression and anxiety, can express it. Even better results occur in those with a positive attitude toward the surgery.

A good communication, education, and informed consent of issues of what patients could go through, what loss of function to expect, and how to cope with pain and disability lead to improved outcome. A C-L psychiatrist in the team could assist patient in being aware and cope with anticipated problems in the postsurgical state.

Psychodermatology

Connecting the boundary between psychiatry and dermatology is a complex interplay of neuroendocrine and immune systems, described as neuroimmunocutaneous system (NICS). It has been reported that psychological stress agitates the epidermal permeability barrier homeostasis, precipitating inflamm-atory disorders like atopic dermatitis and psoriasis. About a third of dermatological patients have an underlying psychological distress that could cause or exacerbate the skin disorder. Patients with psoriasis have increased suicidal ideation. The course of many skin disorders is influenced by stress and psychological events.

Psychocutaneous disorders can be:
- Psychosomatic disorders wherein the course of the skin disease is influenced, precipitated or exacerbated by emotional stress and/or anxiety, e.g., psoriasis and atopic dermatitis.
- Psychiatric disorder with dermatological symptoms which is either self-induced or secondary to the primary psychiatric illness, e.g., delusional parasitosis, trichotillomania, skin excoriation, and obsessive-compulsive disorder (OCD).
- Disfiguring skin conditions leading to psychological symptoms: Skin conditions like ichthyosis, acne conglobata or vitiligo, have fear, depression or suicidal thoughts as a consequence.

All of these illnesses require the dual management with both the specialists addressing the dermatologic and psychological aspects. The psychological interventions include cognitive behavioral psychotherapy, psychotherapeutic stress management techniques, and psychotropic drugs. Choosing the drug requires close interaction between both specialists. The chronicity of several skin diseases imposes a burden on many patients that can benefit from therapy by the C-L psychiatrist.

Transplantation Issues

Transplant surgery has vastly increased over the past decade and C-L psychiatrists have been playing an important role in helping patients and families in dealing with the many psychosocial issues involved.

Psychiatric issues in transplantation:
- Which patients on a waiting list will receive organs and when will it happen?
- Anxiety about the procedure(s)
- Fear of death
- Organ rejection
- Expenses involved
- Adaption to life after successful transplantation.

These issues can be supervised and discussed by C-L psychiatrists in group sessions with transplant recipients and their caregivers, who can support one another and share information and feelings about particular stressors related to the disease. One-fifth of transplant patients develop depression, suicidal thoughts or an adjustment disorder within a year of transplant, and this requires to be addressed. Assessment and counseling of the organ donor too is an important responsibility of the C-L psychiatrist. The donor needs to be well aware of his volunteered loss and be mentally stable. If the donor and recipient are from the same family, they are usually counseled together. Some recipients of cadaver transplants have reservations that need help in resolving.

Psycho-oncology

It is accepted that cancer impacts psychological functioning and that psychological and behavioral variables affect cancer risk and survival. Studies have shown that psychological interventions have played a role in influencing the course of cancer illness with lower morbidity, mortality and recurrence.

About half of all cancer patients have mental disorders, with majority (68%) having adjustment disorder. Apart from tumors of the central nervous system (CNS), the cancer that causes high psychiatric morbidity is pancreatic in origin. Depression (13%) and delirium (8%) too are common. The knowledge of having contacted cancer can lead to fear of death (not always unrealistic), fear of disfigurement and disability, fear of abandonment and loss of independence, fear of disruption in relationships, role functioning and financials stress and denial, anxiety, anger and guilt. Suicidal thoughts are frequent.

Psychiatrists should make a careful assessment of the psychiatric and medical issues and also pay special attention to family factors which could assist in the total management of the patient.

Pain, End of Life Care and Palliative Medicine Units

There are a number of issues related to patients with terminal illness. Management of these patients is quite challenging. Communicating bad news, issues related to prognosis, and care and problems related to palliative care and management of pain are well known to become problematic. Care is focused on providing patients with relief from the symptoms, especially pain and stress of a serious illness irrespective of the diagnosis. The goal is to improve the quality of life for both the patient and the family. Patients may display anxiety, depression, hopelessness, and helplessness. Suicidal ideation and behavior are to be watchfully looked for and handled. Staff that provides care to these patients, may display frustration and a sense of failure.

The psychiatrist working in palliative care should focus on increasing the quality of life using psychological interventions and psychotropics wherever appropriate. However, undertreating the pain and psychiatric symptoms in palliative care seems to be the norm. Psychiatrist as a part of palliative care focuses on comprehensive pain management as well as increasing the quality of life of the patients. Other interventions include reducing the fear of dying and preparing the family for bereavement.

Consultation liaison psychiatrist needs to handle both patients and staff in alleviating symptoms and distress and most importantly enhancing morale through counseling patients, relatives and staff.

MEDICAL ISSUES IN PSYCHIATRIC PATIENTS

Persons with severe mental illness have an excess mortality at adult ages, being two or three times as high as that in the general population, of which about 60% is because of physical illness. Persons with mental illness such as schizophrenia, bipolar disorder, and depression are at increased risk of being obese. The metabolic syndrome is highly prevalent among treated patients with schizophrenia.

There is increased prevalence of diabetes mellitus, cardiovascular risk disease, HIV positivity, and both Hepatitis B and Hepatitis C virus, suggesting both communicable and noncommunicable diseases are more prevalent. The severely psychiatrically ill may miss to identify the symptoms, fail to report them on their own or may not pay heed to the importance of medical treatments, all of which contribute to the mortality.

Increased morbidity and early mortality among the psychiatrically ill can be caused by:

- Poor nutrition
- Reduced physical activity
- Poor self-care and hygiene
- More often involved in high risk sexual behavior and substance use
- Adverse effect of psychotropic
- Genetic factors

Capacity and Consent

Obtaining valid consent prior to assessment and treatment of a patient is a fundamental tenet of medical practice. In the past, physician beneficence was the primary aspect of medical ethics. Today, patient autonomy has assumed greater importance; therefore taking informed consent has become an essential part of treatment protocol.

Valid consent is that which is based on sound information, is freely given and obtained from a patient with "capacity". Physicians make at least an informal decision on a continual basis regarding the patient's ability to give informed consent. The process of consultation involving prescribing medicines and advising the patient on issues related to his illness and recommending follow-up assumes that he is able to comprehend instructions. Patient may have to give consent for medical procedure, treatment or advance directives. Physician may have to assess patient's ability to drive or handle finances. Those patients, who are confused, refuse treatment or suffer from mental illness raise questions about their capacity. The medical team will often ask for psychiatric opinion as to a patient's capacity to make treatment decisions. Though all doctors need to be aware of these issues and be skilled in assessment of capacity and to make decisions regarding consent, they usually "outsource" this to psychiatrists. Liaison psychiatrists are often consulted on matters of capacity as they frequently assess mental disorder, abnormal mental states and have a better knowledge of the applicable law.

The terms "competence" and "capacity" are often used interchangeably and erroneously. Competence, a legal decision, refers to the ability to handle personal affairs and make decisions. Only a judge may declare a person incompetent for specific functions or global incompetence. A determination of capacity, i.e., ability to make informed decisions may be made by any registered practitioner.

Capacity is neither an "all or none" phenomenon, nor a permanent one. The patient may have capacity for some functions but not for others. The capacity to make decisions fluctuates with the patient's condition. In addition to the ability to give consent, other aspects of capacity include the ability to care for self-independently at home or to make financial decisions. There is also the ability to leave against medical advice or refuse treatment.

Physicians are more likely to question a patient's ability to refuse recommended treatment than to question their ability to consent to the recommendations. This is because physicians assess the final decision only, not the patient's rationale for the decision.

CONCLUSION

Consultation-liaison psychiatry is the bridge between psychiatry and the rest of medicine. The rapid progresses in medical illnesses require newer skills and techniques by psychiatrists to handle novel challenges. C-L psychiatry is already divided into various subspecialties to accommodate this expansion. Psychosomatic medicine, though old in practice, has a new role in the art of medicine. With newer advances in biomedical knowledge, this subspecialty will provide the biopsychosocial elements of comprehensive patient care and clinical research to improve clinical outcome and to enhance quality of life.

TAKE-HOME MESSAGES

- Psychiatric disorders are highly prevalent among medically ill patients, and as many as 38.6% of outpatient medically ill suffer from psychiatric illness in India. Psychiatric disorders in the medically ill are generally underdiagnosed and undertreated.
- The C-L psychiatry is a subspecialty of psychiatry that incorporates clinical service, teaching, and research at the borderland of psychiatry and other clinical specialities.
- This subspeciality deals with patients suffering concurrently from both physical and psychological illnesses, requiring collaboration of both specialists in provision of care.
- The C-L psychiatrist renders services as a consultant, providing expert advice on the referred patient on how his or her mental health is affecting care and treatment.

- The psychiatrist may also liaise as part of the medical/surgical team, providing care to the patients and makes suggestions about patient care which may not be evident to the team.
- The focus is on early recognition, early intervention, and prevention of chronicity and disability.
- The scope of C-L psychiatrist involves evaluation, treatment, and management of both the medical and psychiatric conditions, educational functions, and administrative, legal, and research functions.
- Both pharmacological and psychological therapies are useful in treating these patients with both medical and psychiatric illness.
- There are special situations such as in ICUs, hemodialysis, surgical, palliative, end of care units, managing illnesses such as cancer and pain as well as issues of informed consent which pose a challenge to the C-L psychiatrist.

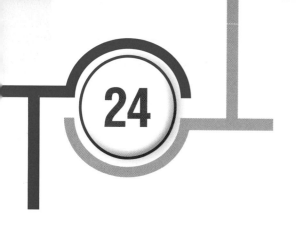

Suicide and Psychiatric Emergencies

Lakshmi Vijayakumar, Vinayak Vijayakumar

INTRODUCTION

In the Oxford dictionary, "Emergency" is defined as "a sudden state of danger requiring immediate action". In the case of a patient, the implication is that without treatment, the patient's life is threatened. This is applicable for both physical and psychiatric illnesses. There is a common misconception that there are no real emergencies in psychiatry. Contrary to this notion, it has been found that psychiatric emergencies are the third most frequent kind of emergency faced by a physician. Only emergencies related to surgical and internal causes occur more frequently. Overall, psychiatric emergencies represent 10% of all the emergencies faced by physicians. Suicidal behaviors and severe behavioral disturbances are two commonly faced conditions in the emergency department (ED). This chapter will look at these challenging clinical situations along with few other common psychiatric emergencies.

SUICIDE

Epidemiology and Definitions

Approximately 75% of all suicides occur in the lower and middle-income countries (LAMIC). In these countries, pesticide poisoning, hanging, and self-immolation are the most common methods used to attempt suicide. The highest rates of suicide are usually seen in the younger age group (<30 years of age). The suicide rate is nearly twice as high in males as compared to females with a ratio of 2:1 in LAMIC (1.4:1 for the Indian population).

According to WHO's definition, suicide is a deliberate act to end one's life. Shneidman defined suicide as "a conscious act of self-induced annihilation, best understood as multidimensional malaise in a needful individual, who defines an issue for which suicide is perceived as the best solution". There are four broad categories of suicidality:

1. Suicide
2. Attempted suicide
3. Suicidal ideation
4. Self-harm

Attempted suicide can be defined as a nonfatal, self-inflicted potentially injurious behavior with an intent to die as a result of the behavior. *Suicidal ideation* merely describes the harboring of suicidal ideas. *Self-harm* can be explained as a self-inflicted potentially harmful behavior with the individual having no intent to die as a result of the behavior such as to affect external circumstances or affect internal state.

Other definitions:
Suicide pact: Agreement or pledge between two or more individuals to take their lives simultaneously.

Physician-assisted suicide: Death caused by the actions of a physician who agreed with the patient's intent to die and acted directly to bring about it.

Double suicide: Two people dying together following a pact. Usually results from one person with depression instigating another who has no psychiatric problem. Sometimes, the depressed patient may commit homicide before suicide.

Copycat suicide: Suicide stories from various outlets (news/entertainment) can provide as role models for a person on the verge of committing suicide. This imitation effect can be explained by the social learning theory of deviant behaviors. A string of such suicides brought into focus the role of media in reporting and the portrayal of suicide.

Suicide counters: Factors that inhibit suicidogenic tendencies are called suicide counters. These factors may arise from economic, personal, family, religion, ethical, and social domains.

Suicidal intent: Defined as the degree to which the individual wished to die at the time of the attempt.

Lethality of a suicidal attempt: The seriousness of the physical consequences of or the risk posed to life by the suicide attempt.

Risk and Protective Factors

Numerous studies have looked at the association between various clinical, biological, and environmental factors and suicide. Based on these studies, certain factors have been associated with a higher risk for suicide (risk factors), while certain factors were found to be associated with a lower rate of suicide (protective factors).

Risk Factors

The risk factors for suicide may be broadly divided into three categories (National Strategy for Suicide Prevention: Goals and Objectives for Action 2001):

Biopsychosocial risk factors
- Presence of mental disorders; alcohol or substance use disorders
- Hopelessness
- Aggressive tendencies
- A history of trauma or abuse
- Major physical illnesses
- A family history of suicide
- Previous suicide attempts

Environmental factors
- Job and financial losses
- Relational or social losses
- Easy access to lethal means
- Local clusters of suicide that have a contagious influence

Sociocultural factors
- Lack of social support and sense of isolation
- Stigma associated with help-seeking behavior
- Barriers to accessing healthcare, especially treatment for mental health and substance abuse
- Certain cultural and religious beliefs (for instance, the belief that suicide represents a noble resolution of a personal dilemma)
- Exposure to, including through the media, and the influence of others who have died by suicide

Protective Factors

- Effective clinical care for mental, physical, and substance use disorders
- Restricted access to highly lethal means of suicide
- Easy access to a variety of clinical interventions and support for help-seeking
- Strong connections with and support from the family and community
- Support through ongoing medical and mental healthcare relationships

- Skills in problem-solving and conflict resolution, and nonviolent handling of disputes
- Cultural and religious beliefs that discourage suicide and support self-preservation

Presentation of the Suicidal Patient

A potentially suicidal patient can present to the ED in the following ways:

- Overtly suicidal patients who either come on their own or are brought by others in search of help
- Patients who have just attempted suicide
- Those presenting with other psychiatric or substance abuse disorders

The third category of patients might also include covertly suicidal patients who come to the ED complaining of various problems. Such patients may present with a confusing array of signs and symptoms. Assessing them can be quite challenging and their potential to commit suicide often goes unassessed. They could present with somatic complaints or have an undiagnosed underlying psychiatric disorder, such as depression or panic disorder. Thus, when evaluating vague or unexplainable physical complaints, the clinician must ask about depression, panic attacks, and the potential for suicide. Similarly, patients presenting with psychotic symptoms or symptoms of depression, anxiety, panic attacks, or drug withdrawal could also be covertly suicidal and must be asked about such feelings.

Assessment of Suicidal Behaviors

Interviewing a Suicidal Patient or Patient Presenting after a Suicidal Attempt

A popular myth that should be quelled immediately is the idea that asking questions about suicide would introduce the idea to the client when no such idea existed previously. Research has shown that most suicidal patients are willing to discuss their thoughts if asked, but only one in six clinicians enquires into the matter. The purpose of the initial interview is not only to collect important information but also to establish a bond with the patient and provide emotional support. However, the initial interview could be challenging due to the patients clinical condition (e.g., drowsiness) or the unfavorable setting (e.g., intensive care unit). In these conditions, the patient might not be very cooperative and might even deny having attempted suicide. Therefore, the patient's fragile mental state should be kept in mind, and efforts should be made to make them feel at ease and slowly establish a rapport. The intensity of questioning should be increased gradually and only when a strong rapport is established that further potentially stressful questions should be presented. This hierarchical approach will reduce the patient's anxiety and apprehension.

A sequence of useful questions is:
- Do you feel unhappy and helpless?
- Do you feel desperate?
- Are you unable to face each day?
- Do you feel that life is a burden and not worth living?
- Do you feel like committing suicide?

It is important to ask these questions in a secure and supportive environment.

In countries like India where the EDs are often crowded and physicians have time constraints, patients who seem suicidal should be gently asked to wait in a quiet room, not left alone, and be assured that the clinician would like to spend more time with them.

Areas of Assessment

The assessment process must include:

- A thorough psychiatric examination with a special focus on identifying risk and protective factors. Special attention must also be paid to identify modifiable risk factors
- Specific enquiry about suicidal thoughts, plans, and behaviors
- Establishing the level of the risk of suicide: low, moderate, high
- Determining the treatment setting and plan

Assessment must also include examination of personality factors and the presence of psychiatric illnesses **(Table 24.1)**. Disorders such as mood disorders, alcohol and substance use disorders, psychotic disorders, anxiety disorders, and personality disorders (especially borderline and antisocial personality) are associated with an increased risk of suicide **(Box 24.1)**.

Determining Suicidal Risk

Establishing the level of suicidal risk is one of the most important parts of the assessment. It is based on a comprehensive assessment of the risk factors for suicide and the warning signs, as well as an appraisal of the protective factors that could mitigate the risk. A simple checklist **(Table 24.2)** could be used to make this assessment in the ED within 20–40 minutes.

Managing the Suicidal Patient

The main goals in managing patients with suicidal behaviors are:

- To protect the patient from self-abuse until the suicide crisis has passed
- To anticipate and treat the medical complications of a suicide attempt
- To define and solve, if possible, the acute problem that precipitated the crisis
- To diagnose and arrange treatment for the underlying problem predisposing the patient to suicidal behavior
- To deal with the acute grief reactions of the bereaved family members of suicide victims

Providing safety and security should be first step in the management of patients with suicidal behaviors. Based on the initial assessment, the clinician has to

Table 24.1: Areas to evaluate in the assessment of suicidal behaviors.	
Current presentation of suicidality	Suicidal or self-harming thoughts, plans, behaviors, and intent
Symptomatic presentation	Evidence of hopelessness, impulsiveness, anhedonia, panic attacks, or anxiety
Psychiatric illness	Current signs and symptoms of psychiatric disorders. Look for comorbidities in particular
History	• Past history of psychiatric illness • Past medical history/surgical history • Family history of suicidal behavior and mental illness, including substance use • Past history of suicidal behavior
Psychosocial situation	• Acute or chronic psychological stressors • Cultural and religious beliefs about suicide • Social support systems
Individual factors	• Personality traits • Past responses to stress • Coping skills

decide whether or not the patient needs hospitalization. If involuntary admission is being considered, the physician should be

aware of the necessary legal requirements. Factors such as psychological factors, support system, living arrangements, good outpatient facilities will decide whether or not hospitalization is required **(Box 24.2)**.

Once the patient has been hospitalized, the treating team must ensure (1) The patient is constantly monitored by the hospital staff; (2) The patient has no access to means of self-harm (removing potentially lethal objects, such as scissors, needles, and pesticides, from the area immediately around the patient; removing objects that one can use to hang themselves; preventing the patient from jumping out of the window or down open stairwells); (3) Immediate treatment

Box 24.1: Warning signs of suicidal behavior.

Warning signs of suicidal behavior according to the American Association of Suicidology
- Hopelessness
- Rage, anger, seeking revenge
- Acting reckless or engaging in risky activities, seemingly without thinking
- Feeling trapped, as if there is no way out
- Increasing alcohol or drug abuse
- Withdrawing from friends, family, or society
- Anxiety, agitation, inability to sleep, or sleeping all the time
- Dramatic changes in mood
- Seeing no reason for living, having no sense of purpose in life

Table 24.2: Checklist to determine degree of suicidal risk.

	Low risk	Medium risk	High risk
Suicide plan details	Vague	Some specifics	Clear
Availability of means	Not available	Available, has access to them close by	Has them in hand
Time	No specific time	Within a few hours	Immediately
Lethality of method	Pill, slashing wrists	Drugs and alcohol	Gun/hanging/pesticides
Chance of intervention	Others present most of the time	Others available if called upon	No one nearby, isolated
Previous suicide attempt	None or one of low lethality	Multiple of low lethality/one of medium lethality	One of high lethality or multiple of moderate lethality
Stress symptoms	None	Moderate	Severe
Coping behavior	Daily activities continue as usual with little change	Some daily activities disrupted	Gross disturbance of daily functioning
Depression	Mild	Moderate	Severe
Resources	Help available	Help available but inconsistent	Help unavailable or hostile environment
Communication aspects	Direct expression of feelings and suicidal behavior	Interpersonalized suicide goal ("they will be sorry-I will show them")	Very indirect or nonverbal expression of internalized suicide goal (guilt, worthlessness)
Personal life	Stable relationships and personality	Acute but short term/psychosomatic illness	Chronic debilitating or acute catastrophic illness
Medical status	No significant medical problems	Acute but short term/psychosomatic illness	Chronic debilitating or acute catastrophic illness

Strongly consider hospitalization:
- Prior attempt of high lethality
- Well-thought-out plan
- Access to lethal means
- Uncommunicative
- Recent major loss
- Social isolation
- Hopelessness
- History of impulsive, high-risk behavior
- Active substance abuse or dependence
- Untreated mood, psychotic, or personality disorder

May consider outpatient management:
- No history of potentially lethal attempts
- Lack of plan/intent; cooperative family member or other adult
- Removal or lack of availability of lethal means
- Communicative
- Availability of intensive outpatient care
- Good social support
- Hopefulness

of the medical consequences of suicide; (4) Repeated assessments to determine the patient's level of suicidal risk on a daily basis.

As suicide attempts by ingestion of pesticides is very common in India, the clinicians should receive basic training on how to manage pesticide poisoning (especially in rural areas). The basic treatment should comprise the following:

▪ Intravenous administration of atropine (2–4 mg in adults and 0.05–0.1 mg/kg in children every 15 minutes till atropinization is achieved) if signs of cholinergic poisoning develop.

▪ Intravenous administration of diazepam should be considered if patient develops seizures.

▪ Oral fluids and forced emesis are not recommended.

"No Suicide Contracts" and Safety Plan

A "no suicide contract" is a clinical contract (not a legal one), usually written, between a patient and a clinician. Here, the patient gives an undertaking that he will not harm himself. The patient provides a "guarantee of safety" along with a "promise" to call specified individuals if there is an increase in suicidal ideation. The contract is based on the principle that the patient will respect the promise made to the physician. However, such a contract should never be a substitute for an informed clinical judgment based on a systematic assessment of risk. It is not recommended for agitated, psychotic, impulsive, intoxicated, and cognitively impaired patients or for adolescents.

The goal of a safety plan is to empower persons in situations that have the potential to precipitate a crisis and to help them manage such situations. The safety plan should be developed before the patient leaves the clinic.

The safety plan basically consists of a sequenced set of instructions including the following:

▪ Identify the source of the low mood (identify the behavior in advance). Engage in activities that make you feel better or distract you (e.g., go for a walk, go to the cinema, call a friend, and/or play music).

▪ If the suicidal thoughts continue, call (1) A support person (previously identified), (2) A physician or mental health professional, (3) A suicide hotline (if one is available, the number should be provided to the patient), or (4) Emergency services.

The details of the individualized safety plan along with the relevant phone numbers, can be written on a small card which the patients can carry with them.

Pharmacological Treatment

Treatment of the underlying psychiatric disorders should also be started simultaneously. Though, there is a risk that the patients may use the recommended medications to attempt suicide, they should not be denied the benefits of medications. Antidepressants are necessary for the treatment of depressive patients. Electroconvulsive therapy is also recommended if rapid results are required, as in the case of patients at high risk of suicide. Mood stabilizers and antipsychotic medication are useful in the treatment of bipolar patients and those with psychotic depression. Lithium is also recommended for use in patients with a high risk of suicide independent of any specific diagnosis. Clozapine also has strong antisuicidal properties when used in patients with schizophrenia and schizoaffective disorder. Recently, Ketamine (as a single bolus or intravenous infusion) has been found to be useful in EDs to reduce acute suicidal ideation/cognition.

OTHER PSYCHIATRIC EMERGENCIES

Psychiatric emergencies other than suicidal behaviors can present in the ED in the form of:

- Aggressive/violent patient
- Anxious patient
- Drug/alcohol intoxication and/or withdrawal
- Grief reaction
- Rape and disaster victims
- Emergencies seen in special populations (children, elderly and women)

A detailed description of the management of each condition may be beyond the purview of this chapter. Kindly refer to the previous chapters for management of anxiety disorders and substance intoxication or withdrawal. This chapter will focus on the management of suicidal behaviors, violence, grief reactions, and disaster victims in the emergency settings.

General Principles in the Management of any Psychiatric Emergency

The first and foremost principle is *"Primum non nocere"*, which means above all, do no harm. Other important principles in managing any psychiatry emergency are:

- Always ensure safety of your own self and of other staff members.
- Always rule out organic causes for any psychiatric presentation **(Table 24.3)**.
- If conditions do not allow you to maintain doctor-patient confidentiality, then take the necessary legal steps.
- If experts are not available for a particular problem, make arrangements to get to the patients as soon as possible.
- Always make sure the assessment includes questions that might be important but difficult to ask.
- Try to use multiple sources to confirm the information collected.
- Do not hesitate to consult a senior colleague when you find yourself with a difficult decision to make.
- Document all the assessment and treatment decisions taken by you and your colleagues.

Managing Patients with Severe Behavioral Disturbances

Aggression is usually the feature in 10% of all psychiatric emergencies. However, it should be stated here that people with mental illness are more likely to be victims of violence than perpetrators. Aggression, violence, psychomotor excitement, and agitation can be the clinical presentation of many underlying conditions, ranging from organic disease to a variety of mental illnesses **(Box 24.3)**. Aggression and violence is most commonly associated with substance abuse and psychosis.

Table 24.3: Psychiatric presentations in medical disorders.

Etiology	Diagnosis	Psychiatric presentation
Infections	Herpes simplex encephalitis	Behavioral changes, cognitive decline, aggression, disinhibition
	Human immunodeficiency virus encephalopathy	Early-onset, rapidly progressive dementia
	Progressive multifocal encephalopathy	Clumsiness, weakness, visual changes, speech difficulty, behavioral changes
	Syphilis	Personality disorder, psychosis, delirium, dementia
	Typhoid fever and other endemic infections	Acute confusion, psychosis, anxiety, depression (rare)
Pharmacological withdrawal	Alcohol	Agitation, hallucinations, persecutory delusions, self-mutilation
	Benzodiazepines	Sleep disturbances, irritability, anxiety, panic attacks, perceptual changes, acute psychosis
	Opiates	Anxiety, agitation, irritability
	Cannabis	Weakness, hypersomnia or insomnia, anxiety, depression, restlessness
Acute metabolic	Hypoglycemia	Confusion, anxiety, nervousness, nightmares
	Central pontine myelinolysis	Behavioral changes, psychosis, cognitive disturbances
Autoimmune	Systemic lupus erythematosus	Cognitive dysfunction, mood disorders, acute confusion, psychosis, paranoia, auditory or visual hallucinations
	Multiple sclerosis	Anxiety, depression, acute psychosis, adult-onset tic disorder
Traumatic	Subarachnoid hemorrhage	Personality changes, intellectual impairment, mood disorders, akinetic mutism, confabulatory amnesia, acute psychosis
	Subdural hematoma	Cognitive impairment, withdrawn behavior, blunted affect, catatonia
Central nervous system disease	Huntington disease	Episodic psychosis
	Parkinson disease	Episodic psychosis, visual hallucinations, mood disorders, apathy, executive dysfunction
	Temporal lobe epilepsy	Depression, fear, anxiety, déjà vu, flashbacks, paranoid delusions, depersonalization, derealization
	Stroke	Confusion, altered mental status

Risk Assessment for Aggression and Violence

Along with the general assessment of the patient's history and mental status, specific focus on certain factors can help determine nature and magnitude of the risk of violence. Young males, criminal peer group, unemployment, past violence, childhood abuse, personality disorders, psychosis with comorbid substance use disorders and low IQ and various other factors to be associated with violence and aggression are factors

Box 24.3: Common causes of aggression and violence in the emergency setting.

Psychiatric causes:
- Schizophrenia—paranoid and nonparanoid
- Mania, hypomania, depression
- Alcohol abuse and withdrawal
- Drug abuse and withdrawal
- Hallucinogens, phencyclidine (PCP)
- Benzodiazepine withdrawal
- Organic mental disorder and brain damage, epilepsy, and dementia
- Personality disorder (particularly antisocial, impulsive, and borderline)
- Learning disability
- Child and adolescent behavior disorders
- Post-traumatic stress disorder
- Dissociative states

Nonpsychiatric causes:
- Criminal, e.g., drug dealing
- Spousal, child abuse
- Child abuse
- Economic

Box 24.4: Risk factors associated with violence.

Demographic factors:
- Male
- Young age
- Socially disadvantaged neighborhoods
- Lack of social support
- Employment problems
- Criminal peer group

Background history:
- Childhood maltreatment
- History of violence
- First violent at young age
- History of childhood conduct disorder
- History of nonviolent criminality

Clinical history:
- Psychopathy
- Substance abuse
- Personality disorder
- Schizophrenia
- Executive dysfunction (problems with planning, multitasking, organization, emotional control)
- Noncompliance with treatment

Psychological and psychosocial factors:
- Anger
- Impulsivity
- Suspiciousness
- Morbid jealousy
- Criminal/violent attitudes
- Command hallucinations (e.g., voices telling the patient to die or kill himself/herself)
- Lack of insight

Current "context":
- Threats of violence
- Interpersonal discord/instability
- Availability of weapons

Environmental risk factors in the emergency department:
- Poor staffing levels and poor patient-staff interactions
- Lack of privacy and overcrowding
- Poor physical facilities

that have been associated with aggression and violence (**Box 24.4**). Symptoms such as delusions of persecution, command hallucinations, suspiciousness, restlessness, and the presence of substance use have been found to be associated with a more imminent risk of violence.

Steps in Management

The general principles in managing any psychiatry emergency (described above) must be adhered to in the management of aggressive patients as well (**Flowchart 24.1**). A few steps should be highlighted as they are particularly important when dealing with violent patients in the ED: (1) *Safety first*—ensure that you and others are not at risk. Ensure that the patient does not have access to any weapons. (2) *Share*—try and built rapport with the patient. Talk calmly and avoid confrontations. (3) *Step back*—do not encroach on the patient. Avoid confrontation.

Initial Step—Nonpharmacological ("Talking Down")

Use nonpharmacological techniques such as *"talking down"* to diffuse the situation. Encourage the patient to talk and listen attentively. Rapport could be built with even an aggressive patient if you devote time, remain calm, and listen.

Flowchart 24.1: Management of aggressive patients (adults).

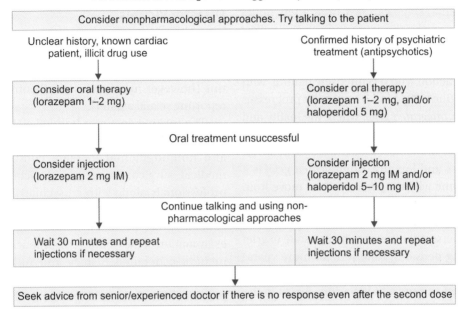

If Talking Down Fails or If the Situation is Escalating

If it is felt that drugs are needed (or mentally ill patients), try to persuade the person to take oral medication. Try and convince the patient that you are trying to help and insist that the purpose of treatment is to improve the situation for the patient first. Take care to avoid unnecessary treatment involving restriction.

If the Patient Refuses Oral Medication and is Still in Need of Sedation

Administer rapid tranquilization. Preparation is key here. One person should be in-charge and has to guide the rest of the team. The drugs should be prepared by the person who will be injecting them. There should be sufficient people to hold one limb each, and another person to administer the prepared injection—a minimum of five people. Once the person has been sedated, he should be routinely monitored.

Planning for the Future

A single treatment will only address the immediate situation. A long-term treatment plan must be made with the patient and their family. Consider making a contract with the patient (not legally binding) on the management of future episodes where rapid tranquilization may be required. This may allow the patient to feel like he is more involved in the treatment process.

Grief Reactions in the Emergency Setting

The terms "bereavement" and "grief" refer to either the state of having lost someone to death, or the response to such a loss. Grieving is a fluid process that is dependent on various factors. It could be described in three different stages: (1) Shock and denial (disbelief, numbness), (2) Acute anguish (withdrawal, anger, guilt, aimlessness, waves of somatic distress, preoccupation), and (3) Resolution (resumption of old roles, return to work, re-experiencing pleasure). The shock and denial stage can last from a few hours to a few weeks, the acute anguish stage a few weeks to a few months and the resolution stages could take months to years. An *acute grief* reaction which is intensely painful, with disruption of normal life, usually progresses into an *integrated grief*, where the reality and the meaning of the death is assimilated and thoughts of the deceased are associated with sadness and longing. *Complicated grief* is a syndrome where a person fails to move from the stage of acute grief to integrated grief. *Pathological grief* reaction may be diagnosed if the person continues to be in a state of grief for long period of time (one or more years) without any improvement.

Grief can present in various forms in the emergency setting. Acute anxiety attacks, severe depression with suicidal ideations, and dissociative states are some of the common presentations. Offering support should be the first and foremost step in such situations. Some basic principles while offering support include: (1) Acceptance of the patients behaviors as "normal reactions", (2) Using language that's consoling, (3) Facilitating release of emotions, and (4) Setting limits to control extreme reactions and self-destructive behaviors.

Medications may be necessary when the bereaved person is in a highly agitated, anxious, aggressive or psychotic state. Short-acting benzodiazepines (lorazepam) and antipsychotics (haloperidol) can be used to manage the situation. Some patients with depression, anxiety or psychosis may require a long-term management plan that may include regular medications. Once the acute crisis has been handled in the ED, if there is no contraindication, the patient can be referred for grief counseling.

Managing Sexual Assault and Disaster Victims

Sexual assault cases presenting to the ED has been steadily increasing over the last decade. Both, women and men can be affected by this (however men are less forthcoming in reporting sexual assault).

The treating doctor or hospital staff must ensure that they are supportive, reassuring, and nonjudgmental. A team comprising medical, surgical, forensic, and social work professionals along with a psychiatrist may be needed to handle such cases. Informed consent must be taken before beginning examination of the victim. Assessment should include a detailed history and full body (including genital) examination. The whole process of the history taking and examination must be done in a sensitive manner without making the victim feel humiliated. The examination itself may be very stressful for the victim as it may trigger flashbacks of the sexual assault. The complete history and examination must be documented in detail. The role of psychiatrist would be to: (1) Provide a nonjudgmental environment to allow the victims to ventilate their feelings, (2) Restore a sense of psychological safety as victims of sexual assault are likely to feel that they are in danger and at risk of further assault, (3) Decide regarding the judicious and short-term use of benzodiazepines, (4) Form a treatment plan that includes following-up the victim (especially to assess for post-traumatic stress disorder), (5) Liaising with the other departments (medical, surgical, forensic, social work) involved in the treatment of the victim and (6) Referral to support groups and specialized psychiatric services, if needed.

Victims of disaster (earthquake, floods, riots and terrorism) also go through a sudden, unexpected, and overwhelming stress.

They can present to the ED with symptoms of guilt, numbness, anger and confusion. A psychiatrist's role in managing such victims in the ED would be very similar to what has been described for victims of rape.

CONCLUSION

The incidence of mental illness, alcohol, and substance abuse and suicidal behaviors is on the rise, and this had led to a proportionate increase in patients presenting with psychiatric emergencies to the ED. Managing patients with suicidal and violent behaviors could be very challenging and anxiety-provoking for health professionals. In India, paucity of resources and support for clinicians during emergencies adds to the difficulties. It is crucial for clinicians to develop the competence to handle suicide attempts, violent behavior, and other psychiatric emergencies so as to improve the level of care offered to the patients.

TAKE-HOME MESSAGES

- Emergency has been defined as a sudden state of danger requiring immediate action. From mental health perspective, the conditions which fall in this category are suicidal ideation and attempts, panic attacks, aggressive and violent patients, intoxication and withdrawal states, pseudo-seizure episodes, grief reactions, sexual assault cases, and disaster victims, etc.

- Suicidality includes suicide, attempted suicide, suicidal ideation, and self-harm cases of various types. A balance of risk factors and protective factors determine the ultimate outcome of cases of suicide.

- Warning signs for suicide include hopelessness, rage, acting reckless, feeling trapped, increasing alcohol or drug abuse, withdrawing from friends and family, anxiety, inability to sleep, seeing no reason or purpose for living.

- Management of a suicidal patient would include general medical measures, treatment of any coexisting psychiatric disorder, psychosocial management or even electroconvulsive therapy.

- It is crucial for clinicians to develop the competence to handle suicide attempts, violent behavior and other psychiatric emergencies.

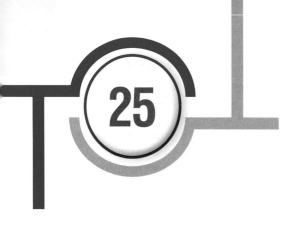

25

Culture-bound Syndromes

PK Dalal, SK Kar

INTRODUCTION

Culture has significant influence on human beliefs and behavior. An individual born in a specific culture, internalizes the cultural values, adopts them and responds in specific ways which are again culturally colored.

Culture-bound syndromes refer to disorders involving psychological or somatic distress, that is produced in a person of specific culture, where the distress is related to the specific cultural beliefs and is recognized as abnormal by the people of that culture. Various other synonyms (culture-specific disorders, folk illnesses, cultural concepts of distress, ethnic neuroses and exotic psychoses) have been used to describe this entity. Yap (1969) had coined the term *"culture-bound syndrome"*. Before the introduction of "culture-bound syndrome" to the conventional international classificatory systems of psychiatry, an attempt had been made to define culture-bound syndrome. The definition proposed for culture-bound syndrome was—*"a collection of signs and symptoms (excluding notions of cause) which is restricted to a limited number of cultures primarily by reason of certain of their psychosocial features"*.

The **Figure 25.1** above represents that culture-bound syndromes are largely influenced by specific cultural characteristics, linked with specific psychiatric disorder

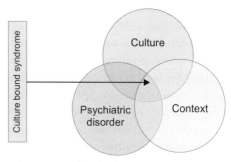

Fig. 25.1: Model of culture-bound syndrome.

by virtue of its clinical characteristics and triggered by contextual factors. This model also attempts to answer the following questions:

- Why somebody develops a culture-bound syndrome (linked to the context)?
- How it causes distress/impairment (linked with psychiatric disorder)?
- What cultural concepts attribute to its development (linked with cultural concept)?

CULTURE-BOUND SYNDROMES IN PSYCHIATRIC DIAGNOSTIC SYSTEMS

Culture-bound syndromes were introduced to the psychiatric diagnostic system in the 10th edition of International Classification of Diseases (ICD-10) and 4th edition of Diagnostic and Statistical Manual of Mental Disorders (DSM-IV). The ICD-10 describes culture-bound syndromes under the category of "Other specified neurotic disorders" and has been assigned the code F48.8. However, ICD-10 does not give any detailed description of the individual culture-bound syndromes. It describes the cultural beliefs that attribute to development of psychopathology as nondelusional. DSM-IV describes culture-bound syndromes in the glossary section and describes them to be independent of different DSM–IV diagnostic categories. The recent edition (5th edition) of Diagnostic and Statistical Manual of Mental Disorders (DSM-5) describes culture-bound syndromes as "Cultural Concepts of Distress" and kept it under the "Glossary section". Long debates are going on over past few decades regarding the independent existence of culture-bound syndromes as distinct diagnostic entities. Many researchers argue that culture-bound syndromes are distinct culture specific manifestation of common psychiatric disorders (depression, somatoform disorder or stress related disorders). Evidences also exist regarding manifestation of the same entity in different cultures in different forms and getting labeled by different culture specific names. The number of entities described under culture-bound syndrome in ICD-10 and DSM-IV has been reduced in DSM-5. The number of culture-bound syndromes described in DSM-IV-TR (25 syndromes) is reduced in DSM-5 (9 syndromes).

DESCRIPTION OF INDIVIDUAL CULTURE-BOUND SYNDROMES

Ataque De Nervios

It is seen among individuals of Latin America. Individuals present with symptoms of emotional disturbance (sadness, anxiety, and anger), crying, shouting, screaming, trembling, aggressive behavior and unusual sensations in chest that rise to head. The individual may also have dissociative symptoms such as amnesia, stupor, pseudoseizure (nonepileptic seizures), depersonalization and derealization. The individual often has a sense of being out of control. The symptoms may or may not be associated with stressful conditions. Similar conditions seen in other Caribbean countries are known by the names—*Indisposition* (in Haiti), *Blacking out* (in Southern United States) and *Falling out* (in West Indies). The symptoms have close link with panic disorder, anxiety disorders, intermittent explosive disorder, dissociative disorder and stress related disorders.

Dhat Syndrome

It is commonly seen in South Asia. The term had been coined by Prof NN Wig in 1960s. It refers to a range of psychosomatic symptoms that the patient attributes to semen loss. Often patients present with anxiety, sadness, worry, apprehension, lack of concentration, lack of energy, reduced appetite, lethargy, fatigability, weakness, sexual dysfunction and burning micturition. Patients report passage of whitish, semen like substance in urine. Attributions also go to loss of semen during masturbation, nocturnal ejaculation and during defecation.

In the South Asian cultures, emphasis is given on the preservation of semen as it is believed to be the "Elixir of Life" in the ancient literatures. Semen is believed to be formed from food extracts by a complex, multistep process of ultracondensation; hence its loss is considered to be a significant threat to the vitality of the individual. It is commonly seen in young, unmarried or newly married males from low socioeconomic status. A similar entity is also increasingly discussed in females, where females express their undue concern for the nonpathological vaginal discharge and attribute loss of genital secretion to similar kind of symptoms seen in males. Dhat syndrome is having similarity with other culture-bound syndromes like— *Koro* (South East Asia) and *Shen-k-uei* (in China). It has phenomenological similarity with major depressive disorder, dysthymia, somatoform disorder, generalized anxiety disorder and sexual dysfunctions.

Khyâl Cap

It is also known as "Khyâl attack" or "wind attacks". It is reported in Cambodian population. The word "Khyâl" refers to a wind like substance. The belief in this disorder is that—a wind like substance will generate in the body along with blood, which may be detrimental to the health of the individual. Often patients present with panic attacks, breathing difficulties, dizziness, palpitation and symptoms of autonomic arousal. The symptoms usually present episodically and the episodes mostly occur unanticipated. Similar conditions do occur in other cultures and known by different names—*pen lom* (Laos), *hwa-byung* (Korea) and *vata* (Sri Lanka). It has clinical resemblance with panic attack, panic disorder, phobia (agoraphobia), generalized anxiety disorder, somatoform disorder and post-traumatic stress disorder.

Kufungisisa

It is seen among the Shona of Zimbabwe. The term "Kufungisisa" refers to "thinking too much". Patients often present with excessive worries related to ill health. The symptoms are mostly anxiety, depression and various somatic complaints, irritability and panic like symptoms. Certain cultures harbor believes that too much thinking is hazardous for the mental and physical health of the individual. Similar entity also exists in certain other cultures like—Africa, East Asia, Caribbean and Latin America, where too much thinking is considered to be pathological. In the African culture, similar entity is known as "*Brain Fag Syndrome*", where the symptoms are attributed to studying too much. The symptoms of Kufungisisa have resemblance with psychiatric disorders like—major depressive disorder, generalized anxiety disorder, dysthymia, post-traumatic stress disorder, obsessive compulsive disorder and grief (bereavement) reaction.

Maladi Moun

Literally, it refers to "humanly caused illness". It is seen among people from Haitian community. There is a popular cultural belief that due to strained interpersonal relationship, people send various psychiatric disorders to harm their enemies. The cause of depression, psychosis and academic failure with acute onset are often explained on the basis of the above explanatory model. People who are intelligent, beautiful or rich, if develop such symptoms in a shorter time frame, then the suspicion about being caused by people out of jealousy is often considered in that culture. It is also observed in many other cultures across the world, where people believe that physical/mental illnesses are caused by envy or social conflicts with people with "*evil eye*". The symptoms often resemble with psychiatric disorders like—delusional disorder and schizophrenia.

Nervios

It refers to a state of "vulnerability" to challenging life circumstances and experiences. It is seen in Latinos of Latin America and United States. Patients commonly present with mood symptoms (anxiety, sadness and irritability), somatic symptoms (pain, headache, gastrointestinal disturbances and trembling sensation) and impairment of functioning. The patients frequently also manifest with dissociative symptoms, sleep disturbances, concentration difficulties and dizziness. Similar entity is also prevalent among Sicilians and Greeks of North America. The symptoms often resemble with depression, anxiety disorders, dissociative disorders, somatoform disorders and schizophrenia.

Shenjingshuairuo

It refers to "weakness of the nervous system". It is seen among the Chinese Mandarin. *Shenjingshuairuo* is characterized by weakness, emotional disturbance, excitement, nervous pain (headache) and sleep disturbances. At least three symptoms from the above five symptoms must present for the diagnosis of this entity as per Chinese Classification of Mental Disorders, 2nd Revised Edition. Here, weakness refers to loss of vital energy due to overstraining and mental fatigue due to excessive worry. Association with family stress or occupational stress or interpersonal stress is often present. Similar conditions also exist in various other cultures of the world in the form of neurasthenia-spectrum of disorders, brain fag syndrome, chronic fatigue syndrome and burnout syndrome. The symptoms of *Shenjingshuairuo* resemble with depression, anxiety disorders, stress related disorders and somatoform disorder.

Susto

It refers to "fright". It is commonly seen among Latinos of Latin America and people living in Central America, South America and Mexico. There is a belief in this culture that the soul leaves the body of the individual following days to years after a frightening event, which results in distress, difficulty in functioning and

playing social roles. The common symptoms presented by people affected by *Susto* are: low mood, loss of appetite, disturbed sleep (decreased or increased or with night mares), low self-esteem, decreased motivation, feelings of worthlessness and multiple somatic complaints. The frightening event can be related to natural calamities, animals, supernatural agents or difficult interpersonal circumstances. Similar culture-bound phenomena are also evident in various other cultures globally. The clinical manifestations of *susto* resemble with depression, stress related disorders and somatoform disorder.

Taijin Kyofusho

It refers to a disorder resulting from "interpersonal fear". It is seen among the Japanese. The individual often experiences anxiety for avoiding interpersonal situations, as he/she perceives his/her behavior or appearance in the social interaction to be unpleasant or inadequate. The individual's concern may be related to body odor, facial blushing, use of inappropriate gestures and eye contact. Anxiety and avoidance of social situations are the core clinical manifestations. Similar manifestations are also seen in Korea, United States, New Zealand and Australia. The clinical manifestation of *taijin kyofusho* resembles with social anxiety disorder and obsessive-compulsive disorder, delusional disorder.

The above nine culture-bound syndromes are described in DSM-5. There is phenomenological resemblance between various culture-bound syndromes. Hence, it is believed that similar entities in different cultures should be given similar names across different cultures. **Table 25.1** summarizes about various other culture-bound syndromes prevalent worldwide.

Table 25.1: Other culture-bound syndromes seen worldwide.

Name of the culture-bound syndrome	Distribution	Clinical characteristics
Koro	Malaysia and Some East Asian countries	• Sudden onset, episodic anxiety of severe kind associated with the belief that penis (in males) or vulva and nipple (in females) are shrinking to be merged with the body • Fear of death present
Latah	Malaysia and Indonesia	• Sudden onset frightening behavior • Features like echopraxia, echolalia, dissociative or trance like behavior may present
Black out	Caribbean region and Southern United States	• Characterized by episodes of fainting with or without preceding dizziness • A sense of inability to move body parts or see despite having normal body functioning
Ghost sickness	American Indians	• Present with—weakness, feeling of insecurity, anxiety, fear, nightmares, fainting, confusion, dizziness, hallucinations and worthlessness
Amok	Malaysia, Laos, Philippines, Papua New, Guinea and Puerto Rico	• Precipitated by interpersonal conflicts (insult, perceiving oneself to be unimportant) • Period of worrying/threatening followed outburst of violent, aggressive and homicidal behavior • Often accompanied by ideas of persecution, amnesia and exhaustion • The individual gets back to the premorbid level after the episode
Bouffee delirante	Haiti and West Africa	• Sudden episodes of aggressive behavior, confusion and psychomotor excitement • May be accompanied with hallucination (visual or auditory) and paranoia
Brain fag syndrome	West Africa	• Seen among students in response to study related challenges • Characterized by anxiety, getting fatigued, difficulty in concentrating, memory difficulties, pain in head and neck, visual difficulties and feeling of tightness, pressure and burning
Pibloktoq	Subarctic Eskimos	• Sudden onset dissociative symptoms associated with extreme excitement accompanied with seizure like activity or stupor may present • Shouting and screaming behavior, tearing of clothes, disruptive, and disorganized behavior may be observed during the episodes • Amnesia about the event may present
Shen-k'uei	Taiwan and China	• Marked anxiety (panic) symptoms accompanied with somatic symptoms (bodyache, dizziness, fatigability, sexual dysfunction), insomnia and nightmares • Complaints of passage of "white turbid urine" are reported. • Symptoms may be attributed to loss of semen
Shin-byung	Korea	• Characterized by anxiety, fear, sleep disturbance, dizziness, loss of appetite, gastrointestinal disturbances followed by dissociative features (possession by spirit)

Contd...

Contd...

Name of the culture-bound syndrome	Distribution	Clinical characteristics
Spell	African-Americans and European-Americans	• Characterized by a trance like state in which the affected individual communicates with deceased relatives or spirits • May be having brief episodes of change in personality
Zar	Ethiopia, Somalia, Egypt, Sudan, Iran, North Africa and Middle East	• Characterized by dissociative features like spirit possession (laughing, shouting, singing, weeping and head banging) • Other features such as apathy, withdrawal behavior, food refusal, refusal to carry out daily routine
Bilis and Colera	Latino group of population	• Characterized by acute onset nervous tension, screaming, trembling, headache, gastrointestinal disturbances and loss of consciousness (in severe cases) • The cause is attributed to strongly experienced anger or rage
Windigo	United States and Canada	• Characterized by dissociative features such as being possessed by the cannibal monster "Windigo" • Fear of becoming a cannibal is present

Various other culture-bound syndromes are discussed in literature worldwide. Paris syndrome is a brief disorder (cultural shock) seen in Japanese tourists visiting Paris. It is characterized by delusional state, depersonalization, derealization, hallucinations, anxiety, dizziness, sweating and tachycardia. Similarly, Stendhal syndrome (also called as Florence syndrome or Hyperkulturemia) is reported in tourists visiting Florence. It is characterized by confusion, dizziness, fainting and even hallucination after seeing beautiful arts of personal significance. Similarly, eating disorders (anorexia nervosa and bulimia nervosa) are considered to be the culture-bound syndrome of western culture by many.

In India, other than Dhat syndrome, various other culture-bound syndromes are also seen **(Table 25.2)**. They are: Gilhari syndrome, Possession syndrome, Jhinjhinia, Bhanmati Sorcery, Suchi-bai and Ascetic syndrome. Epidemics of *Koro* have also been reported in different parts of India. Even literature suggests about coexistence of *Koro* and *Dhat syndrome*. These syndromes produce significant impairment in life.

MANAGEMENT OF CULTURE-BOUND SYNDROMES

Culture-bound syndromes are often mis-diagnosed or underdiagnosed due to comor-bid psychiatric disorders, phenomenological similarity with other psychiatric disorders and sometimes ignorance or unawareness of cultural concepts on the clinician's part. Patients with culture-bound syndromes undergo significant psychological distress. They carry various cultural myths. The management often focuses on resolving the cultural myths through culture specific educational interventions and relieving the symptoms by means of pharmacological as well as psychological interventions.

Various pharmacological interventions are often used in the treatment of distressing symptoms of culture-bound syndromes. Antidepressant medications are useful in treating depressive symptoms, anxiety and somatic symptoms. Short-term use of benzodiazepines may be helpful in management of anxiety and insomnia. Rarely patients may need low dose antipsychotic medications, when the symptoms include psychotic like pattern or marked aggression.

Table 25.2: Culture-bound syndromes (other than Dhat syndrome) unique to India.

Culture-bound syndrome	Distribution	Clinical features
Gilhari syndrome	Rajasthan	• Fear of Gilhari, experiences a form of lizard, crawling under the skin • Intense anxiety and apprehension; fear of death
Possession syndrome	Across Indian states	• Brief episodes of trans (possession) like state during which the individual behaves as if it is possessed by spirit or is under the spell of witchcraft
Jhinjhinia	Assam, North-East states of India, West Bengal	• Presence of dissociative features like paresthesia, loss of sensation, trembling sensation and bodily discomfort
Bhanmati sorcery	Sothern states of India	• Symptoms like somatoform disorder or conversion disorder with cause attributed to evil spirits
Suchi-bai	West Bengal	• Also called purity mania • Refers to excessive concern toward cleanliness in personal life patterns.
Ascetic syndrome	Across Indian states	• Indulgence in strict religious practices and living a life of celibacy through sexual abstinence, social withdrawal and rigorous physical activities

Evidences suggest that addressing the myths through psychoeducational intervention, relaxation exercises, supportive psychotherapy and cognitive behavior therapy (CBT) are found to be useful in the management of several culture-bound syndromes. There is scarcity of research in this area. There is no defined management guideline for treatment of culture-bound syndrome till date.

FUTURE IMPLICATIONS OF CULTURE-BOUND SYNDROMES

Recent years are witnessing an ultrarapid process of urbanization, globalization and modernization resulting in mixing of cultures. It further causes sharing, attenuation, transformation or amalgamation of cultural values. These changes in cultural milieu are likely to influence the manifestation, prevalence as well as outcome of culture-bound syndromes in future. These factors may cause change in the prevalence of culture-bound syndromes, worldwide. Attempts have been made to validate the categories of culture-bound syndromes by comparing them with psychiatric disorder categories. DSM-5 has developed a set of 16 questions (cultural formulation interview) to explore about the influence of culture in causation and manifestation of psychiatric disorders. Cultural formulation interview (CFI) attempts to gather information about:

▪ Individual's cultural identity
▪ Conceptualizing the distress in the light of cultural values
▪ Cultural understanding of vulnerability, resilience and stressor
▪ Cultural understandings about the individual and clinician
▪ Global cultural assessment.

CONCLUSION

Culture-bound syndromes indicate that cultural beliefs and myths significantly produce psychological distress.

Understanding the cultural beliefs and their implications will help in thoughtful management of these conditions. Resolving the cultural myths in a culturally accepted way may be helpful in dealing with patients of culture-bound syndromes.

TAKE-HOME MESSAGES

- Culture-bound syndromes are often centred on specific cultural concepts. There are a large number of such syndromes seen in almost all societies of the world.

- Culture-bound syndromes are important diagnostic entities that often resemble with various other psychiatric disorders or present with a mix of symptoms in different combinations.

- The clinicians need to understand the cultural characteristics of the individual to be able to fully understand the presenting psychopathologies or the syndromes.

- Culture-bound syndromes are managed by resolving cultural myths through psychological interventions as well as pharmacological interventions for symptom control.

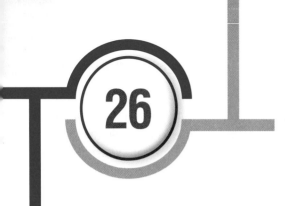

Miscellaneous Other Syndromes of Clinical Interest

Amlan Kusum Jana, Neelanjana Paul

INTRODUCTION

A "syndrome" has traditionally been defined in clinical medicine as a cluster of symptoms and signs that characterize a particular condition, and which are manifestations of certain other diagnosable "diseases". The term "disease" is used for conditions, for which the cause and pathogenesis is known, and where the clinical picture, treatment response, and natural history have been comprehensively described. However, in psychiatry, despite significant advances in our understanding, the etiology, the pathogenesis, clinical manifestations, and diagnostic implications of behavioral abnormalities are still uncertain. Hence, the elaborate classificatory systems of mental "disorders" mainly describe syndromes in their diagnostic criteria, after collating a certain number and pattern of signs and symptoms through extensive field research. This makes diagnosis of mental illnesses challenging more so due to the absence of clear-cut laboratory and radiological investigations. Hence, it is important to rely on clinical methods in psychiatry, properly elucidate the signs and symptoms, and distinguish between different syndromes.

In this chapter, we describe in brief, some of the psychiatric syndromes that have not found place in the diagnostic categories included elsewhere in this book. These syndromes often have a historical or a clinical importance and can help us to understand the nuances of behavioral abnormalities better. Many of the following syndromes are used in both scientific and lay literature for descriptive purposes, and it would be pertinent for junior students of psychiatry to be aware of them, other than the real possibility of them being included in entrance examinations. Each description includes a note on the origin of the epithet, its common manifestations, relevance in current psychiatric nosology, probable etiopathology, related diagnoses, and management.

The various syndromes have been listed in alphabetical order, and hence the sequence does not reflect their clinical importance. The group of syndromes that may be classified as behavioral addictions (BA) is mentioned here in this chapter due to their hitherto uncertain standing in our systems of classification.

ALICE IN WONDERLAND SYNDROME

This name was coined in 1955, by a British psychiatrist John Todd, to label various perceptual distortions, often described by sufferers of migraine that are similar to the dreamy adventures experienced by Alice, the 7-year-old protagonist of an 1865-novel authored by Lewis Carroll. Hence, other synonyms of Alice in Wonderland syndrome (AiWS) are *Todd's syndrome*, or *dysmetropsia*.

Patients have "sensory distortions", i.e., a constant real object is perceived in an altered manner due to a change in the intensity, quality, or spatial form of the stimulus. There may be abnormalities in visual perception, e.g., *micropsia* (objects looking smaller than they actually are), *macropsia* or *megalopsia* (objects appearing bigger), *pelopsia* (objects appearing to be closer than they are), or *teleopsia* (objects appearing farther away). There may also be distortions in perception of time, of sound, the size of external objects, and that of own body parts, as perceived through other sensory modalities, leading to the so-called *Lilliputian hallucinations*, similar to the descriptions in the novel "Gulliver's Travels", written by Jonathan Swift, in 1726. AiWS probably occurs due to alterations in blood flow of brain areas that process information received from external stimuli to reproduce a subjective perception of the outer world. Though named a syndrome, this is actually a symptom that may occur in migraine, brain tumor, with use of psychoactive substances and antiepileptic drug such as topiramate, and is more commonly seen in children. The condition is best managed by treating the underlying cause.

BEHAVIORAL ADDICTION

Dependence is the technically preferred term for addictive behaviors in current classificatory systems, where psychoactive substances are used excessively and uncontrollably with disruption of socio-occupational functioning, tolerance and withdrawal symptoms. These disorders have been shown to occur due to neuroadaptation of dopaminergic and opiate circuits, which constitute the reward system in the brain. Increasing intrusion of technology into our day-to-day life is leading to certain new patterns of activity, which influence the brain reward systems in a similar way in vulnerable individuals. These are being conceptualized as Behavioral Addiction (BA), which are in many ways similar to substance use disorders as regard phenomenology, natural history, and neurobiology. However, they have not yet been classified as a disorder due to serious concerns about medicalizing a "bad" or "socially undesirable" behavior. The following conditions may become the focus of clinical attention, and are being investigated as various types of BA.

- *Pathologic gambling* is the subtype of BA that has been included as a distinct syndrome in DSM-5, and includes impulsive and risky gambling ventures with inability to stop, and which causes harmful long-term consequences. Sufferers often magnify their gambling skills, hold superstitious beliefs and have deficits in working memory, inhibition, planning and other executive functions.

- In *compulsive shopping*, individuals have frequent, irresistible, and senseless shopping sprees, when they clearly buy more than what is necessary or can be afforded. They are often distressed by the buying sprees, which significantly interfere with their work or social functioning.

- *Internet addiction disorder* refers to compulsive overuse of internet, craving, and withdrawal symptoms of irritability or mood fluctuations when deprived of internet availability. There is associated impairment, distress in social settings, decreased participation in real life communication, relationship problems, and deterioration of academic and occupational achievements. The behavior does not occur exclusively with periods of hypomania or mania or other psychiatric condition. Internet addiction may occur in various forms, e.g., computer/game addiction, information overload (or web surfing), net compulsions (e.g., online gambling or online shopping), cyber sexual addiction (i.e., online pornography or online sex addiction), and cyber-relationship addiction (to online relationships).

- *Sexual addiction disorder (compulsive sexual behavior or hypersexual disorder)* includes compulsive masturbation, affairs, use of prostitutes, pornography, cybersex, voyeurism, exhibitionism, sexual harassment, and even sexual offending.

Our understanding of phenomenology, diagnostic criteria, epidemiology, and neuro-biology of BA is still incomplete. However, there are reports that medications used for treating chemical dependency may be successful in treating nondrug addictions, e.g., naltrexone, nalmefene, n-acetyl-cysteine, modafinil, and topiramate.

CHARLES BONNET SYNDROME

Named after the Swiss neurologist, who first described it in 1760, patients with Charles Bonnet syndrome (CBS) have complex visual hallucinations, in background of impaired visual acuity, without any other psycho-pathology or alteration of consciousness. Thus patients have "hallucinations", which is a false perception of objects which are not there. Here, they occur in the visual mode, and are usually complex, i.e., mostly consist of human figures, less frequently of animals, plants and inanimate objects, and may often change position and glide through the room. CBS mainly occurs in the elderly, and with complete or partial disturbance of central or peripheral vision. Subjects usually know that the experience is "unreal" and can modify the phenomena by voluntary control such

as closing the eyelids. The attacks may last for days to years, and often brain pathology cannot be identified. Hence, CBS is explained as the phenomenon of visual release hallucinations (or phantom visual images), and is similar to the musical hallucinations that may occur in a deaf person.

COTARD'S SYNDROME OR WALKING CORPSE'S SYNDROME

Initially described by neurologist Jules Cotard in 1880 as *Le délire des negations*, or "Delirium of Negation", this syndrome is characterized by prominent nihilistic delusions. Incidentally, although this early name mentions "delirium", the condition is very different from our current understanding of delirium as a disorder of consciousness and attention.

A delusion is an abnormal, illogical and unrealistic belief, which cannot be shaken by contrary evidences and which is not shared by persons belonging to his sociocultural background; thus delusions are abnormalities of thought that also influence the patients' emotions, behaviors and interpersonal reactions. Persons with nihilistic delusions believe that either some of their body parts do not exist, or they themselves do not exist, or in extreme cases the world does not exist. There may be an associated delusion of enormity, e.g., where the person thinks that his body size or physical capabilities are of gigantic proportions, like, an ocean (of urine) would be formed if they micturate, or their head would touch the stars if they stood up. Ultimately, patients may neglect their personal hygiene and physical health, leading to emaciation or death.

Initially Cotard's syndrome was thought to represent a unique diagnosis, but subsequently it was found to be commonly seen in depression. According to current classificatory systems, it will be subsumed as a somatic delusion, as a part of "severe depression with psychotic symptoms", or other primary psychotic disorder. It is common in late adulthood with a clear female preponderance. Treatment involves treating the underlying condition.

COUVADE'S SYNDROME

Derived from the French verb "*couver*" meaning "to brood or hatch", the term "couvade" was coined by anthropologist Edward Burnett Tylor in 1865 to refer to certain rituals observed by expectant fathers in ancient cultures like that of Egypt and Cantabri. Hence, opinion differs regarding whether this should be considered a cultural phenomenon or a pathological entity. In Couvade's syndrome, the expectant father develops symptoms like that of his pregnant partner, including nausea, cramps, food cravings, weight gain, tiredness, constipation, and vomiting; the symptoms often develop during the 3rd month of the pregnancy, worsen before birth, and disappear after the birth of the baby. There may be associated gastrointestinal disturbances like morning sickness and indigestion, emotional changes like anxiety, nervousness or irritability, and even an abdominal swelling resembling pregnancy. Various psychological theories have been proposed to explain this poorly-understood condition, like parturition envy, rivalry with the unborn child for maternal attention, a pathological transition to fatherhood, an abnormal reaction to being socially marginalized, and also to paradoxical increased attachment to the fetus. Currently, this condition would be classified as a psychosomatic disorder, which usually does not require treatment as it is self-limiting. However, symptomatic treatment may be started if the depressive or anxiety symptoms are too severe or distressing.

DE CLERAMBAULT'S SYNDROME OR DELUSION OF LOVE

This is a variation of erotomania, where the woman harbors a delusion that a man, commonly belonging to a higher social status and with whom she has no or very limited social contact, has fallen in love with her. The French psychiatrist Gaetan Gatian de Clerambault described this condition in 1942, naming it *psychose passionelle*. The condition is seen usually in females and only one case among those reported by de Clerambault was a male. Patients require antipsychotic medications and supportive psychotherapy in management.

DIOGENES' SYNDROME OR SENILE SQUALOR'S SYNDROME

First recognized in 1966, this syndrome has been named after the Greek philosopher of 4th century BCE, who believed in being content irrespective of his material possessions, and reduced his earthly needs to the bare minimum by begging and living in a barrel. The condition is usually seen in the elderly, and characterized by extreme self-neglect, domestic squalor, social withdrawal, apathy, hoarding of garbage and animals, and lack of shame. This is not a separate disorder as per current nosology, but is commonly seen in frontotemporal dementia, and is thought to originate from neurocognitive impairments in executive function and motivation.

DELUSIONAL MISIDENTIFICATION SYNDROMES

Delusional misidentification syndromes (DMS) may present in acute, transient, or chronic forms. DMS may be seen in paranoid schizophrenia as well as in various organic conditions such as drug intoxication and withdrawal, encephalitis, epilepsy, head injury, brain tumor, Alzheimer's disease, dementia with Lewy bodies, multiple myeloma, and migraine. Various theories have been used to explain DMS such as right temporo-limbic-frontal disconnection, interhemispheric disconnection between cortical areas and cognitive deficits in face recognition. Investigations and treatments are directed at identifying and managing the underlying disorder.

Delusional misidentification again includes the following discrete but related syndromes, each having the most common theme of abnormal belief in "doubles".

- *Capgras's syndrome* was first described in 1923 by a French psychiatrist Joseph *Capgras* and his colleague Jean Reboul-Lachaux, in a French woman, "Madame Macabre", who complained that her husband had been replaced by an exact double. Patients with this syndrome believe that the physical identity of the "double" or the imposter is the same as the original person with whom they usually have close emotional ties; but the psychological identities are different. It may occur in all age groups and is more common in females.
- *Fregoli's syndrome* was first reported by P Courbon and G Fail in a 1927 paper "Syndrome d'illusion de Frégoli et schizophrénie". It is named after a famous Italian actor Leopoldo Fregoli, who had an exceptional ability to change his appearance so quickly during his stage performances that spectators would be fooled into thinking that there were different actors. Here, patients misidentify strangers as some familiar person, who is often a persecutor; and insist that the psychological identity is the same, even though they know that the physical identity is different.

- *Syndrome of intermetamorphosis* a rarer condition where patients believe that someone close to them has been transformed into someone else suggestive of changes in both the physical and psychological characteristics.
- *Syndrome of subjective doubles* is the belief in existence of physical doubles of one's own self, where the "duplicates" are usually thought to have differing psychological identities.
- *Reduplicative paramnesia* (RP) is a similar syndrome of "doubles" first reported by Arnold Pick in 1903, where patients believe that a place has been duplicated, existing in at least two locations simultaneously, which may be familiar, or unfamiliar. The variant he initially described was of "place reduplication", where the person believes that two places with identical features exist simultaneously, but are geographically distant. In "chimeric assimilation", the two places become combined, e.g., the hospital where the patient is in, is believed to be actually his home that has somehow been transformed into the hospital. In "extravagant spatial localization" patients believe that their current location is actually some other location, which is again familiar to them. RP has been mainly reported in cerebral diseases such as dementias and head injury, and patients often have associated cognitive deficits in memory, visuospatial skills, and executive function.

EKBOM'S SYNDROME

Described in 1937 by Swedish neurologist Ekbom, this condition is characterized by a delusion that one's body has been infested by parasites, or small but macroscopic organisms. There may also be tactile hallucinations, where the individuals vividly speak of sensing that the organisms are crawling over, or just under the skin, and sometimes even moving around in different body parts. They typically give detailed descriptions of the parasites and often preserve and present skin fragments and other debris as evidence of their illness. Ekbom's syndrome is classified as "internal" where the parasites are believed to be in the various internal organs or blood, and "external" where the parasites are believed to be in the skin or hair. It is more common in females in their fourth decade. If presenting solely with this delusion, the condition is classified as delusional disorder. However, this delusion can also be a feature of other disorders such as schizophrenia or psychotic depression. Delusions of infestation may be seen in organic brain syndromes like delirium tremens, cocaine dependence, cerebrovascular disease, or dementia, and attributed to occur in thalamic lesions. Treatment includes use of antipsychotics, individual psychotherapy and rarely—electroconvulsive therapy.

GANSER'S SYNDROME

First described by Sigbert Ganser in 1897, in four prisoners, this is the syndrome of approximate answers, that is where individuals give wrong answers to very obvious questions but the answers appear very close to the correct one, as if they have deliberately selected the wrong response, e.g., saying "two plus two" equals three. The condition is also characterized by clouding of consciousness, conversion symptoms and hallucinations, and being subsequently amnesic about their abnormal behavior. Ganser's syndrome was initially considered to be a type of hysterical phenomenon, while recent studies suggest that it occurs due to a transient disturbance in the language functioning of the left hemisphere. However,

current understanding doubts if this deserves any distinct nosological status as a disorder.

MUNCHAUSEN'S SYNDROME

This was first described by Richard Asher in 1951 and named after Baron Karl von Munchausen, a fictional German nobleman who described his fantastic and impossible achievements as a sportsman, traveler and a soldier, in flowery and lengthy language. In this condition, a person deliberately feigns or simulates physical and/or psychiatric disorders, or induces injury or signs of disease to gain clinical attention; the aim is different from malingering where perpetrators feign illness specifically to gain reprieve or leave. Currently classified as factitious disorder, the presentation can be with predominant physical or psychological symptoms or it can be a combination of both. Pathological lying, also known as *pseudologica fantastica* is a key component of this disorder. The condition is uncommon and is seen usually in persons with experience of hospitalization in early age, a significant relationship with a physician in the past, or in cases of organic brain disorder.

Another related condition is induced factitious disorder or Munchausen's syndrome by proxy, where physical or psychological symptoms are deliberately produced or feigned in another person who is under the index person's care, usually in a child by a mother. The syndrome is considered to be a form of child abuse. Psychotherapy is the mainstay of treatment in both Munchausen's syndrome and Munchausen's syndrome by proxy.

OTHELLO'S SYNDROME

Named after the Greek mythological character, which was made even more famous by Shakespeare in his novel, this illness is characterized by delusion of infidelity. The patient believes his/her spouse/sexual partner is cheating on him/her. If this delusion is the only or central characteristic feature of the condition, it would be called a delusional disorder according to the current nosological system. However, it can also be seen in other conditions such as schizophrenia, bipolar disorder or alcohol induced psychosis. This condition is usually seen in the fourth decade of life, mostly in males and subjects often take recourse to violent actions to settle the issue. Management includes use of antipsychotics and cognitive behavior therapy. Treatment of associated substance use disorder (mostly alcohol) is equally important.

STOCKHOLM'S SYNDROME AND LIMA'S SYNDROME

Stockholm's syndrome is seen in the victim, characterized by sympathy, love, and loyalty toward the victimizer with whom the victim is often willing to cooperate. This is commonly described in relation to hostage abduction, though it can also be seen in cases of rape and abuse. The condition was formally named in 1973 after hostages were taken during a bank robbery in Stockholm. Current nosology does not give this condition the status of a separate disorder and management usually involves psychotherapy.

Lima's syndrome is a similar condition where the abductors develop sympathy for the hostages. However, though described in connection with Stockholm's syndrome because of its similarity, this condition is yet to gain proper attention of researchers and clinicians.

VAN GOGH'S SYNDROME

Named after the famous Dutch painter who mutilated his own ear, this condition is typically characterized by repetitive self-mutilation and can be seen in Lesch Nyhan's syndrome, schizophrenia, bipolar disorder, psychoactive substance abuse, and Munchausen's syndrome. Treatment of the underlying disorder is the mainstay of management.

CONCLUSION

To conclude, most of the above syndromes are actually technical terms used in behavioral medicine, and each has varying diagnostic implications. Many are rare, while others are likely to become more common in the context of modern technological and socio-political changes. Hopefully, younger students of psychiatry will be interested enough in these miscellaneous conditions, to research further and finally help to decide whether they are to be relegated to psychiatric history, or are valid clinical entities with clear explanations, differential diagnoses, and treatment.

TAKE-HOME MESSAGES

- A "syndrome" has traditionally been defined as a cluster of symptoms and signs that characterize a particular condition. In psychiatry, a number of unusual clinical syndromes with characteristic features have been described.
- Alice in Wonderland syndrome, Charles Bonnet syndrome, Cotard's syndrome, Couvade's syndrome, De Clerambault's syndrome, Diogenes syndrome, Delusional Misidentification syndromes, Ekbom's syndrome, Ganser's syndrome, Munchausen's syndrome, Othello's syndrome, Stockholm's syndrome, Lima's syndrome, and Van Gogh's syndrome are some of the important names in this category.
- Behavioral addiction is the latest entry into this category and includes pathologic gambling, compulsive shopping, Internet addiction disorder, sexual addiction disorder, etc.

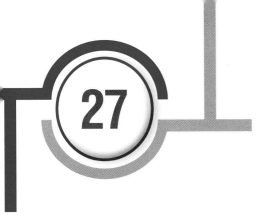

Psychiatry and Law

S Nambi

INTRODUCTION

There exists a dynamic relationship between psychiatry and law. The interface between psychiatry and law is well acknowledged and documented and that is why there is a subspecialty in psychiatry known as forensic psychiatry. Persons suffering from severe mental illness (SMI) often get involved in legal matters. Persons with SMI are vulnerable for both civil and criminal law-suits. The civil matters include issues related to their marriage, property, writing a will, etc. Persons with SMI often do not know as to what they are doing is right or wrong. Their delusion, hallucination, and other behavioral problems such as hostility, suspicion, and impulsivity make them vulnerable to indulge in crime. All persons suffering from SMI are not violent; only some persons are at risk of becoming so. Mental health legislation of each country governs the care and protection of their mentally ill persons. In India, the recently enacted Mental Healthcare Act 2017 is an important milestone in regulating the matters related to persons with mental health problems. Hence, not only psychiatrists but also other medical practitioners should know some basic facts about the interaction of psychiatry and law. Legislation forms an essential component in the delivery of mental healthcare in society. These matters are discussed under the rubric of the subspecialty of forensic psychiatry. It is a subspecialty of psychiatry in which scientific knowledge and clinical experience is applied to legal issues in legal context, embracing civil, criminal, correctional or legislative matters. The forensic psychiatry operates at the interface of two relatively unrelated disciplines, viz.: psychiatry and law.

However, there is an increasing awareness regarding the relationship between psychiatry and law due to:
- Increasing awareness about mental health and its problems
- The influence of urbanization, industrialization, migration, and disturbed family system
- Increasing awareness of the rights of the mentally ill
- The advocacy groups, the lawyer's interventions, etc.

The patients who require expert psychiatric opinion in the judiciary are:
- Those who may do harm to themselves and harm to others in the society
- Those who may not look after themselves, the welfare of their family and property
- Those who may turn out to be dangerous if they act upon their abnormal thinking and perception
- Marital disharmony due to mental illness in one spouse and their seeking help of judiciary for separation or divorce.

Forensic psychiatry can be discussed under the following headings:

- Mental health related legislations
- Crime and mental illness
- Civil issues (responsibilities) in psychiatry

Mental Health Related Legislations

- Mental Healthcare Act, 2017
- Rights of Persons with Disabilities Act, 2016
- Juvenile Justice Act (Care and Protection of Children), 2015

Crime and Mental Illness

- Criminal responsibility
- Domestic Violence Act
- Narcotic Drugs and Psychotropic Substances Act (NDPSA)
- Protection of Children Against Sexual Offences Act (POCSO)

Civil Issues (Responsibilities) in Psychiatry

- Marriage and mental health legislation
- Testamentary capacity
- Witness
- Contract
- Transfer of property
- The right to vote and the right to stand in the election.

MENTAL HEALTH RELATED LEGISLATIONS

Mental Healthcare Act, 2017

In 2017, a new law called 'Mental Healthcare Act (MHCA 2017) has been enacted, which has replaced the previous Mental Health Act of 1987. This Mental Healthcare Act 2017 is an act to ensure provision of mental health services to all, including promotive and preventive services, as well as to protect and preserve their rights. It has now come into force throughout the country. Some of its salient features, which include many new provisions, are given below:

1. Every person has a right to access the mental health care and treatment services funded by the government.
2. There is provision for providing free treatment for the poor and homeless patients.
3. Person with mental illness is considered competent to take treatment decisions despite mental illness unless his capacity to make mental healthcare and treatment decisions is judged to be impaired.
4. Person with mental illness has a right to make advance directive specifying the way he/she prefers to be cared for. They can declare a 'Nominated Representative' to take health-related decisions.
5. Suicide has been decriminalized and is treated as indicative of severe stress.
6. Provides for a wide variety of rights to mentally ill persons, which includes right to confidentiality of health care, right to community living, right to protection, right to legal aid, right to non-discrimination, right to respect and dignity, right to basic amenities of life and a safe and hygienic environment, etc.
7. Mental health establishment and mental illness have been clearly redefined.
8. Admission and discharge procedures of a mentally ill person from psychiatric hospital have been redefined.
9. Only modified ECT is permissible as a mode of treatment.

This act gives a clear definition of mental illness. "Mental illness means a substantial disorder of thinking, mood, perception, orientation and memory that grossly impairs judgment, behavior, capacity to recognize reality or ability to meet the ordinary demands of life; mental conditions associated with the abuse of alcohol and drugs. But it does not include mental retardation."

According to this act, mental health establishment means all the places where persons suffering from mental illness are kept, other than domestic units, for purposes of treatment, convalescence or rehabilitation. It includes psychiatric hospital/nursing homes, including allopathic (Modern medicine), Ayurvedic, Siddha, Unani centers and also includes general hospital psychiatric units.

MHCA 2017 has adopted a humane, progressive and rights-based approach. It aims to provide support and facilities to the persons suffering from mental illness. There is much greater emphasis on protection of the rights of the mentally ill which have been expanded and broadened. Protection of human rights of the mentally ill is much emphasized in the act with a positive intent.

Rights of Persons with Disabilities Act, 2016

This Act replaces the Persons with Disabilities (Equal Opportunities, Protection of Rights and Full Participation) Act, 1995. It fulfills the obligations to the United National Convention on the Rights of Persons with Disabilities (UNCRPD), to which India is a signatory. The purpose of this Act is to fix responsibilities on the central and state government to ensure that disabilities of any kind do not prevent an individual from living a full, meaningful and productive life and thereby making full contribution to the society in accordance with his or her ability. In addition to other physical disabilities like poor vision, hearing loss, locomotor and other physical disabilities, mental illness, and mental retardation have also been included in the list of disabilities for the purpose of disability-related benefits, concessions, and reservation in jobs.

Juvenile Justice Act (Care and Protection of Children), 2015

This Act replaces the previous Juvenile Justice (Care and Protection of Children) Act, 2000 and aims to provide for the comprehensive care and protection, treatment, development, and rehabilitation of neglected or delinquent juvenile. Juvenile means a child who has not completed age of 18 years. Children with conduct disorders or juvenile delinquents are to be treated with compassion and humane approach when they are found to have committed a crime which is proved so in the juvenile justice board. He will not be sent to prison but shall be sent to correctional homes. However, the Act of 2015 has a provision that the children aged 16–18 years may be tried as an adult if they are found to have committed a heinous crime in the opinion of the board.

CRIME AND MENTAL ILLNESS

Criminality has often been associated with mental illness for a long time. However, often it is a matter of chance association. Crime committed by a mentally ill person may not always be directly related to his current diagnosis; it also depends on the basic personality of the individual and the social setting.

Psychiatric causes of crime: Among psychiatric conditions which are associated with crime, most often it is a severe mental illness such as given below:

- Schizophrenia
- Alcohol and drug-related problem
- Bipolar affective disorder-mania
- Organic mental disorders, e.g., behavioral problems due to epilepsy, head injury, etc.
- Impulse control disorder and antisocial personality disorder.

Criminal Responsibility

Everyone is equal and the same before law. Therefore, liabilities for acts of omissions and commission should be the same. However, law provides certain relief to the mentally ill person. If a severely mentally ill person commits a crime, and there is evidence that at the time of crime, he was suffering from a severe mental illness, then he will not be given punishment like other individuals without such illness. This is as per section 84 of Indian Penal Code which states that "nothing is an offence which is done by a person who, at the time of doing it, by reason of unsoundness of mind, is incapable of knowing the nature of the act, or that he is doing what is either wrong or contrary to law". This act is derived from the famous M'Naghten Rule propounded in Britain.

Domestic Violence Act

The protection of women from Domestic Violence Act 2005 is an act to ensure the rights of women and to empower them. It covers victims of violence of any kind occurring within the family. The main causes of such violence occurring within family are because of a spouse suffering from any psychiatric or personality disorder, marital conflict or the husband being an abuser of alcohol or other substances. The provision for punishment for the offender under this Act is severe. Domestic violence is a human rights violation.

Narcotic Drugs and Psychotropic Substances Act

The association of alcohol and other drug abuse and crime is unquestionable. The magnitude of crime committed by addicts is quite substantial. The punishment (imprisonment and penalties) is very severe under this Act and has been clearly defined.

Protection of Children Against Sexual Offences Act

Child sexual abuse refers to offences committed for sexual gratification using children for this purpose by an older adult or elderly who is more powerful. It produces lot of psychiatric disturbances in affected children. It appears that child sexual abuse is increasing in society day by day. With regard to India, child sexual abuse appears to be far more prevalent than society is willing to acknowledge. To ensure protection of children against such offences, the parliament passed the "Protection of Children from Sexual Offences" Act in 2012, which has many stringent provisions. It has also made reporting of any information of such offences mandatory by law. The act is child friendly.

CIVIL ISSUES (RESPONSIBILITIES) IN PSYCHIATRY

Marriage and Mental Health Legislation

Severe mental illnesses often interfere with proper execution of roles within the institution of marriage. Because of such mental illnesses, which are not accepted by the spouse and their families, the chance of breaking down of such relationship becomes probable.

In the modern stressful world, the number of persons suffering from marital conflict is increasing day by day. To tackle these marriage-related problems such as divorce, family courts are established; whether marriages are made in heaven or not, often marriages get dissolved in the family courts in the modern times.

There are two key words in the legal terms about marriage:

1. *Nullity of marriage*: It means that the marriage is held null and void due to prior presence of severe mental illness along with some other reasons. Nullity in other

words means that the marriage did not take place at all.

2. Divorce means that the marriage was a valid one, but the relationship cannot be continued. Following the divorce order, the individual becomes eligible for remarriage.

Unsoundness of mind as a ground for divorce: As per the Hindu Marriage Act, if one of the spouses has been incurably of unsound mind or has been suffering continuously or intermittently from mental disorder, the other spouse can apply for divorce.

As per Hindu Marriage Act, divorce can be sought by a petitioner:

- If the spouse is suffering from incurable mental illness or has been suffering from continuous or periodic mental disorder.
- If the spouse suffering from mental disorder, exhibits abnormality to such a kind and to such an extent that the petitioner cannot reasonably be expected to live with him/her.

Just because a person is suffering from some mental health problem, the court will not grant divorce.

In India marriage and legal aspects are covered by several laws:

- Hindu Marriage Act, 1955
- The Special Marriage Act, 1954
- Dissolution of Muslim Marriages Act, 1939; the Muslim Personal Law (Shariat) Application Act, 1937
- Parsi Marriage and Divorce Act, 1936
- The Indian Christian Marriage Act, 1872
- The Indian Divorce Act, 1869.

Testamentary Capacity (Testament = Will)

As per section 59 of the Indian Succession Act, 1925, "Every person of sound mind, not being a minor, may dispose of his property by will".

A will can be declared invalid if it is proved that at the time of making the will, the testator (the person writing a will):

- Was of unsound mind
- Did not have the mental capacity to understand the consequences of the act.

Witness

Under the Evidence Act, 1872, a mentally ill person is incompetent to enter in to give evidence in a court of law if he is unable to understand the questions asked or to give rational answers to them by virtue of mental illness.

Contract

Under the Indian Contract Act, 1872, every person to be competent to contract must be a major and of sound mind, i.e., he is capable of understanding the contract and of forming a rational judgment as to its effect upon his interests. Severe mentally ill persons cannot enter into a valid contract.

Transfer of Property

Under the Transfer of Property Act, 1882, only persons competent to contract are authorized to transfer property. Hence, person suffering with severe mental illness cannot transfer his/her property to others.

The Right to Vote and Right to Stand for Election

No person of unsound mind can contest an election or exercise the franchise of voting.

Informed Consent is Essential for the Following Conditions

- Admission to a psychiatric hospital on a voluntary basis
- Procedures such as psychosurgery, brain stimulation techniques, etc.
- Narco-analysis, hypnotherapy
- HIV screening

- Some drug treatments, e.g., disulfiram
- Administration of any research drug (clinical drug trials)

CONCLUSION

It is universally accepted that the persons, who are mentally ill, require different sets of rules in relation to their rights, responsibilities and liabilities. Not only the society and other individuals should be protected from the mentally ill, but such mentally ill persons should also be protected against neglect, exclusion, stigma, and abrogation of their rights. They should be given the advantage of due care and concern of the society. Of course, the emphasis has varied from time to time and from region to region. It has depended on the state of prevailing knowledge (and ignorance) and the values of the society.

TAKE-HOME MESSAGES

- There exists a dynamic and inevitable relationship between psychiatry and law, because they both deal with human behavior.
- With increasing complexity in society and changing cultural values, the principles and practices of forensic psychiatry is gradually becoming more and more important.
- Some of the important acts which are of direct relevance to psychiatry are Mental Healthcare Act, 2017, Rights of Persons with Disabilities Act 2016, Juvenile Justice Act (Care and Protection of Children) 2015, Narcotic Drugs and Psychotropic Substances Act (NDPSA) 1985, Protection of Children Against Sexual Offences Act (POCSO) 2012.
- Other issues of life related to mental disorders, which fall within the jurisdiction of forensic psychiatry are criminal responsibility, domestic violence, marriage and divorce, testamentary capacity, witness, contract, transfer of property, the right to vote and the right to stand in the election.

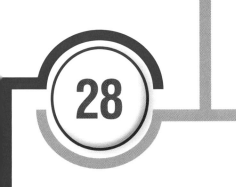

Psychopharmacology and Physical Methods of Treatment

Varghese P Punnoose

INTRODUCTION

Treatments for psychiatric disorders can be broadly classified into either somatic or psychosocial interventions. Somatic methods of treatment include pharmacological treatment and other physical methods such as electroconvulsive therapy (ECT) and others. Psychosocial treatments include various types of psychotherapies, behavior therapy, and rehabilitation. In most psychiatric disorders both somatic and psychosocial treatment are needed for better outcome. The priority and relative importance to be given to the chosen treatment depends on the diagnosis and the individual circumstances of the patient **(Flowchart 28.1)**.

Psychopharmacological Treatment

Why medicines are prescribed to treat psychiatric disorders?

Medicines are prescribed in psychiatric disorders not just as sedatives, hypnotics or tranquillizers. Most of the psychiatric disorders are associated with abnormalities in brain chemistry in terms of altered neurotransmission. Psychopharmacological agents are used to correct the abnormal neurotransmission underlying mental disorders.

Flowchart 28.1: Treatments in psychiatry.

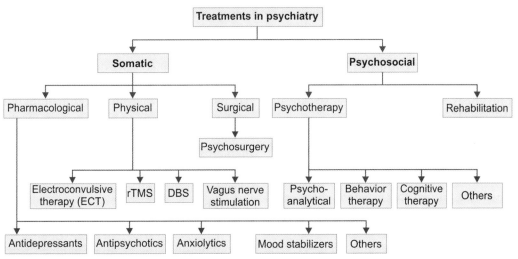

(rTMS: repetitive transcranial magnetic stimulation; DBS: deep brain stimulation)

Psychopharmacological agents can be classified based on their clinical use into:

- Antipsychotics
- Antidepressants
- Anxiolytics and hypnotics
- Mood stabilizers
- Others—stimulants, anticraving agents, antidementia drugs, etc.

Antipsychotics

Antipsychotics are pharmacological agents used as the mainstay of treatment in psychotic disorders such as schizophrenia, delusional disorders, acute and transient psychotic disorders, and schizoaffective disorders. They are also used along with mood stabilizers in the manic episode and mixed states in bipolar disorder. When depression is associated with psychotic features, antipsychotics, especially the atypical ones are used along with antidepressant medications. Antipsychotics also have a role as augmenting agents in the treatment of depression and obsessive compulsive disorder. In hyperactive delirium and in emotional and behavioral symptoms of dementia small dose of antipsychotics for a brief period may have a role. Behavioral stereotypes and self-injuring behavior in autistic spectrum disorders may respond to small dose of antipsychotics such as risperidone or aripiprazole. The term neuroleptics or major tranquillizers used previously in pharmacology texts are not favored **(Flowchart 28.2)**.

First Generation Antipsychotics (Conventional Antipsychotics)

The first antipsychotic agent discovered was chlorpromazine. French psychiatrists Delay and Deniker are credited with the discovery of this molecule in 1951. The efficacy of chlorpromazine in relieving

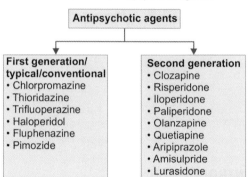

Flowchart 28.2: Antipsychotic agents.

agitation, restlessness, delusions, and hallucinations led to active search for similar other agents and inaugurated the era of modern psychopharmacology. Haloperidol, thioridazine, trifluoperazine, fluphenazine, perphenazine, pimozide, etc., were soon introduced to clinical practice.

Mechanism of action of first generation antipsychotics (FGAs): The common mechanism of action is the blockade of dopamine type 2 (D2) receptors. It has been found that the potency of antipsychotic action is proportionate to the D2 receptor binding profile of the molecule. It is estimated that 70–80% D2 binding is needed for effective antipsychotic action. Haloperidol has got high D2 binding whereas, chlorpromazine and thioridazine are having relatively weak binding on D2 receptors. D2 blockade in mesolimbic dopaminergic pathway is believed to be important for the antipsychotic effect, whereas the D2 blockade in nigrostriatal tract and tuberoinfundibular tract leads to extrapyramidal and endocrine (hyperprolactinemia and galactorrhea) side-effects respectively.

Chlorpromazine: This molecule belongs to the phenothiazine group with an aliphatic side-chain. In addition to the desired D2 receptor antagonism, this molecule interacts with several other neurotransmitter systems, such as acetylcholine, noradrenaline, histamine, and serotonin. Because of these multiple actions chlorpromazine produces a lot of adverse effects like dry mouth, constipation, blurring of vision, orthostatic hypotension and sedation in addition to the extrapyramidal and endocrine side-effects. Uncommon side-effects include cardiac arrhythmias, seizures, paralytic ileus, and precipitation of acute narrow angle glaucoma. The dosage of chlorpromazine for remission of the acute phase is around 800 mg/day given in divided doses, more of the dosage to be given in the evening, considering its sedative properties. In the maintenance phase the dosage requirement is much less, being in the range of 50–400 mg/day. Route of administration is oral. It is available as 50 mg, 100 mg, and 200 mg tablets. It is also available as injection but used very infrequently nowadays.

Haloperidol: Belonging to the butyrophenone group, haloperidol has very potent antipsychotic action. This fact along with its easy availability, favorable side-effect profile and safety in parenteral administration makes it the preferred antipsychotic in acute care settings. The therapeutic dose is 15–20 mg/day. During the acute phase it is given in divided doses but in maintenance phase, it can be given as single bedtime dose. The common side-effects are extrapyramidal symptoms (EPS). It may manifest as tremors, acute dystonia, parkinsonian syndrome or akathisia. It is available as 0.25 mg, 0.5 mg, 1.5 mg, 5 mg, and 10 mg tablets and injections (1 mL ampoule of 5 mg). Haloperidol can be given both by intramuscular (IM) or intravenous (IV) route. Haloperidol is also available as depot injections.

Trifluoperazine: Trifluoperazine is an antipsychotic with medium potency. It is a phenothiazine with piperazine side-chain. The therapeutic dose is 30–40 mg/day. It is available as 5 mg and 10 mg tablets. The adverse effects are the same as that of haloperidol, although relatively less severe.

First generation antipsychotics though effective in relieving the positive psychotic symptoms such as delusions, hallucinations, and disorganization of speech, they were soon found to have adverse effects such as EP (parkinsonian) symptoms, and long-term problems such as development of abnormal involuntary movements (tardive dyskinesia). Furthermore, the FGAs were not that useful in treating the negative symptoms and cognitive symptoms of schizophrenia, the domain of symptoms so crucial in rehabilitation and recovery.

Dosage equivalent of first generation anti-psychotics and potential for extrapyramidal reaction is given in Table 28.1: Treatment with FGAs, especially with the high and medium potency, necessitates the use of anticholinergic agents such as trihexyphenidyl or benzhexol to manage extrapyramidal adverse effects. However, the long-term use of anticholinergics may increase the risk of developing relatively irreversible movement disorders such as tardive dyskinesia. Adverse effects such as acute dystonia are treated by anticholinergics

Table 28.1: Drugs and its dosage equivalent of first generation antipsychotics and extrapyramidal reaction.

Drug name	Therapeutic equivalent (mg)	EPS potential
Chlorpromazine	100	++
Thioridazine	100	+
Trifluoperazine	5	++/+++
Haloperidol	2	+++
Fluphenazine	2	+++
Pimozide	1.5	+++

(EPS: extrapyramidal symptoms)

or agents such as promethazine (phenergan) which is available as parenteral preparation. If akathisia develops during treatment, propranolol or benzodiazepines are the treatments of choice. Temporary withdrawal of antipsychotics and change over to either the ones with lower potency (chlorpromazine) or atypical agents (olanzapine) is a useful strategy if extrapyramidal adverse effects occur.

Neuroleptic malignant syndrome (NMS): It is a rare but potentially lethal adverse effect resulting from treatment with dopamine receptor antagonists. Symptoms include severe muscle rigidity, hyperthermia, akinesia, mutism, confusion, agitation, tachycardia and elevation of blood pressure. Leukocytosis, elevation of creatine phosphokinase (CPK), elevation of liver enzymes are the laboratory findings. Rhabdomyolysis can lead on to renal failure. Mortality can be as high as 20–30%. When NMS is suspected the dopamine antagonists should be stopped immediately. Anticholinergic agents, skeletal muscle relaxant dantrolene, dopamine agonists such as bromocriptine or amantadine are useful in treating NMS. Use of high potency agents and depot preparations increase the risk of NMS.

Second Generation Antipsychotics (Newer or Atypical Antipsychotics)

Psychopharmacologists were in search of molecules which were devoid of parkinsonian adverse effects and tardive dyskinesia and this search resulted in the development of several such agents generally referred to as atypical antipsychotics. The commonly used ones include clozapine, risperidone, olanzapine, quetiapine, aripiprazole, and amisulpride. The less commonly used are paliperidone, iloperidone, ziprasidone, blonanserin, zotepine, and lurasidone.

Mechanism of action of second generation antipsychotics (SGAs): In addition to the dopamine antagonism, they act on the serotonergic receptors, especially the 5HT2A, as well. Hence, they are referred to as the serotonin-dopamine antagonists (SDAs). Dopamine receptors other than D2 are also targeted. The binding of these agents with the DA receptors is weak and short-lasting unlike the typicals. These pharmacological properties translate clinically as less extrapyramidal side-effects and better efficacy in the domain of negative symptoms. Though EPSs are less frequent with SGAs, the chance of developing metabolic syndrome (weight gain, insulin insensitivity-type 2 diabetes mellitus, and dyslipidemia) is higher. This may be mediated through the histaminergic and 5HT2C receptor blockade.

Clozapine: Clozapine is the most efficacious of all antipsychotics. This agent is practically devoid of extrapyramidal side-effects. Despite these advantages clozapine is not used as a first-line antipsychotic because of some serious adverse effects. They include agranulocytosis (approximately 1%), seizures (usually in doses above 400 mg/day), and myocarditis. Metabolic syndrome, sedation, and sialorrhea are other adverse effects which limit the use of clozapine. Considering these, especially the risk of agranulocytosis, clozapine is started in small doses (12.5–25 mg/day) and slowly titrated in increments of 25 mg to reach its therapeutic dose (400–600 mg/day) with close monitoring of blood count. Once the therapeutic dose is reached the monitoring of total blood count and differential count is done on a weekly basis for the first 6 months, thereafter every 2 weeks till 1 year. Monthly monitoring of blood count is desirable as long as the patient is continued on clozapine. Monitoring of blood sugar, lipid levels, and body-mass index once in every 6 months is recommended for patients on clozapine. Apart from being the agent of choice in treatment resistant schizophrenia, clozapine is indicated in schizoaffective and bipolar disorders which do not respond to first-line treatments. Clozapine is also useful in tardive dyskinesia.

Olanzapine: Olanzapine is one of the most frequently used first-line antipsychotics. The fact that this molecule possesses significant mood stabilizing properties makes it a desirable agent in the treatment of bipolar mood disorders as well. Olanzapine has a role as an effective augmenting agent in the treatment of depression. The limiting side-effect is weight gain and its adverse effect on glycemic control. So patients on treatment with olanzapine should be monitored regularly on these parameters. Dosage is 15–20 mg/day. It is available as 5 mg and 10 mg tablets and oral solutions. Short-acting and long-acting injections are also available though not widely used.

Risperidone: Risperidone is the most potent dopamine 2 receptor antagonist among the atypical antipsychotics. So the risk of developing EPS is relatively higher for risperidone (especially in doses above 4 mg/day) when compared to other agents in this group. The alpha adrenergic action of risperidone increases the risk for postural hypotension. Apart from the conventional use in schizophrenia and bipolar disorders, risperidone is also used in the treatment of behavioral stereotypes and self-injurious behavior in autism and intellectual disability (mental retardation). Risperidone is started at a dose of 1 mg twice daily on the 1st day, 2 mg twice daily on the 2nd day and increased to 3 mg twice daily on the 3rd day. The therapeutic dose of risperidone is 6–8 mg/day, though doses up to 12 mg are tried in cases which do not respond well. Monitoring of body mass index (BMI), blood sugar, and lipid levels are recommended. It is available as 1 mg, 2 mg, 3 mg, and 4 mg tablets. Oral solutions are also available. Depot preparations (long-acting injections) may be suitable for patients with poor adherence.

Quetiapine: This molecule has a receptor profile which is very similar to clozapine but efficacy wise inferior. Apart from its use in schizophrenia it is useful in the treatment of bipolar disorders, especially bipolar depression. Though sedation is a limiting side-effect with quetiapine, its anxiolytic and mood stabilizing properties and low EPS risk, makes it a preferred choice for many clinicians who use it in the treatment of schizophrenia, bipolar disorders, and schizoaffective disorders. Dosage is 400–800 mg/day for the acute phase and 100–400 mg/day for the maintenance phase and for antidepressant action.

Ziprasidone: In addition to the D2 and 5HT2 A antagonism, ziprasidone acts as serotonin and norepinephrine reuptake inhibitor. This may make ziprasidone a suitable agent for treating depressive symptoms in psychotic disorders. Concerns about QTc prolongation have limited the use of ziprasidone. Dosage range is 80–160 mg/day.

Amisulpride: At low doses it blocks the presynaptic dopamine D2 and D3 auto-receptors, thereby enhancing dopaminergic transmission. At higher doses it antagonizes these receptors in the postsynaptic membrane thereby reducing dopaminergic transmission. This differential effect of amisulpride may be responsible for its effectiveness in relieving positive symptoms in acute phases (400–800 mg/day) and efficacy against negative symptoms in maintenance phase (50–300 mg/day).

Aripiprazole: In addition to the D2 and 5HT2A receptor antagonism, this molecule also has a partial agonist action at D2 and 5HT1A receptors. The partial agonism results eventually in a functional decline of dopamine activity. It is indicated in the treatment of schizophrenia and acute mania. It is also useful as augmenting agent in the treatment of depression and irritability associated with autistic disorder. Its dosage is 5–30 mg/day.

Use of Depot Antipsychotic Preparations

Adherence to treatment is a very important consideration in psychopharmacology. Several factors like poor insight, adverse effects (such as sedation, akathisia, parkinsonian side-effects, sexual side-effects, weight gain, etc.), health beliefs, stigma, and cost-availability factors might lead to poor adherence. Poor adherence to medication is the most important cause of relapses and recurrences. So every effort should be made to educate patients and their families regarding the need for good compliance with treatment. Use of depot antipsychotics is an effective method of tackling the issue of nonadherence.

The commonly used preparations are:
- Fluphenazine decanoate
- Haloperidol
- Risperidone
- Flupenthixol
- Zuclopenthixol
- Olanzapine

The advantage is that medications can be administered under supervision once in 2–4 weeks. This ensures good adherence and thereby decreases the risk of relapse and recurrences. The disadvantage is the risk of persistence of side-effects throughout the period of slow release of drug. Use of typical antipsychotics in depot form may also increase the risk of development of tardive dyskinesia in long-term.

General Principles in the Use of Antipsychotics

- Use antipsychotics only when clearly indicated and necessary by adhering to the principles of evidence-based practice.
- Start low and go slow in both uptitrating as well as tapering off. Loading dose may be needed in some acute cases (e.g., acute mania). Abrupt cessation may be needed if adverse events like agranulocytosis or other life-threatening events occur.
- Prefer the drug which was effective and tolerated well in the previous episode.
- Use optimum doses. Use adequate therapeutic dose in acute phase and optimize the dose to minimum effective dose during maintenance.
- Watch for adverse effects. Carefully watch for EPS and tardive dyskinesia, especially if the patient is getting FGAs or depot preparations. Monitor and record BMI, total cholesterol, blood sugar, lipid profile, ECG, etc., especially if SGAs are being used.
- Use them for adequate duration. The use of antipsychotics in conditions such as schizophrenia or delusional disorder is indefinite, perhaps life-long. Premature discontinuation may lead to relapse. On the other hand the use, especially of FGAs, in bipolar disorders may be limited only to the acute manic phase.
- Minimize the long-term use of adjuvants like anticholinergics and benzodiazepines.
- Minimize the frequency of usage.
- Always consider cost. The medicines prescribed should be affordable and available.
- Precautions regarding over dosage and deliberate self-harm must always be kept in mind.

Antidepressants

The rationale of using pharmacological agents in the treatment of depression is based on the monoaminergic hypothesis. According to this hypothesis the pathologically low mood, anhedonia (inability to experience pleasure) and other features which define depression are related to a dysregulated brain chemistry involving neurotransmitters such as serotonin (5HT), norepinephrine (NE), and dopamine. Antidepressants act by optimizing the monoamine neurotransmission by inhibiting reuptake or by modulating the receptors or by inhibiting the enzymes metabolizing them. This results in increased synaptic concentration of these neurotransmitters that initiate a series of reactions which correct the abnormal signal transduction in depression (**Flowchart 28.3**).

Tricyclic antidepressants (TCAs): The group name derives from the tricyclic ring structure of all the drugs which belong to this group. Imipramine, amitriptyline, desipramine, nortriptyline, and dothiepin (dosulepin) are the more commonly used drugs of this group. They act by blocking the reuptake of serotonin and NE from the synaptic cleft. TCAs are considered to be the gold standards for antidepressant efficacy. Apart from their action on 5HT and NE, these agents act on the cholinergic, histaminergic, and alpha-adrenergic receptors. These actions result in anticholinergic side-effects like dryness of mouth, urinary retention and constipation;

antihistaminergic side-effects such as sedation and weight-gain and antiadrenergic side-effects like postural hypotension and cardiac rhythm abnormalities. Dosage of imipramine and amitriptyline is in the range of 75–225 mg/day, which may be given as a single bedtime dose. They are available as 25 mg, 50 mg, and 75 mg tablets. Clomipramine is particularly useful in the treatment of obsessive compulsive disorder attributed to its rather high serotonergic action compared to other TCAs.

Monoamine oxidase inhibitors (MAOIs): Inhibiting monoamine oxidase, the enzyme which catabolizes monoamine neurotransmitters increases the synaptic concentration of NE and 5HT. This results in improved signal transduction. This is the proposed mechanism of action of these medications. MAO inhibitors include phenelzine, isocarboxazid, and tranylcypromine. MAO-B inhibitors such as selegiline do not have significant antidepressant action. Though MAO-A inhibitors are effective antidepressants but their potential serious side-effects like hypertensive crisis limits their widespread use in clinical practice. Food items containing amino acid tryptophan, if taken concurrently with these medications, can result in such type of reaction (cheese reaction). So also is the case of interaction with other drugs such as TCAs. A drug free (wash out) interval of at least 2 weeks should be allowed before

Flowchart 28.3: Antidepressants.

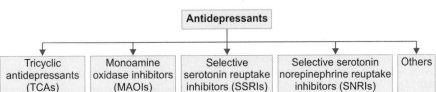

switching over to or switching over from a MAOI. Using a reversible MAOI, such as moclobemide may reduce this risk. MAO inhibitors are especially useful in the treatment of atypical depression and phobias.

Selective serotonin reuptake inhibitors (SSRIs): Selective inhibition of the serotonin transporter in the presynaptic membrane, resulting in more efficient serotonergic transmission, is believed to be the mechanism of action of SSRIs. The commonly used agents include fluoxetine (the first of such molecules), citalopram, escitalopram, sertraline, paroxetine, and fluvoxamine. SSRIs have emerged as the most commonly used antidepressants because of their efficacy which is comparable to TCAs but has better tolerability. SSRIs are relatively devoid of troublesome side-effects such as sedation, dryness of mouth, constipation, weight gain, postural hypotension, cardiac arrhythmias, etc. Common adverse effects with SSRIs are gastrointestinal dyspepsia, diarrhea, etc. Sexual side-effects like anorgasmia, erectile failure or ejaculatory problems such as dry ejaculation or retrograde ejaculation and delayed ejaculation may be a problem in a proportion of patients. The dosage schedule is given below in **Table 28.2**.

Serotonin-norepinephrine reuptake inhibitors (Dual acting antidepressants): They act by preventing the reuptake of both NE and serotonin in a selective manner. Venlafaxine and its isomer desvenlafaxine, duloxetine and milnacipran belong to this group. They are usually prescribed as second-line antidepressants (when there is a poor response to first-line SSRIs) or when physical symptoms such as pain or sensory symptoms predominate the clinical picture. Usually they are well-tolerated such as SSRIs. They should be used with caution in patients with systemic hypertension. Blood pressure monitoring is recommended with serotonin-norepinephrine reuptake inhibitors (SNRI) use. *Dose*: Venlafaxine 75–225 mg/day, desvenlafaxine 50–100 mg/day, duloxetine 40–80 mg/day.

There are several other drugs used in the treatment of depression, which may be of use in resistant cases or with special populations. Mirtazapine (noradrenergic and serotonergic action), trazodone, bupropion (noradrenergic and dopaminergic action) and melatonergic agents such as ramelteon and agomelatine may be useful in such situations.

General Principles of Antidepressant Use

- Select a single antidepressant–either SSRI or TCA—as the first-line agent. Most treatment guidelines recommend SSRI.
- Effectiveness in a previous episode or a positive family history of good response to a particular antidepressant is a good guiding principle in the choice of an antidepressant.
- Start in small doses, step up slowly and carefully; watch for improvement or emergence of side-effects.
- Use adequate and optimal dose aiming for full remission.

Table 28.2: Drugs and its dosage schedule.	
Drugs	*Dosages*
Fluoxetine	10–40 mg/once daily (up to 80 mg in OCD)
Citalopram	20–40 mg/day
Escitalopram	10–20 mg/day
Sertraline	50–200 mg/day
Fluvoxamine	100–200 mg/day
Paroxetine CR	12.5–37.5 mg/day

(CR: controlled release; OCD: obsessive compulsive disorder)

- Wait for 2–4 weeks for the antidepressant effect to appear. Almost every antidepressant has a lag period for the antidepressant action to manifest. This has to be explained to the patient at the time of initiating the treatment.
- If the monotherapy with antidepressant does not give satisfactory response, augmentations, substitutions and combinations can be tried in a systematic fashion as laid down in treatment guidelines.
- Continue the therapeutic dose till the natural cycle of the episode is likely to be over, i.e., 9–12 months, if it is a first episode. If frequent recurrent episodes occur, antidepressants should be continued indefinitely.
- Antidepressants should be tapered off slowly, over a period of several weeks after the treatment is completed.
- Safety precautions should be adhered to with utmost vigilance, especially when antidepressants are prescribed on outpatient basis to a depressed patient with high risk of suicide.
- Always consider cost. The medicines prescribed should be affordable and available.

Mood Stabilizers

Mood is the pervasive and persisting state of feeling tone, which colors a person's thoughts and perceptions. In biological terms, mood is a brain function which is very finely regulated by neural activity. Monoaminergic neurotransmission and hypothalamo-pituitary-adrenal axis are believed to be the biological bases of mood regulation. Pathological dysregulation of mood results in elevation of mood as seen in mania or lowering of mood as seen in depression or mood instability as seen in bipolar disorders.

The fact that chemical agents can favorably influence mood regulation, is the basis for pharmacotherapy in mood disorders. Commonly used medicines which come under this category include lithium, sodium valproate, carbamazepine, oxcarbazepine, and lamotrigine. They are mainly used in the treatment of acute phase and maintenance phase of bipolar mood (affective) disorders. Other indications in psychiatry include their use in treatment of schizoaffective disorder, in treatment of depression as augmenting agents and in treatment of substance related disorders either in withdrawal states or as anticraving agents.

Lithium: Lithium carbonate is one of the first-line mood stabilizers approved for use both in the acute manic phase and in the prophylaxis of bipolar disorder. Several mechanisms of action are suggested to explain the mood stabilizing property of lithium. They are alterations in ion transport, effect on inositol phosphatase second messenger system, on neurotransmitters and neuropeptides and signal transduction pathways.

Lithium is commonly available as 300 mg and 400 mg (sustained release) tablets. During acute mania lithium is initiated in doses of 600–900 mg/day in divided doses. It is slowly uptitrated over a period of 1–2 weeks to achieve a therapeutic level of 1–1.2 mEq/L. Lithium has got a relatively slow onset of its antimanic or mood stabilizing action. Because of this, adjuvants such as antipsychotics or benzodiazepines or combination with valproate may be needed in the acute phase. Once the remission of acute phase is achieved, the dose of lithium can be reduced to keep the serum levels between 0.4–0.6 mEq/L. Prophylactic treatment with lithium brings down relapses and recurrences considerably. Though effective and economic, lithium has got a host of adverse effects.

They include neurological side-effects such as tremor, memory difficulties, and lowering of seizure threshold, endocrine adverse-effects such as hypothyroidism, goiter and hyperparathyroidism, and cardiac problems such as sinus node dysfunction and renal side-effects such as polyuria (nephrogenic diabetes insipidus), concentrating defect, reduced glomerular filtration rate (GFR) and renal tubular acidosis. Dermatological problems such as acne, exacerbation of psoriasis or gastroenterological side-effects such as altered taste, nausea, loss of appetite, and weight gain may be a problem in some. Monitoring of thyroid, renal, and cardiac functions are recommended during lithium treatment.

Since lithium has only a narrow therapeutic index, when a patient is started on lithium, he has to be monitored closely for development of toxicity. Lithium toxicity may be manifested by vomiting, coarse tremors, dysarthria, ataxia, neuromuscular irritability, seizures, and coma. It may be precipitated by inadequate fluid intake or conditions which promote dehydration like fever, diarrhea, and vomiting. Drug interactions may also precipitate lithium toxicity. For the same reason, drugs such as nonsteroidal anti-inflammatory drugs (NSAIDs), thiazide diuretics or angiotensin-converting enzyme (ACE) inhibitors should be used with caution if the patient is on lithium. Mild levels of toxicity may be treated by measures such as discontinuing lithium, adequate hydration, and sodium supplementation. If there are features of severe toxicity, hemodialysis is the treatment of choice.

Valproate: Valproate is the most useful drug in the treatment of a manic episode. The fact that it has got a rapid onset of action and is relatively well tolerated which has made it the most widely prescribed mood stabilizer.

Valproate has less pronounced action in the depressive phase of bipolar disorder. Postulated mechanisms of action include enhancement of gamma aminobutyric acid (GABA) activity, modulation of voltage-sensitive sodium channels and action on extrahypothalamic neuropeptides.

Various formulations of valproate are available—as valproic acid, valproate, divalproex, etc. Once daily preparations and controlled/extended release preparations have made the administration easier, the therapeutic efficacy is achieved when serum concentrations of 50–100 µg/mL is reached and maintained.

Though valproate is relatively well-tolerated, side-effects on liver function and pancreas should be watched for. Hepatotoxocity is more common in pediatric age group and in those with liver diseases. Acute pancreatitis is rare. Other serious-effects include hyperammonemia induced encephalopathy and thrombocytopenia. Teratogenic potential of valproate is also a concern. Risk of neural tube defects is up to 3–5%. So valproate should be avoided in pregnancy. Use of folic acid supplementation has shown to reduce the risk of neural tube defects. Other common side-effects include gastrointestinal (GI) problems such as nausea, vomiting, and dyspepsia and dermatological problems such as hair loss. Nervous system side-effects such as sedation, ataxia, dysarthria, and tremor are self-limited and may wane off with dose reduction.

Carbamazepine and oxcarbazepine: Carbamazepine and its analog oxcarbazepine are considered as second-line mood stabilizers. As with valproate, they are more useful in the acute manic phase than in the depressive phase of bipolar disorder. The mechanism of action is through its binding on the voltage-dependant sodium channels which in turn reduce voltage-dependant calcium channel activation and thus synaptic transmission. Other proposed mechanism of mood stabilization is its action on N-methyl-D-aspartate (NMDA) glutamate receptor channels and potentiation of catecholamine neurotransmission. Carbamazepine is available as 100 and 200 mg immediate release tablets, 200 mg, 300 mg, and 400 mg controlled release tablets. Oxcarbazepine is available as 150 mg, 300 mg, 450 mg, and 600 mg tablets. Start with small doses (200 mg) of carbamazepine and slowly uptitrate to 600–1,200 mg/day over a period of 1–2 weeks. Slow up titration is necessitated by the autoinduction of cytochrome (CYP450) 3A4 enzyme system. Dosages in the range of 800–1,200 mg/day may be needed for the acute manic phase, whereas only lower dosages (400–800 mg/day) may be sufficient for the maintenance phase. In doses which result in more than 9 μg/mL of plasma concentrations, ataxia, and drowsiness may occur. Though carbamazepine is relatively well tolerated, serious dermatological side-effects such as exfoliative dermatitis, toxic epidermal necrolysis (TEN) and Stevens–Johnson's syndrome, blood dyscrasias such as agranulocytosis and aplastic anemia and hepatitis should be cautiously watched for. Other rare adverse effects of concern are decreased cardiac conduction, syndrome of inappropriate production of antidiuretic hormone (SIADH) and teratogenic effects such as cleft palate, microcephaly and neural-tube defects.

Lamotrigine: Lamotrigine is an anticonvulsant mood stabilizer that appears to "stabilize mood from below" in the sense that its clinical effect is most pronounced in the treatment of depressive component of bipolar disorders. It is observed that lamotrigine is more useful in lengthening the intervals between depressive episodes than manic episodes. Lamotrigine is also useful in rapid-cycling bipolar disorders (more than four mood episodes per year). Blockade of voltage—sensitive sodium channels which in turn modulates the release of glutamate and aspartate—is believed to be the mechanism underlying the mood stabilizing action of lamotrigine. Inhibition of serotonin receptor may be contributing to its antidepressant actions. It is available as 25 mg, 50 mg, and 100 mg tablets. Delayed release (once daily) preparations are also available. The principle of "start low and go slow" should be adhered to in initiating treatment with lamotrigine. Starting dose may be 12.5–25 mg/day, which is titrated to the therapeutic dose of 100–200 mg/day over a period of 3-4 weeks. The slow titration is necessitated by the risk of developing serious skin rashes like TEN or Steven–Johnson's syndrome which is estimated to occur in 1 out of 5,000 patients.

Other mood stabilizing agents which are rarely used include anticonvulsants such as phenytoin and calcium channel blockers such as nimodipine and verapamil.

General Principles in the Use of Mood Stabilizers

- Choice of mood stabilizer should be evidence based. For example, a patient with irritable mania and comorbid substance use is most likely to respond to valproate than lithium. A patient with euphoric mania, positive family history of bipolar I is likely to respond to lithium. Rapid cycling (more than four episodes per year) may respond better to valproate or lamotrigine than lithium.
- Proper patient education should be done before and throughout the course of treatment.

- The chosen mood stabilizer should be used in optimum doses. Subtherapeutic doses of mood stabilizer may lead to inadequate response and may lead to unnecessary polypharmacy.
- Proper monitoring at regular intervals as recommended for each agent and documentation should be adhered to. *Example*: Serum lithium monitoring, thyroid screening and monitoring, cardiac monitoring, and renal function monitoring in a patient on lithium.
- Mood stabilizers should be used for adequate period of time. Premature discontinuation should be avoided.
- Combinations of mood stabilizers should be done only if definitely indicated. Drug—drug interactions should be monitored vigilantly during combinations. For example, when valproate is added to a patient on lamotrigine the risk of developing serious dermatological side-effect should be monitored very closely.
- Interactions with medications used for treatment of medical conditions should be warned to the patient and informed to other physicians who are treating the patient.
- Most mood stabilizers have significant teratogenic potential. For example, use of sodium valproate in first trimester of pregnancy carries 2% risk of neural tube defects. So patients should be well informed to take decisions regarding pregnancy planning.
- Mood stabilizers should not be abruptly discontinued as sudden drop in brain levels may increase the risk of breakthrough episodes. They should be tapered off over several weeks carefully monitoring for any signs of relapse or recurrence.

Anxiolytic and Hypnotic Drugs

Introduction of benzodiazepines was a landmark in the pharmacological treatment of anxiety and insomnia. The first drug of this class was chlordiazepoxide which was approved for medical use in 1960. Several such drugs have been introduced since then. They include diazepam, clonazepam, alprazolam, lorazepam, oxazepam, flurazepam, nitrazepam, temazepam, triazolam, estazolam, and quazepam. The mechanism of action is through benzodiazepine receptors which in turn modulate the GABA receptors, the principal inhibitory neurotransmitter in the central nervous system. Because of the rapid anxiolytic and sedative effect, they are useful in the acute treatment of insomnia, anxiety, and agitation. They also have anticonvulsant and muscle relaxant properties. Though they are effective and safe, the risk of physical and psychological dependence should be considered when prescribing them.

Benzodiazepines are divided into three categories depending on the half-life (Box 28.1).

Four factors should be considered when choosing a benzodiazepine; they are route of administration, half-life, lipid solubility, and hepatic metabolism.

Benzodiazepines in general are well absorbed orally. Mouth dissolving preparations (e.g., clonazepam) make the onset of action faster. Absorption is erratic in the IM route for all benzodiazepines except lorazepam and midazolam. So benzodiazepines are preferably administered

---

Box 28.1: Categorization of benzodiazepines depending on the half-life.

Short half-life (2–3 hours): Triazolam
Intermediate half-life (8–30 hours): Alprazolam, lorazepam, oxazepam, estazolam
Long half-life (30–>100 hours): Diazepam, chlordiazepoxide, flurazepam, clonazepam

by oral route. If parenteral route is needed like in the case of treatment of delirium tremens or status epilepticus, diazepam (5–10 mg) is administered by intravenous route very slowly, closely monitoring the respiration. Lorazepam (1–4 mg) can be administered safely through the intramuscular route.

Half-life and lipid solubility determine the onset and duration of action. The advantages of long half-life molecules over the short half-life ones include less frequent dosing, less plasma concentration variations, and less withdrawal symptoms. The disadvantages include drug accumulation, increased daytime sedation and psychomotor impairment. Molecules with long half-lives may reach steady state plasma concentration only in the 2nd week of initiating the treatment. So a dosage that seemed initially in therapeutic doses may lead on to toxicity after 7–10 days. Anterograde amnesia and rebound insomnia are problems encountered with short half-life agents.

Benzodiazepines in general are having high lipid solubility, but it varies from molecule to molecule. Those with high lipid solubility (e.g., diazepam and alprazolam) are able to cross the blood-brain-barrier easily and thereby reach the brain faster resulting in rapid onset of action. The cessation of action is also faster with these agents as they leave the brain rapidly. Lorazepam has lesser lipid solubility compared to diazepam. This property of lorazepam makes the onset of action slower and duration of action longer even though it has a lesser elimination half-life.

How the liver handles benzodiazepines and their metabolites is another consideration in choosing the right molecule. Most benzodiazepines are first oxidized and then hydroxylated before they are glucuronidated to inactive agents in liver; however, oxazepam and lorazepam undergo only glucuronidation in liver and therefore are more suitable in hepatic impairment.

Therapeutic indications of benzodiazepines:

- Insomnia
- Alcohol withdrawal
- Panic disorder
- Catatonia
- Akathisia
- Social phobia
- Acute mania
- As adjuvant in obsessive compulsive disorder (OCD), bipolar disorder, depression, and stress related disorders.

Though benzodiazepines and nonbenzodiazepine hypnotics are indicated for *insomnia*, they should be prescribed with a lot of caution. In many instances insomnia could be a symptom of depression, anxiety disorders, substance use disorders, stress disorders or even psychotic disorders. Conditioned insomnia, sleep–wake schedule disorders or organic conditions may present with insomnia. In such instances the treatment of primary condition results in resolution of insomnia. However, in primary insomnias and in the initial phase of treatments of conditions such as mood disorder and depression, the use of benzodiazepines is justified. The rapid onset of action for diazepam, alprazolam, triazolam, and estazolam makes them suited for inducing sleep quickly and to calm an episodic burst of anxiety faster. Temazepam, flurazepam, quazepam, estazolam, and triazolam are the benzodiazepines approved for use as hypnotics. Hypnotics should not be used for >7–10 consecutive days without a thorough evaluation of the cause of insomnia. Patients taking benzodiazepines should be warned about possible daytime sedation and slowing of psychomotor responses. They should exert caution in driving or operating machineries. Elderly individuals may develop ataxia and confusion especially at night. This may increase the risk of fall and injuries. Paradoxical agitation and delayed onset of action resulting in daytime sedation are other problems which may occur in geriatric population.

Drugs such as zolpidem, zaleplon, and eszopiclone (usually referred to as the Z drugs) are effective hypnotics which act through nonbenzodiazepine mechanism. They are selective for certain subunits of GABA receptor unlike the nonselective activation of all three binding sites of GABA-A receptor by benzodiazepines. This selectivity explains their rather specific hypnotic action and sparing of anticonvulsant and muscle relaxation effects. Even though, the chance of developing dependence and rebound insomnia are less with Z drugs, it is prudent to exercise caution in prescribing them for long periods.

Benzodiazepines are indicated mainly in three types of *anxiety disorders*—(1) panic disorders, (2) social phobia, and (3) generalized anxiety disorder (GAD). In panic disorder they are useful adjuvants to the specific pharmacological agents such as SSRI. High-potency benzodiazepines such as alprazolam and clonazepam are the preferred ones in panic disorder. They can be tapered after 3–4 weeks once the therapeutic benefits of SSRIs are established. In social phobia clonazepam is the preferred benzodiazepine. Anxiety associated with GAD responds very well to benzodiazepines. Treatment with medications in GAD should be limited to a brief predetermined period if possible. However, being a chronic condition, some patients with GAD may require long-term treatment. In such instances, it should be monitored closely for preventing misuse. It has to be emphasized that medications should always be combined with nonpharmacological techniques such as relaxation therapies, psychotherapy, and behavior therapy in the treatment of anxiety disorders.

The use of benzodiazepines in OCD is mainly for two purpose—short-term use in the initial phase to reduce the anxiety and as an adjuvant or augmentation agent along with SSRIs or clomipramine. Clonazepam has been recommended more frequently for this. In the treatment of post-traumatic stress disorders, acute stress reaction, and adjustment disorders they can be used as adjuvant treatments for short-terms.

Benzodiazepines are useful in *the detoxification phase of treatment of alcohol dependence*. Conventionally, chlordiazepoxide (librium) has been used as the benzodiazepine of choice for this purpose. In fact, any benzodiazepine can be used to treat alcohol withdrawal symptoms. In presence of hepatic impairment, lorazepam or oxazepam may have pharmacokinetic advantages over other agents. Starting benzodiazepines early in a patient who is dependent on alcohol may help to prevent the development of severe withdrawal symptoms such as delirium tremens. Patient's dependant on alcohol may require higher doses of benzodiazepines to contain the withdrawal symptoms in the initial phase (60–120 mg of chlordiazepoxide or 6–12 mg of lorazepam). This is explained on the basis of cross-tolerance between ethanol and benzodiazepines—both acting on the same receptor—GABA-A–benzodiazepine receptor complex. Benzodiazepines should be tapered off within the first 2–3 weeks of detoxification. Continuing benzodiazepines beyond the period of detoxification carries the risk of developing benzodiazepine dependence. The need or demand from the patient to continue benzodiazepines even after the withdrawal symptoms have subsided, should arouse suspicion about presence of a comorbid mood or anxiety disorder. In treatment of other substance dependence such as nicotine dependence also benzodiazepines might be needed as adjuvants for short-term control of anxiety, insomnia and restlessness.

Lorazepam has emerged as a first-line treatment of *acute catatonia* in the recent years. Chronic catatonia may not respond well to benzodiazepines. Catatonia not responding to benzodiazepine may respond to electroconvulsive therapy. Though the first-line treatment of *akathisia* (an adverse effect of treatment with dopamine antagonists characterized by restlessness and agitation) is beta blockers, benzodiazepines are useful in some patients.

In *bipolar disorders* benzodiazepines such as clonazepam and lorazepam used in large doses may be helpful in acute mania. They may also have a place as adjuvants in the maintenance phase along with mood stabilizers such as lithium.

Buspirone is a nonbenzodiazepine anxiolytic which has little hypnotic property. It acts through the 5HT1A receptor. The approved indication for this drug is for the treatment of GAD. Unlike benzodiazepines, buspirone takes 2–4 weeks for showing its anxiolytic effect. It has less effect on the somatic components of anxiety though is equally effective as benzodiazepines in relieving the psychic components. It is also used as an augmenting agent in the treatment of depression. Other uses include SSRI-induced sexual dysfunction, nicotine craving and attention-deficit/hyperactivity disorder (ADHD). Dosage ranges from 15 to 60 mg/day.

General Principles in Treatment with Anxiolytics and Hypnotic

- Insomnia should be evaluated before a pharmacological agent is prescribed.
- Primary causes of insomnia like depression, anxiety disorders, organic conditions and substance use should be considered and treated first.
- Use of benzodiazepines should be limited to brief period in treatment of insomnia or stress related disorders.
- When benzodiazepines are used as adjuvants to antidepressants in conditions such as depression or panic disorders, they should be discontinued after the first 2–3 weeks.
- Benzodiazepines should not be continued beyond the period of withdrawal symptoms of detoxification when they are used in the treatment of alcohol addiction.
- Choice, dosing, and spacing of benzodiazepines should be based on consideration of their half-lives, metabolism, lipid solubility, and coexisting medical conditions such as hepatic impairment.
- Hypnotic prescriptions should not be repeated or refilled without adequate evaluation.
- If the patient is found to misuse hypnotics or is suspected to be dependent, insist to get psychiatric help for managing the problem.

Drugs Used in Treatment of Attention-deficit/Hyperactivity Disorder

Pharmacologic treatment of ADHD includes stimulants and nonstimulants **(Table 28.3)**.

Among these the most widely used are methylphenidate (stimulant) and atomoxetine (nonstimulant).

Methylphenidate: This is the first choice in most cases of ADHD which requires pharmacologic intervention. It is effective in three-fourths of children with ADHD. It

Table 28.3: Pharmacologic treatment of ADHD including stimulants and nonstimulants.

Stimulants	Nonstimulants	Others
• Methylphenidate • Dexmethylphenidate • Amphetamine salts • Dextroamphetamine • Lisdexamfetamine	• Atomoxetine • Clonidine • Guanfacine	• Modafinil • Bupropion

acts by dopamine agonism in the prefrontal cortex (PFC). Enhanced dopamine activity in the PFC improves attention span and reduces hyperactivity and impulse control. It is available as immediate and sustained release tablets of 5–20 mg. The duration of action of immediate release preparations is 3–4 hrs, whereas the sustained release tablets may continue to act for 8 hours. That means the SR preparations need to be given only once morning daily. Other techniques such as osmotic-controlled release oral delivery system (OROS) and application of skin patches have been developed to tackle issues such as multiple dosing during daytime and better control over termination of drug effect. Methylphenidate is usually well-tolerated with only a few side-effects such as anorexia, nausea, stomach aches, headaches, and insomnia. There were concerns whether they might produce growth retardation. Long-term studies have shown that if drug holidays are given in weekends and during vacations these children can make up for the growth.

Atomoxetine: Atomoxetine is a NE reuptake inhibitor. Selective inhibition of presynaptic NE transporter in PFC enhances dopaminergic transmission which translates into clinical effect of improving the attention span and enhancing impulse control. Recommended dose is 0.5–1.8 mg/kg. A short half-life of 5 hours necessitates twice daily dosing. It is usually well-tolerated but side-effects such as reduced appetite, abdominal discomfort, and dizziness may occur in some children. Genetically, determined slow metabolism and drug–drug interactions may lead to toxic levels. The fact that atomoxetine also helps to reduce the comorbid anxiety and depressive symptom, is an advantage in the treatment of ADHD.

Long-acting extended release preparations of alpha-agonists clonidine and guanfacine have been approved for the treatment of ADHD. These centrally acting α2-adrenergic agonists are believed to enhance PF functioning. These agents may be preferred when tic disorders are comorbid with ADHD. Blood pressure monitoring is needed in children who are on these agents.

Bupropion, an antidepressant, with selective reuptake inhibition of NE and dopamine and modafinil originally developed to reduce sleepiness in narcolepsy has been found to be useful in some children with ADHD.

Anticraving Agents

Craving is an irresistible urge to use a psychoactive substance despite knowing the adverse consequence associated with its continued use. Craving is one of the major causes for relapse in addiction disorders. Craving is a biological phenomenon mediated by the reward circuits in the brain. Pharmacological agents which have been found to reduce craving in alcohol dependence include acamprosate, naltrexone, topiramate, baclofen, gabapentin, etc.

Acamprosate is an antagonist at N-methyl-D-aspartic acid (NMDA) receptor. Its anticraving property is probably related to its antagonism of the excitatory neurotransmitter glutamate. It is indicated in motivated persons who have undergone detoxification for alcohol dependence but continue to experience craving. Acamprosate calcium is available as 333 mg tablets. Dosage is two tablets three times daily. Lower dosage should be used in renal impairment.

Naltrexone is an opioid receptor blocking agent. Reduced reward in drinking is expected to reduce craving. 50 mg tablet per day is the usual dosage. Topiramate, an anticonvulsant agent, reduces craving through its GABAergic effects. This agent may be useful in alcohol dependent patients who are overweight. About 50–100 mg/day orally is the recommended dose for anticraving effects.

Disulfiram, popularly known as antabuse, is not an anticraving agent in its strict pharmacological sense. It is a deterrent which leads to aversive conditioning with alcohol use. Since it is used in the treatment of alcohol dependence, it is described here. Disulfiram inhibits aldehyde dehydrogenase, an enzyme which converts acetaldehyde to acetyl CoA. (Acetaldehyde is formed from alcohol by oxidation of ethyl alcohol by alcohol dehydrogenase). Accumulation of acetaldehyde produces a wide array of unpleasant effects such as nausea, vomiting, throbbing headache, flushing, sweating, dyspnea, chest pain, and vertigo. Tachycardia and hypertension can occur. This set of reaction referred to as antabuse reaction may sometimes lead to serious problems such as respiratory depression, cardiovascular collapse, acute heart failure, seizures, and loss of consciousness or even death. Disulfiram is available as 250 mg tablets. After the detoxification, if the patient is motivated to remain abstinent, disulfiram is administered as 500 mg tablet for the 1st week, followed by 125–250 mg/day as maintenance dose. Patient should be warned that even consumption of small quantities of alcohol may lead on to serious reactions. It is unethical to administer disulfiram without patient's consent.

Antidementia Drugs

Pharmacotherapy has a limited, but definite role in the treatment of neurocognitive disorders. No pharmacological agent available today can claim to cure dementia, but they have been demonstrated to improve the cognitive and noncognitive (emotional and behavioral) symptoms of dementia. Long-term follow-up studies have also shown that they slow down the deterioration in dementia and improve the quality of life. The demonstrated delay in the need for placement in a nursing home or full-time supervision by a home nurse or caregiver testifies for the effectiveness of these agents.

Various drugs commonly used in dementia are given in **Table 28.4**. Donepezil and memantine are the most widely pre-scribed agents.

Table 28.4: Drugs used in dementia.

Cholinesterase Inhibitors	Glutamate antagonist	Others (evidence base is weak)
• Donepezil (5–10 mg/day) • Galantamine (8–24 mg/day) • Rivastigmine (3–12 mg/day)	• Memantine (10–20 mg/day)	• Cerebral metabolic enhancers • Calcium channel inhibitors • Ondansetron • Selegiline • Ginkgo biloba • Estrogen replacement therapy • Vitamin E

Cholinesterase inhibitors reduce the inactivation of acetyl choline which in turn enhances the cholinergic neurotransmission. Cholinergic pathway is believed to be very important in memory consolidation and goal-directed thinking. These drugs are most useful in patients with mild-to-moderate severity of Alzheimer's disease who have sufficient reserve of cholinergic network left in the basal forebrain.

Donepezil is the most commonly prescribed molecule. Its relative selectivity on central nervous system cholinesterase inhibition (i.e., sparing of GI tract) makes it more tolerated than other drugs in this group. Increased availability of acetylcholine in hippocampus and cerebral cortex enhances cognitive functions. In long-term use the progression of memory impairment is slowed down. Behavioral and emotional symptoms such as apathy, depression, mood changes, anxiety, and psychotic symptoms improve. The half-life is 70 hours in elderly necessitating only once daily dosing. About 5–10 mg/day is the usual dosage. Starting with lower dose of 5 mg reduces the incidence of GI adverse effects such as nausea, vomiting, and diarrhea. Rarely bradyarrhythmias might occur especially in those with pre-existing cardiac disease.

Memantine acts by blocking NMDA receptor thus reducing the glutamate mediated excitotoxic damage to neurons in Alzheimer's disease. It is approved for use in moderate to severe cases of Alzheimer's dementia. It is available as 5 and 10 mg tablets. The starting dose is 5 mg and the recommended target dose is 20 mg/day with weekly increments of 5 mg. The usual adverse effects are dizziness, headache, confusion, and constipation. It is not recommended in patients with severe renal impairment. Donepezil and memantine can be combined in treatment of Alzheimer's dementia.

PHYSICAL METHODS OF TREATMENT IN PSYCHIATRY

INTRODUCTION AND HISTORY

Physical methods of treatment for mental illness have a long history dating back to prehistoric times. Trephining of skull bones to release evil spirits has been practiced in tribal cultures. Serendipity played a role in the introduction of malarial fever therapy for general paresis in late 19th century. This evoked interest in biological therapies for psychiatric illnesses in early 20th century. 1930s were the time for insulin coma therapy and psychosurgery. In 1934, first catatonic patient was successfully treated with IM injections of camphor to produce seizures. This was based on the observation that a naturally occurring seizure brings relief from psychotic symptoms. In 1938, Lucio Bini and Ugo Cerletti demonstrated the use of electricity to induce seizure in the treatment of a "delusional and incoherent" patient. The safety and success of this therapy led to the popularity of ECT as the first-line therapy throughout 1940s. Later on ECT fell into disrepute mainly because of its indiscriminate use in mental hospitals and adverse media publicity. Over the last 20–30 years, various other physical methods have been used for the purpose of brain stimulation. A list of various methods of physical treatment currently in practice is given in **Table 28.5**.

BRAIN STIMULATION METHODS

Electroconvulsive Therapy

Induction of seizure by application of electricity through electrodes placed over the scalp has proved to be very effective in treating conditions varying from depression

Table 28.5: List of physical treatments currently in practice.

Physical	Surgical
• Electroconvulsive therapy	• Subcaudate tractotomy
• Transcranial magnetic stimulation (rTMS)	• Anterior cingulotomy
• Transcranial direct current stimulation	• Limbic leukotomy
• Cranial electrical stimulation	• Anterior capsulotomy
• Magnetic seizure therapy	• Deep brain stimulation
• Vagus nerve stimulation	
• Implanted cortical stimulation	

to catatonia. Safety and effectiveness made it popular among clinicians in the initial years but the way it was practiced in mental hospitals, by generating a seizure with electrical shock without anesthesia and the exaggerated propaganda by antipsychiatry movement about its "permanent brain damaging effects", led to lot of damage to the reputation of this life saving treatment. Furthermore, the increasing emphasis placed on human rights and informed consent in modern legislative culture has discouraged many clinicians from including ECT into their therapeutic options.

Basic electrophysiology in this treatment is the triggering of seizure activity in normal neurons by application of pulses of current under carefully controlled conditions.

Mechanism of action: The exact mechanism of action is unknown. Positron emission tomography (PET) studies have shown brain metabolism decreases after seizures. Decrease in cerebral metabolism correlated with therapeutic response. ECT affects cellular mechanisms of memory and mood regulation and raises seizure threshold. It causes neurochemical changes and receptor changes such as downregulation of post-β-adrenergic receptors and affects coupling of G-proteins to receptors.

Indications: Severe depressive disorder (Unipolar or Bipolar) with high risk of suicide is the most important indication for ECT. In such cases ECT has the fastest onset of action than antidepressants and very effective in relieving depression and suicidal ideas. Postpartum mood disorders and postpartum psychosis are conditions requiring rapid relief. ECT is effective and safe in such situations. If catatonic syndrome resulting from mood disorder or schizophrenia does not respond to medical interventions, such as treatment with lorazepam, ECT is the treatment of choice. Resistant manic episode is another indication for ECT. ECT is a third-line management of treatment resistance encountered in the management of depression and OCD. Apart from these major indications, ECT is occasionally useful in the management of delirium, NMS, intractable seizure disorders, on–off phenomenon of Parkinson's disease, etc.

Clinical guidelines in the administration of ECT: The present day standard practice is to administer ECT under general anesthesia—the modified ECT. Informed consent is taken in accordance with provisions of Mental Healthcare Act. A thorough physical examination and investigations are done as pre-ECT work up to exclude medical contraindications like raised intracranial tension, recent myocardial infarction, spinal instability, stability of dentures and respiratory infections. Discuss the risk, benefits and alternate treatment approaches. Patient is kept without any oral intake for 6 hours before treatment. Intravenous line is established and bite block is inserted in mouth. Muscarinic anticholinergic drug is given to reduce oral and respiratory secretions and to prevent bradycardia during the procedure. Anesthetic agents such as methohexital or propofol are administered. Muscle relaxants such as succinylcholine are given to minimize bone fractures and other injuries from seizures. Convulsions should be monitored either by electroencephalography (EEG) leads or physically by isolating a limb— that is by inflating a BP cuff at ankle in excess of systolic pressure before administering the muscle relaxant. Adequate airway patency and oxygenation is ensured during the procedure.

Electrode placement: Bilateral (BL) electrode placement with two electrodes being placed one on each side at frontotemporal position is the most common method. This has also shown to be the most effective method. The disadvantage with BL electrode placement is the possibility of causing more cognitive dysfunctions as a side-effect. Right unilateral (RUL) electrode placement with one electrode on frontotemporal position and other just next to vertex over the nondominant hemisphere reduces the cognitive adverse effects but at the cost of reduced clinically efficacy.

Contraindications: There are no absolute contraindications for ECT. Relative contraindications include recent myocardial infarction, intracerebral aneurysm, space occupying lesions or any conditions resulting in increased intracranial pressure. Pregnancy is not a contraindication for ECT.

A course of 6–12 ECTs given with a frequency of two or three therapies per week is usually recommended for depression. Mania and schizophrenia may require more sessions to achieve remission. Cognitive assessment should be done along with the routine assessments after each session. If severe cognitive impairments are noticed, more spacing may be needed and the BL electrode placement may be changed to RUL. Maintenance ECT with a frequency of once a week, once in 2 weeks or once in a month, may be needed for a small group of patients.

Common adverse effects: Confusion, headache, and delirium shortly after seizure while patient is coming out of anesthesia. Transient and usually reversible cognitive impairment and retrograde amnesia may occur in some persons. Tongue bites, compression fracture of mid-thoracic vertebrae are uncommon problems.

Transcranial Magnetic Stimulation

Repetitive transcranial magnetic stimulation (rTMS) involves application of a rapidly changing magnetic field to the superficial layers of the cerebral cortex, which locally induces small electric currents called "eddy" currents. It uses magnetic fields to indirectly induce electrical pulses. Stimulation applied to dorsolateral prefrontal cortex (DLPFC) has significant antidepressant activity. Clinical studies have also suggested rTMS in treatment of schizophrenia, anxiety disorder, OCD, panic disorder, and Tourette's syndrome. Most serious known risk is an unintended seizure.

Transcranial Direct Current Stimulation

Transcranial direct current stimulation (tDCS) is a noninvasive form of treatment that uses very weak (1–3 mA) direct electrical current applied to scalp. It works via polarization and does not affect action potential firing in cortical neurons. Antidepressant effects are noted after anodal polarization of DLPFC. Positive effects in cognitive and motor function are also reported. It has no known serious adverse effects and is usually well tolerated. However, it can cause minimal tingling at site of stimulation and skin irritation.

Cranial Electrical Stimulation

This uses a weak (1–4 mA) alternating current. Stimulation with alternating microcurrent affects the thalamic and hypothalamic brain tissue and facilitates the release of neurotransmitters. It is widely used in treatment in regions of world where medications are not available or are beyond financial reach, for treatment of depression, anxiety, and insomnia. *Side-effects:* Local skin effects, general feeling of dizziness, not advised during pregnancy, those with low BP and those who have arrhythmias or pacemaker.

Magnetic Seizure Therapy

It is a novel form of convulsive therapy. This uses an alternating magnetic field that crosses the scalp and calvarium bone and induces a more localized electrical current in the targeted regions of the cerebral cortex. Aim is to produce a seizure whose focus and pattern of spread may be controlled. It is performed under general anesthesia (GA) with a muscle relaxant. It requires approximately the same preparation and infrastructure as ECT. Magnetic seizure therapy (MST) is still in the stage of clinical trials and is not Food and Drug Administration (FDA) approved. *Side-effects:* Risks associated with anesthesia and generalized seizure may be there; it may also affect hearing due to the clicking noise produced by the magnetic coil.

Vagus Nerve Stimulation

Vagus nerve stimulation (VNS) is the direct, intermittent electrical stimulation of the left cervical vagus nerve via an implanted pulse generator, usually in the left chest wall. The electrode is wrapped around the left vagus nerve in the neck and is connected to the generator subcutaneously. Chronic stimulation of these nerve fibers predominantly changes activity in the brainstem nuclei such as the nucleus of the tractus solitarius and other neighboring nuclei (e.g., Raphe nucleus) that alter serotonergic activity in cortical and limbic structures. *Side-effects*: Voice alteration, dyspnea, neck pain, perioperative infection, small risk of vocal cord paralysis, bradycardia, or asystole.

Implanted Cortical Stimulation

Electrodes are implanted over the surface of the cortex to provide electrical brain stimulation in a targeted superficial region. This approach is being studied for treatment of conditions such as stroke, tinnitus, and treatment-resistant depression.

SURGICAL METHODS

Ablative lesions are made in specific brain areas. Target areas are accessed by magnetic resonance guided imaging and by stereotactic neurosurgical techniques. Surgical intervention is predominantly reserved for patients with severe, incapacitating major depression or OCD who have failed an exhaustive array of standard treatments. Surgery is not approved unless a multidisciplinary committee reaches consensus regarding its appropriateness for a given candidate and the patient renders informed consent. Various relevant surgical procedures are being described here.

Subcaudate Tractotomy

This procedure targets the substantia innominata (just inferior to the head of the caudate nucleus) and interrupts white matter tracts connecting orbitofrontal cortex and subcortical structures. The surgery involves placement of radioactive yttrium-90 seeds at the desired centroid, yielding lesion volumes of approximately 2 cc on each side. Indications for subcaudate tractotomy are major depression, OCD, and other severe anxiety disorders.

Anterior Cingulotomy

The surgery is conducted under local anesthesia and 2–3 approximately 1-cc lesions are made on each side by thermocoagulation through bilateral burr holes. The target is within anterior cingulate cortex (Brodmann areas 24 and 32), at the margin of the white matter bundle known as the cingulum. The indications for anterior cingulotomy include major depression and OCD.

Limbic Leukotomy

The procedure combines the targets of subcaudate tractotomy and anterior cingulotomy. The indications for limbic leukotomy include major depression, OCD, and other severe anxiety disorders. More recently, there is also some evidence that this procedure might be beneficial for repetitive self-injurious behaviors or in the context of severe tic disorders.

Anterior Capsulotomy

The procedure places lesions within the anterior limb of the internal capsule, which impinges on the adjacent ventral striatum, thereby interrupting fibers of passage between PFC and subcortical nuclei including the dorsomedial thalamus. Indications for anterior capsulotomy include major depression, OCD, and other severe anxiety disorders.

Deep Brain Stimulation

The procedure involves placement of small diameter brain leads of approximately 1.3 mm with multiple electrode contacts into subcortical nuclei or specific white matter tracts. Guided by multimodal imaging and stereotactic land marking, the surgeon places the leads in the selected brain areas. Later the pulse generator (pacemaker) is implanted subdermally in the anterior chest wall. This pacemaker is connected to the brain leads by extension wires tunnelled under the skin. By activating various combinations of electrodes flexible modulation of brain functions (neuromodulation) are expected. The parameters to be optimized for individual patient are performed by a trained psychiatrist. Deep brain stimulation (DBS) of ventral anterior limb of internal capsule and adjacent ventral striatum have been demonstrated to benefit intractable OCD. DBS of subgenual cingulate cortex may benefit treatment resistant depression.

CONCLUSION

Use of psychopharmacological agents is the mainstay of treatment in psychotic disorders such as schizophrenia, delusional disorders, and schizoaffective disorders and mood disorders such as bipolar disorders and major depressive disorders. Medications are also indicated as first-line agents in anxiety disorders such as panic disorders, OCD, and GAD. Several stress-related disorders require pharmacological agents as adjuvant agents. The mechanism of actions and pharmacokinetics of individual molecules are beyond the scope of this book, which may be consulted in larger textbooks of pharmacology. However, the general principles in the prescription of each group of agents have been described here. Nonpsychiatrist medical professionals are advised to make themselves familiar with two or three commonly used drugs from each group, e.g., fluoxetine and escitalopram from the antidepressant group.

Electroconvulsive therapy, other brain stimulation techniques, and neurosurgical interventions have a definite place in the management of conditions such as severe and resistant depression, OCD, catatonia, etc. ECT is the oldest but still the most evidence based treatment among these. It is safe, effective, and fast in patients with severe depression with high suicidal risk. More evidence base is needed for the safety and efficacy of other treatments such as rTMS, tDCS, VNS, and DBS to be applied in the routine clinical settings. Cost should constitute another consideration as these treatments with the exception of ECT and tDCS are very expensive. The advances in electrophysiology, neuroimaging, and stereotactic neurosurgical technique are expected to bring up more effective and novel physical treatments for psychiatric disorders.

TAKE-HOME MESSAGES

- Treatments for psychiatric disorders can be broadly classified into either somatic or psychosocial interventions. Somatic methods of treatment include pharmacological treatment and other physical methods such as ECT and others.
- Psychopharmacological agents are generally classified on the basis of their clinical use into various categories such as antipsychotics, antidepressants, anxiolytics and hypnotics, mood stabilizers, and others which include stimulants, anticraving agents, anti-dementia drugs, etc.
- Antipsychotics may belong either to first generation or second generation category. Apart from regular formulations, antipsychotics are also available as depot injectable formulations. Antidepressants may be a TCA, MAOI, SSRI, SNRI or others. Commonly used mood stabilizers are lithium, valproate, carbamazepine and oxcarbazepine. Anxiolytic and hypnotic drugs include benzodiazepines, buspirone and Z group drugs such as zolpidem, zaleplon, and eszopiclone. Anticraving drugs include acamprosate, naltrexone, topiramate and baclofen. Most commonly used antidementia drugs are donepezil and memantine. Pharmacologic treatment of ADHD includes stimulants and nonstimulants, the most common being methylphenidate and atomoxetine respectively.
- Other physical methods of treatment include ECT, rTMS, tDCS, cranial electrical stimulation, MST, VNS, implanted cortical stimulation and various psychosurgical methods. Except ECT, most other interventions of this category require further study and therefore have to be used judiciously.

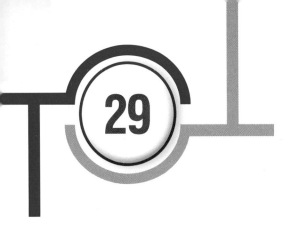

Psychotherapies

Nitin Gupta, Sushmita Bhattacharya

INTRODUCTION

The term psychotherapy is derived from an ancient Greek word, psychē—meaning breath, spirit, or soul, and therapeia or therapeuein, meaning to nurse or cure. English psychiatrist Walter Cooper Dendy first introduced the term "psycho-therapeia" in 1853. The most widely accepted definition of psychotherapy is that given by Wolberg (1967): Psychotherapy is the treatment, by psychological means, of problems of an emotional nature in which a trained person deliberately establishes a professional relationship with the patient with the object of:

- Removing modifying, or retarding existing symptoms,
- Mediating disturbed patterns of behavior, and
- Promoting positive personality growth and development.

A simpler definition is that psychotherapy happens when two persons work together to correct the personality problems of one of them using primarily the functions of communication for this purpose (Cameron 1961). Psychotherapy differs from informal psychological help which one may receive from family, friends or acquaintances, in primarily two significant ways: it is provided by a trained, socially sanctioned person or healer, and it involves use of certain psychological principles and is guided by an articulated theory that explains the patients distress and prescribes method for alleviating them (J Frank, 1961).

Over recent years, mental health practices have seen a paradigm shift with revival of interest in evidence-based psychotherapies. There is increasing evidence for use of combination of selected psychotherapeutic approach with psychotropic medications. This calls for increasing emphasis on psychotherapy training at all levels, so that the future practitioner can appreciate the role of psychotherapeutic treatment in the setting of psychiatry as well as mental health more broadly.

PRINCIPAL APPROACHES

As can be seen from the definition, psychotherapy utilizes the process of communication between the therapist and the patient. It can be conducted through the verbal or nonverbal mode. There are several kinds of psychotherapies. The goal of all forms of psychotherapies is to alleviate the distress and facilitate certain changes in emotions, attitude and behavior. There are different approaches to psychotherapy, which vary considerably in their emphasis in accordance with the primary targets and whether they seek to modify thoughts, emotional states or behavior.

To simplify, the varieties of psychotherapy can be divided into three main groups: (1) supportive therapy, (2) re-educative therapy, and (3) reconstructive therapy. Various types of therapies have crystallized around these three principal approaches. The choice of psychotherapeutic technique used depends not only on the problem at hand, but also on patient, social or environmental factors. It also depends on patient and therapist preference as well as the skill and experience of the therapist. The different broad types of psychotherapies and their objectives are listed below in the **Table 29.1**.

Who should receive psychotherapy? Psychotherapy can be given to anyone in whom psychological factors are believed to be contributing to, or causing distress and disability. It can include those who are suffering with psychiatric illnesses like depression, anxiety, and psychosis and also those who have been disturbed by current life stresses or events like bereavement. It also includes those whose behavior is unruly or upsets others like problem behavior in children, people with antisocial personalities and people who are abusing substances.

Certain patient variables have been identified which have good prognostic value for psychotherapy and these include:

- Strong motivation and willingness to change
- Desire for self understanding and a capacity for reflection
- An ability to understand, appreciate and express one's emotions

Table 29.1: Different broad types of psychotherapies and their objectives.	
Supportive therapy	*Objectives:* • Achieving an emotional equilibrium • Strengthening existing defenses • Elaborating better mechanisms of maintaining control
Re-educative therapy	*Objectives:* Emphasis on remodeling the patient's attitude and behavior. Less emphasis on searching the causes *Includes:* • Behavior therapy • Cognitive therapy • Interpersonal therapy • Rational emotive therapy • Group psychotherapy • Marital therapy • Family therapy • Psychodrama
Reconstructive therapy	*Objectives:* • Emphasis on developing insight into unconscious conflicts, based on the premise that past experiences have retarded the normal psychosocial growth • Efforts to achieve expansion of personality growth and development with new adaptive personalities *Includes:* • Classical psychoanalysis • Psychoanalytically-oriented (Psychodynamic) psychotherapy • Brief dynamic psychotherapy

- Good coping strength
- Presence of positive achievements in the past
- Capacity to form good relationships and presence of at least one strong relationship.

Despite the differences in various psychotherapeutic approaches, there are certain similarities in the therapeutic procedures, which are universal to all forms of psychotherapies. These key therapeutic functions are as follows:

- Emphasis on strengthening the therapeutic relationship between the patient and the therapist.
- Instilling hope in the patient for a better outcome, and shaping his expectations in keeping with reality.
- Providing opportunities for cognitive and experiential learning by providing patient with new information and facts and new possibilities for dealing with problems.
- Enhancing the patient's sense of mastery, competence and self-worth.
- "Working through" the process of change (Sidney Bloch).

TYPES OF PSYCHOTHERAPEUTIC TECHNIQUES

Supportive Therapy

This is a form of therapy, which attempts at alleviating or removing the symptoms so that the patient can function at his normal level. No attempt is made to change the personality structure of the patient. It is usually for a short period but can be long-term depending on problem at hand. Following are some of the principles of supportive therapy:

- *Guidance*—providing active help in form of fact giving and interpretation.
- *Tension control and release*—regulating tension through various modes like relaxation exercises, massage, meditation, biofeedback, and hypnosis.
- *Environmental manipulation*—attempt to identify and remedy defects in living situations that create problems.
- *Externalization of interests*—encouraging patients to resume meaningful activities and develop new recreational or leisure activities.
- Providing reassurance
- *Prestige suggestion*—suggestion delivered by therapist in an authoritative manner having a positive and optimistic bearing on the patient
- Persuasion
- *Ventilation and catharsis*—providing an uncritical and sympathetic ear to the patient
- Inspirational group therapy.

Behavior Therapy

Behavior therapy includes a wide variety of techniques, which are based on the principles of learning theory, aimed at modifying the maladaptive behavior of the patient to reduce the dysfunction, and to improve the quality of life. A behavioral approach involves thinking about problems as learned behaviors and teaching patients to learn new ways of behaving (and sometimes thinking) to reduce symptoms and improve quality of life.

Behavior psychology, or behaviorism, started making inroads into the field of mental health care around early 20th century. John B Watson is known as the father of behaviorism. Joseph Wolpe (who developed a technique known as "systematic desensitization"), Hans Eysenck, MB Shapiro and BF Skinner were some other prominent names that contributed towards the development of behavioral approaches to treat mental health problems.

Majority of the behavior techniques are based upon the principles of classical conditioning (developed by Ivan Pavlov) and operant conditioning (developed by BF Skinner). *Classical conditioning* happens when two stimuli are repeatedly paired; a response which is initially elicited by the second stimulus is eventually elicited by the first stimulus alone (Pavlov's dog experiment; learning by association). *Operant conditioning* model means that the strength of a behavior is modified by the behavior's consequences, such as reward or punishment. The behavior that is followed by a reward is more likely to occur again.

Behavior therapy is typically a short duration therapy (around 6–8 weeks) and quite cost effective. The focus is on current problems and behavior. Initially daily sessions can be planned which can then be conducted in a more spaced out manner later on. A behavioral analysis is usually carried out before planning behavior therapy in order to do a detailed assessment of the problem behavior. There are various structured methods of carrying out behavior analysis; one of the simplest methods being ABC charting, which involves looking at the:

- **A**ntecedent (e.g., circumstances under which the behavior began; who, if any, were present; other details),
- **B**ehavior (description of the behavior in detail), and
- **C**onsequence (what happened after the behavior occurred; what factors helped to maintain behavior).

Some of the important behavioral techniques are described briefly here.

Systematic Desensitization

Developed by Wolpe, systematic desensitization is based on the principle of counter-conditioning, wherein a feared object is paired with an incompatible response. In this form of treatment, the patient overcomes maladaptive (unhelpful) anxiety elicited by any object/situation by gradually approaching the feared situation in a relaxed state that inhibits anxiety (i.e., incompatible with anxiety). The negative reaction of anxiety is inhibited by the relaxed state (reciprocal inhibition).

It primarily consists of three main steps:

Firstly, patient learns to attain a state of complete relaxation via *relaxation training* (described later).

This is followed by *hierarchy construction* in which the patient and the therapist prepare a graded list or hierarchy of anxiety provoking events or situations in descending order of hierarchy provocation.

The last step is the *desensitization of stimulus* by exposing the patient to the stimulus which elicits the anxiety response. The least anxiety provoking stimulus is confronted first. This can be done either with the help of imagery, or in reality (*in vivo* exposure). As the patient experiences anxiety, he is asked to relax. With time, the patient is able to control his anxiety on exposure to the stimulus. Gradually the hierarchy is climbed up till the maximum anxiety provoking stimulus is reached. Hence in this way, the learned relaxation state and the anxiety provoking stimuli are systematically paired so that the stimuli no more cause anxiety.

Systematic desensitization is a treatment of choice in phobias, obsessive-compulsive disorders (OCD) and other anxiety disorders. An example of using systematic desensitization for a patient suffering from fear of heights (acrophobia) is a behavioral program that slowly exposes the person to high situations, while ensuing relaxation techniques, desensitizing them over a period of time and slowly introducing greater heights.

Therapeutic Graded Exposure

This is similar to systematic desensitization except that relaxation training is not involved. Graded exposure to the anxiety provoking stimulus in real life context is provided to learn firsthand that exposure or the resultant anxiety does not lead to any dangerous consequence. For example, patients afraid of dog can be shown a picture of dog and then one can progress to touching a real dog.

Flooding

Flooding is another type of exposure therapy in which patient is exposed to the feared stimuli and escape is made impossible. Also, there is no hierarchy and patient is usually exposed to the most anxiety provoking stimuli. This is usually the method of choice used in the treatment of phobias. It is based on the premise that escaping and avoidance from the anxiety provoking situation reinforces the anxiety through conditioning. The therapist encourages the patient to confront the feared situation directly. The exposure can be actual (*in vivo*) or imaginary. Patient experiences fear and anxiety which subsides gradually. By prolonged contact with the phobic stimulus, anxiety and phobic behavior decreases and patient gains a sense of mastery. An example of flooding therapy is—a person having fear of dog will be straight away put in a room with dog and asked to stroke the dog.

Aversion Therapy

Aversion therapy is used for the behaviors which are pleasant but undesirable by the patient, e.g., substance dependence, sexual deviation, certain other behaviors with impulsive or compulsive qualities (nail biting, trichotillomania, etc.). The underlying principal is that when a noxious or unpleasant stimulus (punishment) is presented immediately after an undesirable behavioral response, the undesirable response is eventually inhibited. Various noxious stimuli that can be used are low voltage electrical stimuli, drugs that produce unpleasant effects like vomiting (disulfiram), social disapproval, or even corporal punishment. Use of aversion therapy has declined in recent times as many clinicians feel that it leads to violation of human rights of the patient.

Relaxation Training

The aim of these therapies is to induce physiological effects opposite to that occurring in anxiety; like slowed heart rate and muscular relaxation. Relaxation techniques are an integral part of a majority of behavior therapies, such as systematic desensitization. Some of the methods used to induce relaxation are:

- Jacobson's progressive muscular relaxation (JPMR): One of the most frequently used and highly effective technique in which patient first tenses and then relaxes group of muscles in a fixed order starting from small muscle groups of the feet or hands and working upwards towards the head, or vice versa.
- Hypnosis (described separately later on).
- *Biofeedback:* Involves use of an instrument (usually electronic), which provides immediate feedback to the patient regarding his physiological status normally not available to the conscious mind, such as pulse rate, blood pressure, electrocardiogram (ECG), electromyography (EMG), and galvanic skin response (GSR). This feedback is through auditory or visual (bar of lights) display. This mechanism is based on the idea that autonomic nervous system can come under voluntary control through learning (operant conditioning). Patients

are instructed to control the parameters, using the feedback as a guide. Relaxation is easily achieved by this method. The other uses of biofeedback include treatment of enuresis and fecal incontinence, migraine and tension headache, idiopathic hypertension, asthma, cardiac arrhythmias, uncontrolled tonic-clonic seizures, and also for neuromuscular rehabilitation.

- Transcendental meditation, Yoga (Pranayama, Vipassana), Zen are some of the traditional methods to attain a state of calmness, which have been used for centuries.

Eye Movement Desensitization and Reprocessing

Eye movement desensitization and reprocessing (EMDR) is a type of psychotherapy which has been shown to be effective in post-traumatic stress disorder (PTSD) in decreasing the effect of distressing memories. Apart from PTSD, it has also been used in phobias and panic disorders. It involves a standardized procedure in which saccadic eye movements are induced while the person is asked to focus on anxiety producing/traumatic thoughts, images or sensations. This has been shown to reduce anxiety associated with the event. The exact mechanism of action of this technique is still under debate.

Assertiveness Training

This is a form of behavior therapy useful for depression, social anxiety, and interpersonal problems. It is based on the principle that difficulty in expressing oneself clearly in an interpersonal situation often leads to anxiety, decreased sense of self-worth and interpersonal problems. These training programs are meant to enable a person to

express in a more direct and honest manner while respecting the dignity of the other person. Assertiveness training also focuses on learning assertive behaviors and practicing these with the help of a therapist.

Social Skills Training

This type of psychotherapy focuses on improving the social skills (verbal and nonverbal communication) of a person by predominantly behavioral (and cognitive) approach. Social skills deficits are commonly seen in patients with schizophrenia and are an important cause of poor overall outcome. Apart from schizophrenia, patients with depression, social anxiety disorder, and autism may also benefit with social skills training. It involves teaching a wide variety of skills such as eye contact, greeting, smiling, showing appropriate emotional response, initiating and sustaining conversation. Depending upon requirement, it can cover areas such as– conflict management, assertiveness training, negotiating and compromising.

Other Behavioral Techniques

Few other behavioral techniques like modeling, reinforcement, family therapy, and marital therapy will be described under the section for "special clinical population".

Cognitive Therapy or Cognitive Behavior Therapy

Cognitive behavior therapy (CBT) is a structured, short-term therapy directed towards resolution of current problems by modifying dysfunctional (inaccurate and/or unhelpful) thinking and behavior. Developed independently by Aaron Beck and Meichenbaum in 1960s, the underlying principal is that the person's perception about an event or a situation influences their mood and behavior (also called as the "Cognitive model"). The Cognitive theory assumes that cognitive dysfunctions (distorted thoughts) are the core cause of psychological distress. For example, in depression the patient will hold a negative view of himself, his future and the world around him (i.e., the cognitive triad). The therapist plays an active role and the goal of therapy is to help patients to identify and evaluate the negative cognitions, to develop alternative and more flexible schemas, and to rehearse both new cognitive and behavioral responses. Changing the way a person thinks can alleviate the psychiatric disorder. The therapy is usually short lasting and consists of 15–20 visits over a period of 2–3 months. This type of therapy can be used for treatment of depression, anxiety disorder, panic disorder, phobias, eating disorders, anticipatory anxiety, and also for teaching problem-solving methods.

The therapy's cognitive approach includes four techniques-eliciting automatic thoughts or cognitions (how a person perceives a situation/event), testing automatic thoughts, identifying maladaptive underlying assumptions, and testing the validity of maladaptive assumptions.

For example, a patient suffering from depression thinks that "I am a failure, I can't do anything right". The therapist identifies that these automatic thoughts contribute to his feeling of sadness and his problematic behavior (social isolation, decreased work output). The therapist helps the patient to identify and test the validity of these automatic thoughts (challenging them and showing that these might not be true). The therapist also helps the patient to identify the underlying assumptions of worthlessness thereby helping to challenge his maladaptive thinking. In this way patient learns to identify the thoughts associated with his/her

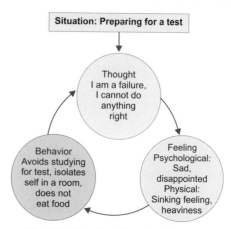

Fig. 29.1: Situation: Preparing for a test.

distressing mood and behavior, and learns to develop more adaptive responses to his thinking.

Cognitive behavioral therapy also includes behavioral techniques such as activity scheduling (making a list of activities to be performed in a structured manner), homework, graded task assignment, behavioral rehearsal, role play, and diversion techniques **(Fig. 29.1)**.

Group Therapy

Group therapy is a modality in which a group of people (usually between 8 and 10) work together towards the attainment of common goals under the leadership of therapist or a professionally trained person. It is a time saving and effective technique usually used in treatment of substance dependence as well as chronic and persistent psychiatric disorders like schizophrenia and affective disorders. Group therapy offers patients (and their relatives) an opportunity to realize that many others have, and share problems, which are very similar to their own problems, and that they are not alone in their suffering. It provides a platform for mutual support and understanding and counters isolation experienced by the patients and relatives.

Typically, sessions are held once or twice a week, with each session lasting 1–2 hours. The patients usually sit in a circle, with equal opportunities for interaction. Group therapy may utilize different psychological approaches such as psychoanalytic, supportive, and transactional or behavioral approaches.

Over the years, many types of self-help groups have emerged comprising of people with similar problems and symptoms [Alcoholics anonymous (AA), narcotics anonymous, gamblers anonymous, and overeaters anonymous]. For a better understanding, AA is described in detail.

Alcoholics Anonymous

It is one of the most popular nontherapist mediated intervention group which offers membership to anyone having a "drinking problem". It also comprises of fellowship of men and women who have had a "drinking problem in past". It was founded by Bill Wilson and Dr Bob Smith in 1935, and has existed in India since 1957. The program consists of 12 steps offering members a way to live life without alcohol. Group discussions and meetings are held in which members communicate with each other and share their experiences. The AA belief system includes the requirement of a searching personal inventory, commitment to a greater power, making amends to other people, and carrying the message to other alcoholics. It also takes in to account motivation enhancement by proximal goals, role modeling, relapse management in terms of alternative activity and new social networks.

Hypnosis

Hypnosis is a state of normal mind in which focal attention is increased and peripheral awareness is diminished. Suggestibility is increased and critical judgment is partially impaired. The state of hypnosis can either be artificially induced, or induced by self. However, not everyone can be hypnotized. The capacity to be hypnotized and, relatedly, the occurrence of spontaneous trance states is a trait/feature that varies between individuals. This can be measured by using tests such as the "eye roll sign" or "hand levitation test", which indicate about the degree of suggestibility of a person. A wide variety of techniques are available for the induction of hypnosis. The hypnotherapist may aid in the achievement of the state and use its uncritical, intense focus to facilitate the acceptance of new thoughts and feelings, thereby accelerating therapeutic change. For the subject, hypnosis is typified by a feeling of involuntariness and movements seem automatic. The person in trance state becomes highly suggestible to commands of the hypnotherapist, without understanding their nature. There is absence of body movements, changed voice quality and retardation of reflexes like swallowing or blinking. It is also associated with partial or complete amnesia for the events occurring during the hypnotic state and time distortion.

Hypnosis helps in facilitating acceptance of new thoughts and feelings making it useful in treating habitual problems and also with symptom management. Some of the indications for hypnosis are smoking, overeating, phobias, anxiety, conversion symptoms, and chronic pain. Hypnosis can also aid in relieving distress notably for posttraumatic stress disorder. It has additionally been used for memory retrieval.

Psychoanalysis and Psychoanalytical Psychotherapy

The term "Psychoanalysis" is virtually synonymous with Sigmund Freud, its founding father. The psychotherapeutic model is based on his vast work in the field of psychoanalysis in the late 19th and early 20th century. Apart from Freud, many other techniques developed by other important workers (such as Carl Jung, Alfred Adler, Erich Fromm, Harry Stack Sullivan, Karen Horney, Melanie Klein, Otto Rank, Wilhelm Reich and many others) are also in use. The work done by Freud is referred to as "classical or orthodox psychoanalysis", in order to distinguish it from the more recent variations known as "psychoanalytic psychotherapy".

Classical Psychoanalysis

Freudian psychoanalysis aims at the recognition and resolution of unconscious conflicts and gaining insight into the intrapsychic events. It aims at structural reorganization of personality with symptom relief being an indirect result. It is a long-term process lasting 3–5 years, and typically needing 3–5 visits/week. The main technique used is "free association" in which the patient is allowed to communicate in an unguided manner (speaking freely whatever comes to mind). The therapist adopts a passive, nondirective approach. The "resistance" of the patient during therapy (unwillingness to discuss a particular topic or opposing the treatment in any form) and "transference" (patient's feelings, behavior and relationship with therapist) is recognized and interpreted. Analysis of the "resistance" and "transference" reveals the unconscious and childhood conflicts and this forms the essence of the psychoanalytic technique. The defense mechanisms (unconscious psychological strategies brought into play to cope with reality) are also identified during this process. During the therapy, the patient typically lies on the couch, with the therapist sitting just out of view. No other therapy is usually used as adjunct. It is suitable for all neurotic disorders like depression, anxiety, conversion disorder,

OCD as well as personality disorders. Certain patient prerequisites like psychological mindedness, capacity for insight, good ego strength, and high motivation are required for this form of therapy to be successful. The use of this technique has become limited due to various reasons—including its long duration leading to economic and time constraints, clinical prerequisites, stringent rules, as well as availability of other effective forms of therapies of a shorter duration.

Psychoanalytically-oriented (Psychodynamic) Psychotherapy

Psychoanalytically-oriented, psychodynamic psychotherapy is a much more direct form of psychoanalysis. The duration of therapy is much briefer. The patient and the therapist may sit face-to-face or else a couch is used. The technique is nearly the same as psychoanalysis; however emphasis on the interpretation of transference, resistance and defenses is less. Advice is given to the patient occasionally and focus is more on the current interpersonal events and transference to others outside of session. Additional modes of treatment, including drug therapy are also allowed.

Brief Psychodynamic Psychotherapy

These are time limited treatments (usually 10–12 sessions) based on psychoanalysis and psychodynamic theory. These include several methods with their essence being dynamic interaction between therapist and patient, active interpretation and use of transference, and early termination of therapy.

PSYCHOTHERAPY FOR SPECIFIC CLINICAL POPULATION

Children and Adolescents

Children are increasingly being referred for psychological intervention for emotional and behavioral disorders (especially problems of inattention, hyperactivity and impulsivity, or problems of conduct). Other reasons for referral include academic problems (learning disorders, etc.), autism spectrum disorders, eating disorders, affective and anxiety spectrum disorders, substance use disorders and deliberate self-harm. Inadequate parental care and neglect are few other reasons which may be underlying the behavior or emotional problems. Individual psychotherapy with children can be done using cognitive, psychoanalytic, or behavioral approaches. Establishing rapport and having a good therapeutic relationship is the hallmark of all forms of therapies. *Play therapy* is a special form of therapy developed for use in children, which utilizes play as a means of communication to understand the child's origin of symptoms. It is particularly useful in preschool children in which language and immature communication skills may impede other types of therapy. Observation of a child's play, the pattern, type of toys used, and interaction during the play can help understand the cause of disturbed behavior. Either a nondirective approach can be used in which unstructured play is allowed in which the child is given various toys (dolls, animals, cars, crayons, sand tray, etc.). The principle behind this approach is that through the play, the child will be able to express one's feelings towards self, others and environment. A more directive approach can also be used in which the therapist guides the child through the play with the aim of facilitating cognitive or behavioral changes. Family therapy and parent training techniques are also commonly used when indicated.

Some special types of behavior techniques commonly used with children for modifying maladaptive behavior are listed below:

- *Positive reinforcement*: Here, the desirable behavior is reinforced by a reward, either material or symbolic.
- *Negative reinforcement*: Here, on performance of the desirable behavior, punishment can be avoided.
- *Modeling*: The person is exposed to "model" behavior and is induced to copy it. This can also be used to avoid certain behaviors.
- *Time-out*: Here, the reinforcement is withdrawn for some time, contingent upon the undesired response. Time-out is often used in therapy with children.
- *Punishment*: Aversive stimulus is presented, contingent upon undesired response (i.e., whenever undesired response occurs, punishment is given).

Family Therapy

In this type of therapy, the aim is to seek change in relational functioning and focus of intervention is on the family as a unit, rather than an individual. The therapist aims to modify the interactions among the family members and improve the functioning of the family as a unit.

Family therapy is indicated whenever there are relational problems in the family (either primarily or secondary to psychiatric illness). It can also be used for improving the family's coping in case of presence of psychosocial stressors, and managing the expressed emotions of family.

There are several varieties of family therapies, such as those based on psychodynamic, behavioral or systemic principles. Components of therapy include problem solving, training in communication skills, writing a behavioral contract, and homework assignments.

Marital and Sexual Therapies

Marital (or couples) therapy aims at resolving the conflicts between the couple over a range of parameters like social, emotional, financial or sexual. It also involves different psychotherapeutic approaches with focus on restructuring the couple's interaction, coping effectively with problems and reducing the distress present in the relationship. Sexual therapy is also primarily intended for couples but can also be used for individuals. Masters and Johnson Therapy (1970) is a widely used and effective therapy for sexual problems.

OTHERS

Numerous others psychotherapeutic approaches have been developed which are being used for specific purposes. Some of them are described briefly.

Abreaction: This form of therapy focuses on reliving the events of a traumatic or painful experience. It is indicated in conversion and dissociative disorders. It is based on the principle that the symptoms are produced due to the repressed emotions related to the traumatic event. Therefore, release and expression of these previously repressed emotions by reliving the event will help in achieving cure. Suggestion and hypnosis may be used in reliving the painful events. This approach is usually used in combination with other psychotherapeutic approaches.

Interpersonal therapy: This form of psychotherapy is based on the premise that interpersonal relations between patient and significant others are important in developing and maintaining psychiatric disorders. It is a time-limited approach with 1–2 sessions/week over a span of 5–6 months. It focuses on improving the quality of interpersonal and social functioning. It is commonly used for treating depression and adjustment disorders.

Psychodrama: Based on use of role play and guided drama for gaining insight into problems and exploring solutions. It requires a group setting in which the patient usually plays the role of protagonist and others play specific supporting roles. It has been seen to be useful in a variety of clinical and nonclinical situations.

Indian Context

In India, the psychoanalytic movement was started by Girindra Sekhar Bose who founded the Indian Psychoanalytic Society in 1922 in Kolkata. He was a pioneer of modern psychotherapy who developed and practiced his concept of psychoanalysis around the same time that Freud was practicing psychoanalysis. Over the next several decades, several workers emphasized the relevance of Indian culture, religion and philosophy in practicing psychotherapy. Gradually, it was established that traditional psychotherapy can be as efficacious as classical psychotherapy, with common therapeutic ingredients in both the approaches. The differences between Indian psychotherapy with its western counterpart were also identified. As compared to western psychotherapeutic approach, the traditional approach is less formal and circumscribed. There is less emphasis on the western concepts of patient autonomy and assumption of equal responsibility. Rather there is dependence on therapist who is considered as a guide and a benevolent senior. It is also believed that most Indian patients, as compared to western patients, are not psychologically minded. Rather than introspection and emotional expression, focus is more on physical symptoms. Also, they are more open to the traditional concepts of karma,

Basic tenets of traditional doctor patient relationship:
- Relationship is all-compassing
- Relationship is filial rather than professional
- The doctor is a family member, a friend, philosopher and guide
- Permits an ongoing multi-model interaction between the doctor and patient
- The doctor is seen as a social leader, a community elder, a benevolent senior
- The relationship is not limited to symptom removal, but also for solving problems of everyday life
- Relationship for development, self-realization and self-actualization
- Doctor is seen as a Guru, a teacher and a specialist of life itself

Source: Reproduced from Psychotherapy in a traditional society: Context, concept, and practice. Varma VK and Gupta Nitin, 2008.

reincarnation, faith healing and often have magical expectations of cure. The basic tenets of traditional doctor patient relationship are given in the following **Box 29.1**.

Traditionally, India has three major psychotherapeutic systems which have distinct philosophies of their own: Yoga, Vedanta, and Buddhism. These have their own particular relevance to our culture, and sometimes, may be more effective than the western psychotherapeutic approach in terms of better acceptability, cost-effectiveness and cultural consistency and ease of self-administration.

Ethical Aspects of Psychotherapy

The four principles of professional ethics—(1) beneficence (doing good and providing maximum benefit to the patient), (2) respect for autonomy (appreciation of persons right to self-determination and promoting independence), (3) nonmaleficence (first do no harm), and (4) justice (providing equal and fair treatment)—are prominent in contemporary psychotherapy. It is of utmost importance that the therapist follows the basic standards of ethical practice.

Informed consent is another important aspect, which involves disclosing all treatment related aspects and empowering the patient to take an informed decision about their treatment. Where ever possible, therapeutic contract (a written document which includes detailed structure of therapy, and rules and responsibilities of both patient and therapist) should be made and effective documentation should be done.

Confidentiality, and the respect for privacy is another vital feature of psychotherapy. *Confidentiality* refers to the therapist's responsibility not to release information learned during the course of psychotherapy to third parties. Confidentiality is an essential ingredient of psychotherapy as it is a precondition for patients to be able to speak freely to therapists and discuss their most intimate details. However, confidentiality must also give way to the responsibility to protect others when a patient makes a credible threat to harm someone.

Boundary issue in psychotherapy is a complex area which presents significant dilemma to the therapist, as often nonsexual boundary crossing can serve the treatment plan. Although, this is still a matter of significant debate as to which behavior on the part of patient/therapist should be seen as boundary violation and should not be allowed. However, sexual behavior of any kind is a clear boundary violation and should not be done/permitted in any context.

CONCLUSION

To conclude, psychotherapy is an attempt to relieve a person's psychological distress and disability by psychological means. A psychotherapist requires years of training and expertise to be able to skillfully practice psychotherapy. There are various schools of psychotherapy which differ in their process and underlying principles, but with the common aim of lessening the emotional discomfort and facilitating greater integrity of personality. Research has shown that psychotherapy alone, or in combination with medication, is a highly successful treatment modality for a wide range of illnesses. Nevertheless, further research is still required to know about the process and outcome of psychotherapy, and its mediating factors.

TAKE-HOME MESSAGES

- Psychotherapy is a collaborative treatment based on the relationship between an individual and a therapist.
- It is indicated for various psychiatric illnesses like depression, OCD, anxiety, phobias as well as other emotional, behavioral and personality problems.
- There are three principal approaches namely supportive, re-educative and reconstructive. Various schools of psychotherapy (supportive, behavioral, cognitive, and psychoanalytic) are based around these principal approaches.
- The type of psychotherapy done depends on patient's problems, therapist's theoretical orientation and expertise, and current research evidence.
- Certain patient, therapist and environmental variables work in combination that determines the therapeutic process and outcome.
- It is a structured and time bound process, which may take months to years; and requires a joint and dedicated effort from both patient and therapist.

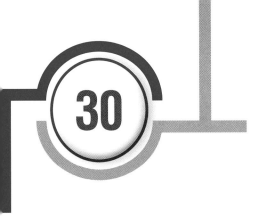

Community and Preventive Psychiatry

R Srinivasa Murthy

INTRODUCTION

During the last three centuries, care of the persons diagnosed with mental disorders has seen major paradigm shifts as to what are the causes and treatments of mental disorders, where they should be cared for, who should care for them, and the rights of the persons diagnosed with mental disorders. The shift can also be seen in the terms used, from bad to mad to sad, and the places of care from jails to asylums to mental hospitals to the community. These changes are a reflection of the advances in the understanding of human behavior, especially that of the functioning of the brain, availability of improved techniques of therapeutic interventions, and the progressive thinking in the field of human rights. The current goal of care is to assure quality life to persons diagnosed with mental disorders in the community. The current situation places a number of challenges and opportunities for medical officers at the primary healthcare facilities.

SCOPE OF MENTAL HEALTH

The mental health needs of the general population can be considered under three broad groups:

First, a group of mental health needs refers to the *psychosocial needs* of the general population, especially in children and youth associated with rapid social change and developmental needs.

In adults, specific groups like women, elderly will have mental health needs arising from their specific life situations. There are other needs related to stress management, rational and healthy use of alcohol and tranquilizers in the general population. There will be specific needs among the persons under severe stress (debt-related suicides, following communal conflict, disasters, etc.). Interventions for this large group of people are more focused on preventive and promotional activities. These can be undertaken at the general population level, through community-level interventions, at the family level, and at the individual level, in settings such as schools, health facilities, and community meeting centers like religious centers, clubs, etc.

The *second* set of needs refers to behavioral changes and the care of *common mental disorders* that are present among those seeking primary healthcare. Most studies, including the recently completed National Mental Health Survey, in 2016, have shown this to be about 10% of the adult general population and about 20–25% general medical clinic population. Most of these disorders are related to psychosocial stress factors in the lives of patients. This group of patients most frequently presents with somatic complaints and is not recognized as having psychological problems by general medical personnel. Nonrecognition often leads to unnecessary investigations, use of nonspecific medicines such as analgesics and vitamins without benefit to the patients. In addition, this group is known to utilize primary healthcare more than those with physical disorders. There is another group including the likes of diabetes, hypertension, and cancer patients, in which psychosocial factors play an important role. In both these groups of patients coming to primary healthcare, a number of interventions are known to be effective. The interventions can range from patient education about the link of physical complaints to life situation (reinterpretation), exercise, listening to music, teaching relaxation techniques, providing opportunities to share feelings and problems, counseling, problem-solving skills, group-work, and use of tranquilizers/antidepressants for limited periods of time. *All of these interventions can be undertaken by both the medical officers and other staff, such as nurses, and health workers at primary healthcare facilities.*

The *third* is a set of conditions related to the *major mental disorders* (schizophrenia, manic-depressive psychosis, depression, substance abuse, epilepsy, mental retardation, etc.) which are known to be prevalent in about 2% of the population. These conditions are important as they contribute to the global burden of diseases (above 15% in 2015) and effective interventions are available to provide care to this group of persons. Early interventions can reduce disability and promote recovery. Care of persons with these disorders can be undertaken both by primary healthcare personnel and the mental health specialists. (Mental health needs of the community are given in detail as an appendix at the end of the chapter).

HISTORICAL DEVELOPMENT OF MENTAL HEALTHCARE

The development of mental healthcare all over the world is best described as a developing process. The World Health Report, 2001 (WHO, 2001) described the changes over the last two centuries, where the shift of care has moved from institutions to the community:

"The care of people with mental and behavioral disorders has always reflected prevailing social values related to the social perception of mental illness. Through the ages, people with mental and behavioral disorders have been treated in different ways. They have been given a high status in societies which believe them to intermediate with gods and the dead. In medieval Europe and elsewhere, they were beaten and burnt at the stake. They have been locked up in large institutions. They have been explored as scientific objects. And they have been cared for and integrated into the communities to which they belong. In Europe, the 19th century witnessed diverging trends. On one hand, mental illness was seen as a legitimate topic for scientific enquiry; psychiatry burgeoned as a medical discipline, and people with mental disorders were considered medical patients. On the other hand, people with mental disorders, like those with many other diseases and undesirable social behavior, were isolated from society in large custodial institutions, the state mental hospitals, formerly known as lunatic asylums. These trends were later exported to Africa, the Americas, and Asia. During the second half of the 20th century, a shift in the mental healthcare paradigm took place, largely owing to three independent factors, namely—(1) psychopharmacology made significant progress, with the discovery of new classes of drugs, particularly neuroleptics and antidepressants, as well as the development of new forms of psychosocial interventions; (2) the human rights movement became a truly international phenomenon under the sponsorship of the newly created United Nations, and democracy advanced on a global basis, albeit at different speeds in different places; and (3) social and mental components were firmly incorporated in the definition of health of the newly established WHO in 1948. These technical and sociopolitical events contributed to a change in emphasis: from care in large custodial institutions to more open and flexible care in the community. Community care is about the empowerment of people with mental and behavioral disorders. In practice, community care implies the development of a wide range of services within local settings (emphasis added)."

International Developments

The World Health Organization, in 2001, in its World Health Report, 2001 (New Knowledge, New Hope) reviewed the developments in mental health and recommended action at the level of countries with differing levels of mental health services. The 10 key recommendations were to integrate mental health with primary healthcare, provision of essential psychiatric medicines, provide care in the community, educate the public and involve communities, families, and consumers, with changes in the areas of policies/legislation, human resources, linkage with other sectors, monitoring and research.

The key issue for the service planners is to determine the optimal mix of services and the level of provision of particular service delivery channels. The absolute need for various services differs greatly between countries but the relative needs for different services, i.e. the proportions of different services as parts of the total mental health service provision, are broadly the same in many countries. Services should be planned in a holistic fashion so as to create an optimal mix.

Figure 30.1 shows the relationship between the different service components. It is clear that the most numerous services ought to be self-care management, informal community mental health services, and community mental health services provided by the primary healthcare staff, followed by psychiatric services based in general hospitals and formal community mental health services, and lastly by specialist mental health services. The emphasis placed on delivering mental health treatment and care through services based in general hospitals or community mental health services should be determined by the strengths of the current mental health or general health system, as well as by cultural and socioeconomic variables.

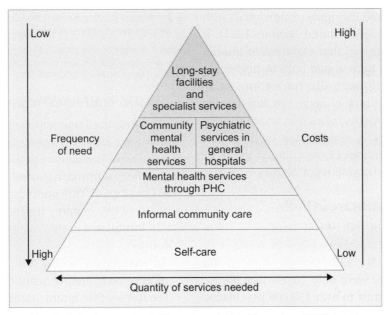

Fig. 30.1: Optimum mix of different mental health services (WHO, 2003). (PHC: primary health care)

In a country like India, where majority of the mentally ill persons are living in the community and where there are vast amount of unmet mental health service needs, it would be prudent to utilize the approaches of self-care and informal care. Most of the past quarter century of mental health planning has been on integration of mental health with general health services. However, there are pockets of self-care, informal care by the families (e.g. mental handicap, schizophrenia) and patient groups (e.g. drug dependence) to point to the value of this approach to mental health care). In order for this to become a reality, there has to be a paradigm shift in the organization of knowledge, dissemination of information and skills, and greater efforts towards empowerment of the community.

Another important development in the recent past occurred in 1991. The United Nations General Assembly adopted the *principles for the protection of persons with mental illness and the improvement of mental healthcare,* emphasizing care in the community and the rights of individuals with mental disorders (United Nations 1991). It is now recognized that violation of human rights can be perpetrated both by neglecting the patient through discrimination, carelessness, and lack of access to services, as well as by intrusive, restrictive, and regressive interventions. A more recent document is the United Nations Convention on Rights of Persons with Disabilities of 2006.

Mental Healthcare in India

At the time of India's Independence, there were almost no mental health services in the country. For a population of about 300 million, there were only 10,000 psychiatric beds, in contrast to over 150,000 psychiatric beds for about 30 million in United Kingdom at that time. The initial period of 1947–1966

focused on doubling of the psychiatric beds, along with development of training centers to train psychiatrists, clinical psychologists, psychiatric social workers, and psychiatric nurses. The period of 1960s and 1970s saw the emergence of general hospital psychiatric units in a big way both as service providers and training centers. The community psychiatry initiatives were taken up initially in the 1970s and in a big way from the 1980s, following the adoption of the National Mental Health Programme (NMHP) in August 1982.

Barriers to implementation of NMHP in India

- *Shortage of trained manpower in the field of mental health*
- *Social stigma and lack of knowledge of psychiatric patients and their families*
- *Negative attitude of general practitioners, primary care physicians, and other specialists*
- *NGO/voluntary organizations do not find this field attractive*
- *Inadequate staff and infrastructure of mental hospitals and psychiatric wings of medical colleges*
- *Uneven distribution of sparse resources limiting the availability of mental healthcare to those living in urban areas*
- *Inadequate funding for mental health, which remains a relatively low priority area*

Source: Annual Report 2006–7; Ministry of Health and Family Welfare, Government of India. New Delhi. p. 140.

National Mental Health Programme (1982)

Recognizing the large gap, in the available professional and institutional resources to provide mental healthcare to the population, alternative community-based approaches were developed. This alternative approach received policy support in the form of the NMHP, formulated in 1982, with the following objectives:

- To ensure availability and accessibility of minimum mental healthcare for all in the foreseeable future, particularly to the most vulnerable and underprivileged sections of population;

- To encourage application of mental health knowledge in general healthcare and in social development;
- To promote community participation in the mental health service development and to stimulate efforts toward self-help in the community.

Approaches to realize the stated programme objectives were:

- Diffusion of mental health skills to the periphery of the health service system;
- Appropriate appointment of tasks in mental healthcare;
- Integration of basic mental healthcare into general health services;
- Linkage to community development and mental healthcare.

Following the formulation and acceptance of the NMHP in 1982, there has been considerable progress in the field. Efforts to integrate mental health with general healthcare started with single PHCs in Raipur Rani (Haryana), Sakalawara (Karnataka), Baroda (Gujarat), Kolkata (West Bengal), and Patiala (Punjab) (1976–1984). This was followed by the Bellary District Mental Health Program (DMHP; 1985–1991). For the next 25 years, the DMHP has been gradually extended to over 300 districts. In addition, the scope of NMHP was enlarged in 2005 and 2012, to include strengthening of departments of psychiatry in medical colleges, setting up of centers of excellence, inclusion of suicide prevention, and school/college mental health.

Other important developments of the last few years have been the formulation of a new National Mental Health Policy in 2014 and promulgation of the Mental Healthcare Act (MHCA) 2017. MHCA states *"Every person shall have a right to access mental healthcare and treatment from mental health services run or funded by the appropriate Government"*.

This is the promise of the State, which has tremendous potential for changes.

COMMUNITY MENTAL HEALTH INITIATIVES

A striking aspect of the developments of mental health services in India is as much the location of the care in the community (where most of the ill persons were already living) as the utilization of a wide variety of resources of the community. For example, in the initial phase, the existing general healthcare infrastructure was the primary focus of integration of mental health services. Soon, the increased use of family members, volunteers, counselors, mentally ill persons, survivors of disasters, parents of children with mental disorders, as well as the education system was put to practice. *In this way, the three principles of community psychiatry— meeting population-based needs, use of range of resources, and accessibility were partially addressed.*

It is important to recognize that there were simultaneously other community mental healthcare initiatives in the country. For example, even as early as the 1950s, various approaches to involving the family members in the care of their ill family members were in operation at centers like Amritsar, Vellore, and Bangalore. A number of other initiatives, especially by the voluntary organizations, have enlarged both the scope of mental healthcare as well as the role of care providers. These initiatives have included setting up of day care centers, half-way homes, long-stay homes, suicide prevention centers, school mental health programs, disaster mental healthcare, community-based programs for the care of the mentally retarded, elderly persons, persons with dementia, and substance abuse. One very India-specific development of significance is the increasing role played by the family members both for self-help, mutual support, and toward advocacy. This development, to a large extent, has occurred with the partnership with the professionals, especially by the voluntary organizations, unlike in some of the western countries where there is this lack of cooperation between patients, families, and professionals.

PREVENTION OF MENTAL DISORDERS

There are a number of mental disorders that can be prevented. An example is prevention of mental retardation by a wide variety of public health measures. These measures include antenatal care, nutrition support to pregnant mothers, supervised delivery, postnatal care, immunization, adequate nutrition for infants, iodine supplementation of salt, early stimulation for low birth babies, prevention of accidents, and treatment of epilepsy.

PROMOTION OF MENTAL HEALTH

There is evidence to show that health promotion programs are capable of increasing resilience and other mental health factors such as self-esteem, problem-solving skills, stress and conflict management skills, feelings of mastery and self-efficacy. Promotion of mental health would include reduction of a range of risk factors such as low birth weight, preterm deliveries, poor parenting behavior, lack of early bonding and parental affection, child abuse and neglect, teenage pregnancies, aggression, and being a victim of regular bullying. Mental health promotion has also social outcomes such as better academic achievement, increase in productivity and reduction in productivity loss, lowering divorce rate, reduction in family violence, reduction in youth delinquency, and reduction in use of social services.

Mental health promotion works as universal input for prevention of mental disorders.

The promotion of mental health should begin in schools on a priority basis, through imparting of the life skills education programs. The religious precepts and practices that are promotive of mental health (e.g. meditation, yoga, prayer, social supports in crisis situations) should be identified and encouraged.

A very important contribution of India, in promotion of health in general and mental health in particular, is the science of yoga. Currently yoga has been widely accepted and practiced internationally. Yoga is a discipline, a system that has evolved in India over several thousand years to facilitate general well-being the evolution of consciousness. It offers a worldview, a lifestyle, and a series of techniques by which changes in human awareness can be brought about. The basic aim of yoga is growth, development, and evolution of mind. The yogic techniques when practiced correctly give rise to certain types of reactions within the person, so that there are qualitative and quantitative changes in awareness. It is hence understandable that the United Nations accorded a formal and special status for yoga declaring 21st June as the International Yoga Day.

There is growing awareness of making mental health skills a part of everyone in the society. Self-care in depression is the most written subject. The shift in self-care is to move mental health from a "deviancy model" to "normalcy model". When mental health is presented not as neutral knowledge/information, but skills that are relevant to the wellbeing of the individual, the acceptance of mental health/mental disorders will be greater. The vulnerability of all human beings to mental health issues and the availability of a wide range of skills (sharing of feelings, listening, taking supports, relaxation, mindfulness, exercise, focus of restful sleep, writing down disturbing feelings, developing mind relaxing activities like listening to music, etc.) can change the way mental health is seen as part of everyone's life. This could be the best "stigma buster". The growth of mobile phones and the internet allows for reaching and remaining in contact with the population to promote self-care for mental health.

CONCLUSION

Development of mental health services all over the world, countries rich and poor alike, have been the product of social developments, specifically the importance society gives to the rights of disadvantaged/marginalized groups. Economically rich countries have addressed the movement from the institutionalized care to community care building on the strengths of their social institutions. India began this process about 50 years back and has made significant progress. There is need to continue the process by widening the scope of the mental health interventions, increasing the involvement of all available community resources, and embedding the interventions in the historical, social, and cultural roots of India. Medical officers at the primary healthcare level are a vital part of the community and preventive psychiatry movement. The current situation presents challenges and opportunities for mental health professionals, primary care doctors, and people in the coming years.

APPENDIX: MENTAL HEALTH NEEDS OF THE COMMUNITY

The mental health needs of the community relate to a wide variety of conditions and situations. These include—*(1) serious mental disorders in the community;* *(2) persons with acute conditions; (3) persons with long-standing (chronic) mental disorders; (4) substance abuse; (5) intellectual developmental disability; (6) rehabilitation; (7) mental disorders in primary healthcare; (8) mental health of women; (9) children and adolescents—school going and out of school; (10) mental health needs of the elderly; (11) special groups like refugees, survivors of disasters; (12) persons attempting suicide; (13) public mental health education; (14) persons in institutional settings; (15) prevention of mental disorders; and (16) promotion of mental health.*

Serious mental disorders in the community: General population epidemiological studies indicate that severe mental disorders like major depression, schizophrenia, bipolar affective disorder, and dementia would be seen in all the populations. In view of the limited services available in the community, especially in the rural areas, it can be expected that there will be a large number of persons with these disorders who have not received either any or only incomplete treatment and/or rehabilitation services, who will be brought for care when services would be made available in the community.

Persons with acute conditions: The fresh episodes of acute psychoses would be *3 per 10,000 population.* Treatment of these conditions is important as they cause significant distress to the ill individual, burden of care to the family, and sometimes social disruption. More importantly, they are all treatable and recovery is possible to a great extent. Equally important is the observation that early interventions give better outcome with less possibility of long-standing illness (chronicity). Most of this treatment can be undertaken as ambulatory care by general medical practitioners with only short-term hospitalization in some patients.

Persons with long-standing (chronic) mental disorders: This group of disorders includes schizophrenia, bipolar affective disorders, and dementia. It is estimated that the point prevalence of this group would be about *5–8 per 1,000 population.* The "chronicity" is mostly contributed by the lack of opportunities for early treatment and absence of rehabilitative services; besides a small group of treatment-resistant patients (e.g. schizophrenia) and progressively deteriorating patients (dementia), also add to the pool of chronicity. The "chronic" patients of schizophrenic illness have demonstrated to be responsive to treatment even in late stages of illness. The treatments are simple to administer. The requirements in these group of patients are regular medication, support of the family, training to the family in caring skills, support in crisis and respite care, rehabilitation, acceptance and integration into the community. The primary healthcare personnel, health workers, and medical officers can provide this care. In bipolar affective disorder, prophylactic treatment can prevent relapses and recovery. In dementia, support to the family, symptomatic treatment, and guidance to accommodate the failing mental functions can reduce the distress, disability, and burden to the family.

Substance abuse: Substance abuse and substance dependence are growing public health problems in India. The abuse includes use of alcohol, drugs of intoxication, and prescription drugs. There is evidence that the prescription drugs are occupying a greater role in substance abuse in the country (GOI, 2004). The public health costs are enormous; interventions need to be addressed both at prevention, early identification, care, and rehabilitation.

Intellectual developmental disability: Intellectual developmental disability (IDD), earlier called mental retardation/handicap, belongs to the class of developmental disabilities (DD), and is also called intellectual disability (ID). These are conditions in which one or more of human capabilities fail to develop adequately from childhood. Apart from MR, other DDs are specific delays in speech and language, in motor skills, in scholastic skills, and autistic-spectrum disorders. Most of them are static encephalopathies, meaning that though they have some significant delay, they continue to improve with the passage of time, albeit at a slower rate. Widely accepted definitions that are currently available stress on three dimensions: the intellectual (IQ <70), developmental (onset before 18 years of age), and thirdly the social (diminished ability to adapt to the daily demands of the normal social environment) criteria. Prevalence of mental retardation in India is around 2% for mild mental retardation and 0.5% for severe mental retardation, inclusive of moderate, severe, and profound categories (defined as IQ <50). The major correlates are excess in males and rural areas. At least one-third of children attending Child Psychiatry OPD's or Child Guidance Clinics have MR. Important interventions are the prevention, early identification, early stimulation, special education, parental training, vocational training, rehabilitation, and long-term care when carers are no more. National Trust specifically addresses the needs of this group of persons.

Rehabilitation: Rehabilitation is an important part of mental health services for a number of reasons. *Firstly,* in a number of severe mental disorders like schizophrenia, bipolar disorder, and substance abuse, there is a definite percentage of affected people who do not fully recover and have limitations in their functioning resulting in disability that needs to be addressed through rehabilitation. *Secondly*, due to the paucity of services in our country, a large proportion of severely ill persons seek treatment for their illness at a time when already certain disability has set in. *Thirdly*, at different stages of the treatment, rehabilitation interventions, such as encouraging activities of daily living, living in a therapeutic community to learn social skills, day care centers, vocational training, sheltered workshops where ill individuals can do productive work under support and supervision, and community care facilities when there are no family members to support the ill person, are generally not available. At present in India, the rehabilitation facilities are very limited and largely the result of efforts of individual persons and voluntary organizations.

Mental disorders in primary healthcare: This group forms the biggest group of persons with mental disorders. In normal circumstances, about 20–25% of those seeking primary care are known to suffer from different mental disorders. This group represents an important group for four reasons. *Firstly*, when not correctly diagnosed, often they are subjected to inappropriate treatments which are nonspecific (vitamins, tonics, etc.) and form a group where investigations are wasteful; *Secondly*, these persons can be effectively cared for by the physicians at the level of primary healthcare; *Thirdly*, by providing care at this level, the stigma of mental disorders is reduced or absent; *Fourthly*, this approach is cost-effective. Specific measures known to be effective to care for this group are—correct diagnosis with explanations; avoiding unnecessary investigations; listening to the patients; relaxation techniques; guidance about daily routines and activities; mobilizing

the family resources; use of medicines for short periods and formation of groups of patients for self-help.

Mental health of women: Women represent a special group for mental health care. The needs of women from mental health point are well recognized in all populations. Though the overall prevalence of mental and behavioral disorders is not different between men and women, anxiety and depressive disorders are more common among women. Almost all studies show that depressive disorders are 1.5–2 times more in women than in men, during the adult life. The reasons for these differences are partly biological, partly social and psychological. In addition, women are more often the victims of domestic violence. Studies in developed countries have shown that women experiencing domestic violence have higher symptoms of psychological distress and greater frequency of contemplation of suicide. From all these perspectives, mental health needs of women are greater, of special nature, and need interventions that are sensitive to their needs. Specific measures to care of this group would include the following strategies—greater number of women health personnel, specific training to health personnel on gender issues, mental health education about self-care for mental health, support to women to form self-help groups, emotional support at individual and family levels, and income generating activities.

Children and adolescents-school going and out of school: Children and adolescents (CAA) form a very important group for mental healthcare. Besides the needs of children in peace conditions, CAA have been exposed and experience intense trauma in form of wars, displacement, disability, and disruption of childhood. In this way, they are especially vulnerable. There are three broad mental health needs requiring urgent attention. *Firstly*, the emotional problems relating to developmental processes seem to affect about 10% of the children. *Secondly*, mental retardation of all severity put together constitute about 3% of the population, whereas the prevalence of more severe types is about 5 per 1,000. This group requires early identification, home-based stimulation, special education, behavioral training for self-care and daily activities, and at a later age vocational training. *Thirdly,* need is for promotion of mental health, for example the life skills education (LSE). LSE not only improves immediate functioning of children, but also has the potential to prevent problems of drug abuse, suicide, delinquency, and risk taking behavior (e.g. HIV/AIDS). These need to be addressed in school going children as well as in the nonschool going children. The latter group requires a lot of innovative approaches, similar to the ones developed for street children in countries like India, Brazil, etc. The most important goal would to be to restore childhood to all children; create conditions for optimal development at home and society; provide healthy adult contacts; facilitate life skills education; crisis support; friendly noninstitutional mental health services, and create an atmosphere of security and hopeful future.

Mental health needs of elderly: As a result of demographic transition, India's elderly population has increased from 12 million in 1901 to 57 million in 1990 and it became 104 million in 2011. From mere 5.1% in 1901 the elderly will become 20% of the population by 2050. Elderly people suffer from the dual medical problems of both communicable as well as degenerative diseases. The two most common mental disorders, that they get afflicted with, are depression and dementia. There is need for prevention, early identification, treatment, and rehabilitation. As over 70% of elderly in urban areas and 34% in rural areas are economically dependent on their families, and almost all the elderly live with their families, support programs for the families are an important area for intervention.

Special groups—refugees, disaster-affected populations: It is well-recognized that refugees and disaster-affected population represent a group of persons with special emotional needs. They have double the rates of mental disorders as compared to the general population. This is because of the extreme disruption that they happen to experience in life and also because of many lost opportunities and obstacle that appear as a consequence. All these people need opportunity to rebuild their lives and reorganize their life goals. Some of the well-recognized strategies are recognition of the special needs by community and health personnel; community based and ambulant mental healthcare facilities; opportunities to share the painful experiences of trauma; formation of self-help groups with common needs; and crisis support and rehabilitative efforts for vocational and social life.

Suicide and attempted suicide: Suicide and attempted suicide represent a "cry for help" in a situation perceived as hopeless. Suicide and attempted suicide rates vary across countries. Organizing services for suicide prevention have the double advantage of preventing premature loss of lives as well as the sensitization of the community to mental health issues as being relevant to all of the population. Experience in other countries have shown that following measures would be effective in addressing the problems of attempted suicide and suicide: recognition of the "normalcy" of suicidal ideation in specific adverse life situations; increasing intra-family communication to share feelings, experiences, and mutual support; life skills education to children and adolescents; early recognition and treatment of mental disorders by general physicians; support for acute crisis through volunteers in crisis centers; support to persons who have attempted suicide to prevent repetition; support to families where suicide has occurred and use of religious centers for mental health education. Voluntary organizations working with small communities can address these needs effectively.

Public mental health education: This need, though not usually seen as part of the services, becomes important because of very limited public awareness in the community about mental health and mental illness. Mental disorders are traditionally very much stigmatized and persons with mental disorders experience many forms of discrimination. This largely arises from lack of information about the importance and nature of the mental health and mental disorders. Specifically, there is need to share with the general population—principles of child growth and development; emotional needs of individuals in different stages of life; response to stress and its presentation in individuals; importance of family in child development; importance of family in crisis situations; the value of social supports in maintaining mental health; adolescent experience and manifestations of adolescent behavior; early symptoms of mental disorders; treatment methods; importance of work in rehabilitation of mentally ill persons; avoidance of mistreatment of persons with mental disorders; what individuals, families, and communities can do to promote mental health, prevent mental disorders, and care for mentally ill persons.

Persons in institutional settings (prisons, orphanages, etc.): Persons in institutional settings have special needs for mental healthcare. Generally, these institutions have greater proportion of individuals with mental health needs. These can be in the form of acute and chronic psychoses, mental retardation, dementia, and drug dependence. In addition, living in an institution, without daily routines, social contacts, and opportunities for fulfillment of one's needs and capacities can result in emotional problems like depression, adjustment problems, and suicidal thoughts. Solutions to these problems have to be found by recognizing the emotional needs of the persons; sensitizing the staff of institutions to emotional aspects of the residents; training the medical staff in mental healthcare; providing coping skills to the residents; creating opportunities for emotional fulfillment through education, hobbies, entertainment, forming relationships, etc.

Prevention of mental disorders: As described earlier there are a number of mental disorders that can be prevented. An example is prevention of mental retardation by a wide variety of public health measures. These measures include antenatal care, nutrition support to pregnant mothers, supervised delivery, postnatal care, immunization, adequate nutrition for infants, iodization of salt, early stimulation for low birth babies, prevention of accidents, and treatment of epilepsy.

Promotion of mental health: The promotion of mental health should on a priority begin in schools through the life skills education program. The religious precepts and practices that are promotive of mental health (e.g. meditation, yoga, prayer, social supports in crisis situations) should be identified and encouraged.

TAKE HOME MESSAGES

- Recent times have seen major paradigm-shifts related to mental disorders as to their causes, modes of treatment, their caregivers, their place of care, and their rights.
- Mental health needs of community can be conceptualized firstly as psychosocial needs, secondly as needs related to care of common mental disorders in primary healthcare, and thirdly as related to care of major mental disorders in specialist services.
- The 10 key recommendations of WHO to develop mental health services were to integrate mental health with primary health care, provision of essential psychiatric medicines, provide care in the community, educate the public and involve communities, families, and consumers, with changes in the areas of policies/legislation, human resources, linkage with other sectors, monitoring and research.

- The community psychiatry initiatives were taken up initially in the 1970s and in a big way from the 1980s, following the adoption of the NMHP in August 1982.
- Other important developments of the last few years have been the formulation of National Mental Health Policy in 2014 and promulgation of the Mental Healthcare Act in 2017.
- In the initial phase, the existing general healthcare infrastructure was the primary focus for integration of mental health services. Soon, the increased use of family members, volunteers, counselors, mentally ill persons, survivors of disasters, parents of children with mental disorders, as well as the education system was put to practice.
- There are a number of mental disorders that can be prevented. Promotion of mental health can be achieved by increasing internal resilience and resistance to stressors, as well as by reduction of a range of risk factors of mental disorders.

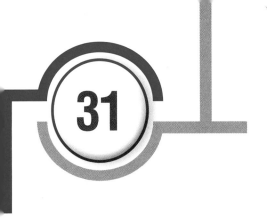

History of Psychiatry

RC Jiloha, Deeksha Elwadhi

INTRODUCTION

History, by its nature, cannot be silent; even the chronicler of ill-recorded times has nonetheless several tales to tell. History is the ultimate elder. It is like the roots of a tree which provide stability for growth. In psychiatry we have traversed the path from the broken soul to the broken brain, from philosophical ruminations to biological conundrums. The vicissitudes of the world brought paradigm shifts within the subject, which is pertinent to be looked in, to learn the evolution of this intriguing subject and evaluate various changes that were embarked upon to reach where we currently are. This chapter attempts to provide basic knowledge of birth and growth of psychiatry and the lessons learnt from the past to show light for the future of the subject.

The word "psychiatry" was first introduced in 1808 by Johann Christian Reil (1755–1820), who argued for psychiatry as a specialty of medicine and outlined the reasons that people who were mentally ill should not be treated by experts of other disciplines, but by physicians. Abnormalities in human behavior have been known and recognized since the beginning of civilization and the ways to cope and understand the causality have evolved from ancient periods to modern times. Medical ideas in general and specifically so in psychiatry are molded by the dominant thoughts of the period and greatly influenced by the reigning philosophies, thoughts, and beliefs as will be clear in the trajectory of evolution of this field.

ANCIENT PERIOD

The belief in supernatural forces was the commonality of all ancient cultures. This period was dominated by magical beliefs, religious rituals, and herbal healing as therapeutic intervention. Preventive measures included the use of amulets and talismans.

Hippocrates and Plato of the ancient Greece, each gave their theories regarding madness and its cure. *Hippocrates* (460–357 BC) refuted the invocation of deities and demons in the causation of disease. He held that diseases are caused by imbalances in the four humors (blood, phlegm, yellow bile, black bile), which led to different types of illnesses like excesses of phlegm caused a form of dementia, yellow bile caused manic rage, and black bile caused melancholia. In the first attempt to explain different temperaments, Hippocratic authors also described the phlegmatic, choleric, and sanguine personalities. *Plato* (429–347 BC) described different types of soul and divided madness according to causality. *Aristotle* (384–322 BC), the famous Greek philosopher proposed the idea of a psyche-part of a human being that is mental and separate from the body. *Galen* (130–200 AD), a Roman physician, consolidated the teachings of Greeks and his treatise "*On the Diagnosis and Cure of the Soul's Passion*", contained how to approach and treat psychological problems.

In the Indian subcontinent, description of mental disorders was detailed in the Vedic texts; the *Atharva Veda* emphasized on the role of divine curses in the causation of mental illness. The Vedas were followed by the *Upanishads* which recognized the supremacy of the mind, describing its various functions, states of consciousness and personality make up in detail. The classical Indian schools of medicine influenced by *Ayurveda* came up in Taxila and Kasi in the 6th century BC, with a shift from magico-religious to rational causation. *Bhut vidya* one of the eight specializations of *Ayurveda* dealt with the treatment of people with mental disorders. The theory of *doshas*, which influenced the personality and propensity to get a disease in a man, was similar to the humoral theory of ancient Greece. Charaka the famous Indian physician defined man as an aggregate of mind, spirit and body, outlining their imbalance as the etiological mechanism of insanity. In the indigenous herbal pharmacopeia there were powerful remedies such as opium, cannabis, brahmi and sarpagandha. *Rauwolfia serpentina* was a popular drug for insanity in ancient India. Other schools of medicine in India like the *Unani* system and the *Siddha* system also talked about various psychiatric illnesses and suggested methods to treat them. These systems still continue to offer help for various forms of psychological conditions and temperaments. Religious practices such as meditation and yoga were regularly used for psychological treatment.

RENAISSANCE PERIOD: ESTABLISHMENT OF LUNATIC ASYLUMS

During the early period of the middle ages demonic possession was still considered as one of the pertinent causes of mental illness, and patients were labeled as witches with elaborate rituals for warding off the spirits.

The spread of the Muslim empire resulted in the setting up of the first asylum in Baghdad followed by Cairo. In 1547, the monastery of St Mary of Bethlehem, London was converted into a lunatic asylum by the king. Soon it became widely known for its deplorable conditions. However, in the following years, a chain of similar asylums came up throughout Europe and other parts of the world. The San Hipolito in Mexico in 1566, La Maison de Charenton in Paris in 1641, a mental hospital in Moscow in 1764, Lunatic's Tower in Vienna in 1784, are some important names in the series.

Paracelsus (1493–1541), the famous physician, refuted the humoral theory and believed in the theory of instincts being influenced by stars. He was a pioneer in several aspects of the "medical revolution" of the Renaissance, emphasizing the value of observation in combination with received wisdom.

Robert Burton (1577–1640) was an English scholar at Oxford University, best known for the classic, "*The Anatomy of Melancholy*", a comprehensive treatise on all previous medical-psychological thought on melancholy which became the most famous book on psychiatry in the 17th century.

In India, Maulana Fazlur-Lah Hakim is reported to have looked after the mental patients in an asylum at Mandu during the reign of Alauddin Khilji (1436–1469) at Dhar.

However, the emergence of lunatic asylums in India is entirely a British concept. After the historic battle of Plassey in 1757, when the East India Company began to exercise its political powers, a chain of lunatic asylums came up along the coat-line of Indian peninsula. The first mental asylum of India was established in 1745 in Mumbai and the second in 1784 in Kolkata, but no trace of these remain. The third mental asylum established in 1794 at Chennai exists at the same location as Institute of Mental Health, Chennai. The first Indian Lunacy Act came up in 1858 after the British Crown took over from the East India Company. This Act laid down guidelines for the establishment of mental asylums and procedures for admitting patients. Several mental hospitals were established along the length and breadth of the country primarily for the custodial care and not much was done regarding the treatment of the patients.

PSYCHIATRY IN THE 18TH AND 19TH CENTURY

William Cullen (1710–1790) in Germany published his own nosology of mental disorders. He used the term neurosis for the first time to describe varied group of mental diseases (including apoplexy, paralysis, dyspepsia, hypochondriasis, epilepsy, and hysteria).

Philippe Pinel (1745–1826) revolutionized care of the mentally ill by liberating over 50 patients from the Bicêtre in France. He propagated a humane approach for the care of the mentally ill patients in his influential book, *A Treatise on Insanity*, and proposed a new classification of mental illnesses: mania, melancholia, idiocy, and dementia, with heredity and environment as the causal factors.

A significant development occurred in the understanding of psychopathology, etiology, and classification of mental disorders during this period. *Jean Esquirol (1772–1840)* coined the term hallucination, differentiating it from illusion. *Benjamin Rush* (1745–1828) the father of American psychiatry wrote a comprehensive book on mental illnesses. *Wilhelm Griesinger* (1817–1868) considered mental diseases to be brain diseases. *Benedict-Augustin Morel* (1809–1873) named and described "Demence Precoce" as a form of insanity caused by inherited "mental degeneration" that became worse from one generation to the next. *Emil Kraepelin* (1856–1926) divided psychoses into two groups on the basis of outcome: Manic-depressive insanity, in which patients usually recovered, and Dementia Praecox which ultimately deteriorated into vegetative state and had early onset.

PSYCHIATRY IN THE 20TH CENTURY

The turn of the 20th century was heralded by the famous book by *Sigmund Freud* (1856–1939), *The Interpretation of Dreams*. Freud the founder of psychoanalysis discovered the manifestations of the unconscious and how to use them in treating psychiatric patients; described infantile sexuality and how it accounted for adult disorders. He emerged as a key player in shaping up the concepts and understanding of psychiatry in the first half of 20th century and continues to intrigue popular culture till date. Subsequently, various schools of psychoanalysis were established by many known as post-Freudians and Neo-Freudians. Of these Carl Jung, Alfred Adler, Melanie Klein, Karen Horney, and Anna Freud are noteworthy.

Eugene Bleuler (1857–1939) coined the term Schizophrenia for Dementia Praecox and added that deterioration was not the necessary outcome. In addition to Hebephrenia, Catatonia and Paranoid described by Kraepelin, he added fourth type, Simple Schizophrenia.

Julius von Wagner-Jauregg (1857–1940) was the first psychiatrist to receive the Nobel Prize in 1927 for discovering malaria therapy for General Paresis of the Insane which is a syndrome caused by late stage syphilis.

Adolf Meyer (1866–1950), a dominant figure in American psychiatry from 1912–1940, conceptualized psychobiological school of psychiatry and viewed the patient as a biological and psychological unity who became ill because of internal pathology and maladaptation's to the environment. He treated patients with medical and nonmedical therapies in community clinics.

Karl Jaspers (1883–1969), in his influential book *General Psychopathology*, delineated different mental states to show the meaningful connections between different thoughts (without looking for an underlying cause), and stressed on the need of using empathy to understand the felt mental state of the patient.

Two Italian psychiatrists, *Ugo Cerletti* (1897–1963) and *Lucio Bini* (1908–1964), devised electro-convulsive therapy (ECT) and used it in Rome in 1938 for the first time to produce convulsions that alleviated symptoms of schizophrenia.

Egas Moniz and *Almeida Lima* pioneered the art of psychosurgery for treatment of psychiatric illnesses. This work earned a Nobel Prize for Moniz in 1949.

The second half of the 20th century saw unprecedented growth in psychiatry with impetus on research, treatments, and the diagnosis and classification of mental disorders along with deinstitutionalization and community care of patients due to concerns of inadequate care within institutions and rising economic burden for the same. The evolution was influenced by two major changes, firstly the development and growth of psychopharmacology and secondly the emergence of antipsychiatry movement.

In 1952, two French psychiatrists, *Jean Delay* (1907–1987) and *Pierre Deniker* (1917–1999), accidentally discovered chlorpromazine which was found to significantly calm down agitated psychotic patients. The following decade saw the unprecedented rise of antipsychotic, antidepressant and anxiolytic drugs, which fundamentally changed the therapeutic paradigms for the treatment of the mentally ill. The 60s witnessed the rise in the antipsychiatry movement led by RD Laing, Thomas Szasz and David Cooper.

In India, the living conditions in the mental asylums had significantly deteriorated due to lack of funds and indifferent attitude of the custodians of these institutions by the beginning of 20th century. In 1905, the government was forced to take steps to improve the condition of the asylums which resulted in central supervision of the asylums. Indian lunacy Act, 1912 came into force which would influence psychiatry in India for a long time to come. Nomenclature of such institutions was changed later from Lunatic Asylums to Mental Hospitals. Administrative control of the hospitals was shifted from the prison authorities to the Directorate of Health Services which assented to the medical status of psychiatry. The First World War saw an unprecedented rise in the number of admissions in mental hospitals, especially of the Bombay Presidency. With the increase in demand for care of the mentally ill soldiers and the English, European Mental Hospital (now called the Central Institute of Psychiatry) at Ranchi was established in 1918 under the charge of Colonel Berkeley Hill who took avid interest in application of recent advances in management of these patients.

Many innovative programs like occupational therapy, hydrotherapy, habit formation chart were started in this institute, which resulted in its stronghold in the field of care of the mentally ill. Central institute of Psychiatry (CIP) became the first center outside Europe to use new therapeutic modalities like cardiazol-induced seizure (1938), ECT (1943) and psychosurgery (1947). Rauwolfia extracts were being used for treatment of psychotic patients in the 1940s.

Girindra Sekhar Bose introduced general hospital psychiatry in India, establishing the first general hospital psychiatric unit at the RG Kar Medical College in 1933. He founded the Indian Psycho-analytical Association in Calcutta in 1921. Colonel Owen Berkeley-Hill, the medical superintendent of European Mental Hospital, Ranchi, in 1929, founded the Indian Association for Mental Hygiene. The two organizations gradually lost steam. In 1946, Dr Nagendra Nath De consulted Major RB Davis and TA Munro to revive the organization and lead to the formation of the Indian Psychiatric Society, the national organization of Psychiatrists in India, in Delhi on 7th January 1947; Colonel Dhunjibhoy being elected the founder President of the Society. Post his migration after independence, the first meeting of the Indian Psychiatric Society (IPS) was convened under the Presidentship of Dr NN De on 2nd January 1948 at Patna.

PSYCHIATRY IN INDEPENDENT INDIA

Post-independence psychiatry inherited an asylum-based mental health system from the British which was custodial in its outlook and financially draining. There was negligible manpower to run the existing system and provide services to the entire population. There was dearth in research literature specifically pertaining to the unique aspects of the Indian subcontinent and the magnitude of the problem in the country.

General Hospital Psychiatry

Girindra Sekhar Bose in Calcutta and KK Masani in Bombay had already taken the lead to establish general hospital psychiatry units (GHPUs) in their respective cities in the fourth decade of 20th century. A psychiatry unit was opened in 1939 at Patna Medical College within the Department of Medicine. S Datta Ray established psychiatry outpatient clinic at Irwin hospital in 1957, which was the first GHPU in Delhi. Clinics at Lucknow and Chandigarh were established with NN Wig's initiative followed by a chain of GHPUs all over the country. It was one of the most influential developments, which integrated psychiatry with general medical stream and proved to be more cost-effective as compared to the asylum system.

Manpower Development

Soon after its formation, the IPS appointed a committee on Postgraduate Psychiatry Education. As per the Bhore committee suggestions, there was an increase in the mental asylums in the early years after independence; "All India Institute of Mental Health" was established in 1954 at Bangalore, which was later renamed as "National Institute of Mental Health and Neurosciences" (NIMHANS) in 1974 as the nodal center for manpower development and research. From 1947–1967 there were only six institutes in India offering postgraduate degrees (MD), and from these centers about 14 psychiatrists qualified every year. The first postgraduate MD degree in psychiatry was awarded by Patna University to Dr LP Varma in the year 1941, which was later retrospectively recognized by Medical Council of India in the year 2008. During the last four decades there has been substantial growth in the facilities available for psychiatry training, still it is very much less than what is required for the country. Today, there are about 8–9 thousand psychiatrists in the country which is very much below what is ideally desirable. The number of other mental health professionals, such as clinical psychologists, psychiatric social worker and psychiatric nurses, is also very much below what is required.

New Mental Health Legislation

The first draft for the Mental Health bill was written in 1949 by RB Davis, SA Hasib, and JJ Roy on the initiative of IPS but took almost four decades to be notified as, "Mental Health Act-1987". However, it has now been replaced by a new act called, "Mental Healthcare Act-2017", to make it aligned with the provisions of the United Nations Convention on Rights of Persons with Disability, to which India is also a signatory. Persons with Disabilities Act-1995 has also been replaced by a new act called Rights of Persons with disabilities Act-2016, in which mental illness has also been included in the list of disabilities.

National Mental Health Program

In the late 1950s Vidya Sagar, at Amritsar Mental Hospital began involving the family members of the patients in their treatments, which heralded a major movement and paved the path towards community psychiatry. Psychiatry in India gradually moved from the shackles of isolated existence in mental hospitals to community with the setting up of the two landmark community psychiatry projects, one in South India at Sakalwara, near Bangalore under NIMHANS and another in North at Raipur Rani near Chandigarh under PGIMER. National Mental Health Program was launched in 1982 with the objective of providing mental health services to all needy, to integrate mental health with the general health services with the community participation.

Research in psychiatry initially focused on individual course of disease and phenomenology, which later grew to give information regarding the epidemiology which was of importance in drafting the policies and programs for the growth of the field. New psychotherapeutic models like *Guru-Chela* Relations model by Dr JS Neki, psychotherapy based on tenets of Bhagwad Gita by Dr Venkoba Rao and Hanuman complex by Dr NN Wig came into clinical application.

Role of the Supreme Court

The 90's saw the intervention of the Supreme Court in response to a number of PILs which ushered the era of judicial activism in the arena of mental health. The Court recognized that the mentally ill have a right to food, water, personal hygiene, sanitation, recreation which is an extension of the right to life as in Article 21. Quality norms and standards in mental health are nonnegotiable. Treatment, teaching, training and research must be integrated to produce the desired results. Obligation of the State in providing undiluted care and attention to mentally ill persons is fundamental to the recognition of their human rights and is irreversible. The Supreme Court declared three mental hospitals autonomous and handed over their monitoring to the National Human Rights Commission, with the following objectives:

- To provide diagnostic and therapeutic facilities for mental patients
- To develop an infrastructure for providing social and occupational rehabilitation to mental patients

- To provide professional and para-professional training in the fields of psychiatry, clinical psychology, psychiatric social work, and psychiatric nursing
- To extend mental health services at the community level by providing training to medical and paramedical personnel in the field
- To conduct research in behavioral sciences.

THE NEW MILLENNIUM

The dawn of the new millennium promised advances in the field of molecular psychiatry and neuroimaging modalities. It began with the conferring of the Nobel Prize to Dr Eric R Kandel, a psychiatrist for his work on the physiological basis of memory.

The World Health Report 2001 with an Indian psychiatrist Dr R Srinivasa Murthy as the editor-in-chief and principal writer provided a new understanding of mental disorders in a comprehensive way, examining the scope of prevention, service provision and planning. It offered ten recommendations for action with relevance in the current times, as follows:
- Provision of treatment in primary care
- Ensuring availability of psychotropic drugs
- Community care
- Public education
- Involvement of communities, families, and consumers
- Establishment of national policies, programs, and legislation
- Human resource development
- Linkage with other sectors
- Monitoring of community mental health
- Supporting research activities

It also brought with it an impetus for change in the classificatory system of psychiatric disorders which partly culminated with the release of diagnostic and statistical manual of mental disorders (DSM-5). The rights-based chapter in psychiatry was embarked on with the adoption of the United Nations Convention on the Rights of Persons with Disabilities in 2006 by the UN general assembly.

INDIAN SCENARIO

In India the beginning of the new millennium was with the disastrous tragedy at Erwadi, that glaringly brought to forefront the pitiable conditions and atrocities faced by the mentally ill in various institutions. However, this also brought in the much needed vigor for the overhauling of psychiatric services with reformed strategy of the National Mental Health Programme (NMHP), development of the new Mental Healthcare Act 2017 and increase in integration of services with manpower training at all levels.

CONCLUSION

Coincidentally, it is interesting to note that taking a good clinical history is a very important part of psychiatry for understanding the disease and formulate a management plan. Understanding the history of psychiatry as a discipline is also very important to take lessons from the past. The past few decades have seen a surge in the knowledge of the subject with increased understanding about multifactorial etiology of psychiatric disorders, stressing on integrative and inclusive approach towards management. Psychiatry has witnessed three revolutions, the first being the era of asylums, followed by psychoanalysis and finally the revolution of community psychiatry. The fourth and final can be the biological revolution, however the research impetus in this field is conspicuously lacking in our country. It took the unfortunate incident of charring of innocent victim-patients at Erwadi for the country to wake up from its slumber, even though history suggests that our scriptures were well endowed with knowledge regarding mental illness. The treatment goal has endured a paradigm shift from avoiding harm to the society to realignment with the society. Even though we have taken significant strides forwards, there is enough left to be explored and done, as in the words of the famous poet, Robert Frost, "there are miles to go before I sleep."

TAKE-HOME MESSAGES

- History is the ultimate elder. History always has a story to tell, it cannot remain silent.
- History of psychiatry has traversed the path from the broken soul to the broken brain, from philosophical ruminations to biological conundrums.
- The word "psychiatry" was first introduced in 1808 by Johann Christian Reil (1755–1820) of Germany.
- First asylum in the Muslim world was opened in Baghdad followed by Cairo. In 1547, the monastery of St Mary of Bethlehem, London was converted into a lunatic asylum by the King.

- The oldest surviving mental asylum in the country was established in 1794 at Chennai which still exists at the same location as Institute of Mental Health, Chennai. The first Indian Lunacy Act came up in 1858.
- *Julius von Wagner-Jauregg* (1857–1940) was the first psychiatrist to receive the Nobel Prize in 1927 for discovering malaria therapy for General Paresis of the Insane. Egas Moniz also received Nobel Prize in 1949 for his work on Psychosurgery.
- *Girindra Sekhar Bose* established the first general hospital psychiatric unit at the RG Kar Medical College in 1933.
- The first postgraduate MD degree in psychiatry was awarded by Patna University to Dr LP Varma in the year 1941.
- The first meeting of the Indian Psychiatric Society was convened under the Presidentship of Dr. NN De on 2nd January 1948 at Patna.
- Psychiatry has witnessed three revolutions, the first being the era of asylums, followed by psychoanalysis and finally the revolution of community psychiatry. The fourth and final can be the biological revolution.

32

Future of Psychiatry

Naren P Rao, Santosh K Chaturvedi

INTRODUCTION

The importance of psychiatry in future is definitely going to increase, both from a clinical as well as research perspective. Many exciting developments await psychiatry, and its practice. It might not be an exaggeration to predict that psychiatry will be an integral part of medical practice. Psychological, social, ecological and environmental factors are identified in many medical diseases. Psychological and emotional reactions to diseases and surgical procedures have long been acknowledged, and these would need to be addressed.

In this chapter, the importance of mental illnesses, psychiatry training, clinical practice and research in near and distant future are discussed. The question whether, psychiatry would be considered as a medical or neurological specialty will continue to be debated in the future. The search for brain involvement in different psychiatric disorders will continue, and the positive discoveries would make one wonder if depression and schizophrenia are neurological diseases with clear evidence of brain dysfunction and abnormalities.

IMPORTANCE OF MENTAL ILLNESS IN FUTURE

Mental disorders, mainly depression and substance use disorders, are a major reason for morbidity and disability throughout the world. In India, mental disorders contribute to a substantial disease burden and as per the recent national mental health survey, lifetime prevalence of mental disorders is 13.7% in individuals above the age of 18. It is important to note that within India there is a significant variation in prevalence of mental disorders between rural areas and urban metros. The prevalence of schizophrenia and other psychoses, mood disorders and neurotic or stress-related disorders (6.93%) was nearly two to three times more in urban metros.

Several factors may be responsible for this higher prevalence of the disorder like:
- Lifestyle
- Higher rates of substance use
- Lack of family support
- Ethnic minority
- Increased rate of infections or
- Other biological and environmental factors, like urbanization.

Another important but neglected area, which will be a focus of attention, is age-related cognitive disorders. With increasing longevity even in our country, age-related disorders are going to be a major concern soon. As is seen in some countries, like Japan, where there are large number of persons above the age of 90 years, newer mental health issues are being noted. As the risk of development of dementia increases with age, the prevalence of dementia is likely to increase in India too. In 2010, there were 3.7 million Indians with dementia and the numbers are expected to double by 2030. In addition, the high burden of cardiovascular risk factors such as hypertension, diabetes, obesity, smoking, alcoholism, as seen in Indian population, is surely likely to lead to a rise in cerebrovascular disease-related vascular dementia and mixed dementias.

Yet another area which will gain prominence will be comorbidity or multimorbidity. Pure, isolated psychiatric disorders, as defined today, may be rare presentation. Psychiatric disorders will have comorbid another psychiatric disorder, personality disorder, alcohol or substance use disorder or one or more of the noncommunicable diseases. This will be a challenge in future, since medical and psychiatric textbooks still discuss and describe medical and psychiatric disorders in isolation. In clinical and practical terms, doctors will have to deal with persons with multiple disorders, which have their own complications and challenges.

INTERNET-RELATED PSYCHIATRIC DISORDERS

Internet addiction disorder is a topic of worldwide concern considering rapid growth of social and entertainment applications of internet. It is a nonchemical, behavioral addiction in which person is preoccupied with the use of internet and has compulsive use of internet for longer than originally intended. This results in investment of significant amount of time in use of computer or mobile phone and results in distress. The problematic computer use comes at the expense of real social interactions and results in extreme retreat to seclusion. Importantly, internet addiction affects adolescent population and poses risks to youths' mental health, and may likely produce negative consequences in everyday life. Individual suffering from internet addiction has difficulties in self-identity, self-image and adaptive social relationships. They often suffer from loss of control, anger, mood fluctuations, low distress and frustration tolerance and social withdrawal. This would affect one's social and family life and result in familial conflicts.

PSYCHIATRY TRAINING

Despite the high prevalence of mental disorders in India, the number of trained human resources is limited. There is a substantial deficit of dedicated human resources for mental health services: 52% of the districts in India did not have psychiatric facilities and there was an acute shortage of psychiatrists (77%), psychologists (97%) and psychiatric social workers (90%) as per a study in 2004 and the condition is more or less the same even today. Hence, people with neuropsychiatric disorders remain largely undiagnosed and even when diagnosed, do not have access to sustainable, affordable treatment and optimal medical care. In addition to the lack of trained manpower, another important concern is the inequitable distribution of available manpower. The available manpower is predominantly located in cities with minimal availability of psychiatric care in rural population. Considering the increasing prevalence of mental illness and age-related cognitive disorders the need for trained manpower is likely to be significant in the future.

Posting of interns in department of psychiatry has become compulsory since the last few years, and Indian Psychiatric Society is demanding a longer clinical posting and separate examination during the medical course. This will ensure medical students to learn psychiatry with greater motivation and interest, as it would also be a great asset for them in their clinical practice.

Problem-based learning (PBL) in medical teaching is the way forward to include psychiatry training in medical institutes. PBL will ensure discussion and orientation toward psychiatric aspects all through the medical course, the right way to understanding and providing holistic care for all medical disorders.

Specialization and superspecialization also have already come to the discipline of psychiatry. There are Doctor of Medicine (DM) courses in child psychiatry, geriatric psychiatry and addiction psychiatry currently. Other DM courses in community psychiatry, rehabilitation psychiatry, perinatal psychiatry and so on may come up, in future.

Another area of concern is lack of trained manpower involved in research in mental illness. According to an estimate by the United Nations Educational, Scientific and Cultural Organization (UNESCO), while there are three researchers for every 1,000 residents in developed countries, the numbers are ten times less in lower middle-income countries three for every 10,000 residents (UNESCO 2002). The number of people involved in research for brain disorders is approximately one per million persons. The number of clinicians involved in research in mental illness is even less. In 1990, the Commission on Health Research for Development estimated that while 90% of the world's health problems are in developing countries, less than 10% of the global health research resources were being applied toward these problems. This imbalance is designated as the "10/90 gap". Within India, there is a disproportionate distribution of trained resources with investment and output being concentrated in few institutes. A mapping of neuroscience research in India revealed that 9.2% of institutions contribute 80.1% of papers.

PSYCHIATRY AS A MEDICAL SPECIALTY: CURRENT STATUS AND FUTURE PERSPECTIVES

With rapid advances in the medical field, the diagnosis and treatment of majority medical diseases are standardized with the etiopathogenesis primarily involving a biological mechanism. On the contrary, the current psychiatric practice follows a holistic approach takes into consideration all three levels—(1) biological, (2) psychological and (3) social in individual assessment and treatment. This makes imperative for the psychiatrist to imbibe a clinical skill that incorporates a humane and psychosocial dimension of care that uniquely sets him apart from other medical disciplines. These skills make the psychiatrist a core member of many multispecialty medical teams where the psychiatrist can apply these skills into medical care termed as "Liaison Psychiatry". While the role of the liaison psychiatry and emphasis on the psychopathology will remain unchanged, the advances in cognitive neuroscience and understanding of molecular mechanisms, advances in investigative modalities and novel treatment options may have impact on psychiatric practice in future.

Psychiatric aspects of many medical disorders are already sprouting as independent specialties. In future, many more will develop. Currently, many of these are subsumed under consultation liaison psychiatry. Some of these are:

- Psycho-oncology
- Psychonephrology
- Psycho-ophthalmology
- Psychosomatic obstetrics and gynecology/psychogynecology
- Psychocardiology
- Psychodermatology
- Neuropsychiatry
- Perinatal psychiatry, and so on.

UNDERSTANDING PATHOPHYSIOLOGY OF PSYCHIATRIC DISORDERS: ADVANCES IN COGNITIVE NEUROSCIENCE

Recent advances in understanding mental illness and advances in neuroscience research have led to a new area of cognitive neuroscience. Major advances in molecular biology and neuroimaging in the last two decades have provided psychiatry with powerful tools which help to understand the biological mechanisms involved in the pathogenesis of various psychiatric disorders. With newer neuroscience techniques, the role of genes, neurotransmitters and neural circuits in specific cognitive functions are better understood. Following these advances, a heuristic model linking the gene with the behavior has been proposed which also allows a two-directional interaction with physical environment and social factors in the environment. A schematic representation of the proposed model is given in **Flowchart 32.1**. As seen in this model, the genetic variation drives molecular mechanisms resulting in changes in the neurotransmitters and intracellular signaling system. The process of gene expression can be influenced by environmental factors, both physical and social, through interaction between gene and environment. These changes at molecular level will in turn influence the way a single neuron and in effect how a network of neurons will work. Functioning of neural circuit will bring about the changes in behavior. Advances in cognitive neuroscience have given important leads for exploring further the genetic, molecular and cellular processes underlying behavior.

Advances in electrophysiology like electroencephalography, neuroimaging like functional magnetic resonance imaging (MRI) have provided insights into the abnormalities in neural circuits underlying psychiatric disorder. These advances will also help to understand the psychiatric symptoms commonly seen in various medical diseases like hypothyroidism, epilepsy, post head injury personality changes, systemic lupus erythematosus, etc. While the biological basis of the psychiatric disorders will facilitate the integration of the field of psychiatry with other specialties in a hospital setting, the skill sets required in psychiatric clinical practice makes them unique among the medical specialties.

FUTURE OF PSYCHIATRIC DIAGNOSIS: USE OF INVESTIGATIVE MODALITIES TO AID THE DIAGNOSIS OF PSYCHIATRIC DISORDERS

The contemporary psychiatric practice is predominantly based on the clinical interview and symptom clusters for the diagnosis of psychiatric disorders. In the absence of an objective marker similar to other medical illnesses, such as fasting blood sugar for diabetes mellitus, makes the diagnosis of psychiatric disorders amenable to be influenced by subjective perceptions of the psychiatrist. This is a major challenge in current psychiatric practice and different

Flowchart 32.1: Genotype to behavior through hierarchical intermediate stages.

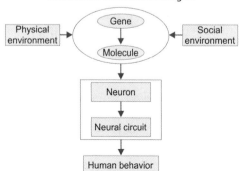

modes of investigations are being evaluated for being used as objective markers. Amongst these possible biomarkers, neuroimaging and neurochemical measures have been promising. Converging evidence from different lines of research suggests structural, functional and connectivity abnormalities in brains of patients with different psychiatric disorders. The following neuroimaging techniques have been examined to be candidate biomarkers for psychiatric disorders.

- Magnetic resonance imaging
- Functional MRI
- Single-photon emission computed tomography (SPECT) and
- Positron emission tomography (PET)

Dementia is an example where neuroimaging modalities play an important role in the diagnosis. Till last decade, the role of neuroimaging modalities like computed tomography (CT) or MRI was limited primarily in ruling out structural lesions of the brain like tumors, abscess or identifying areas of hemorrhage and infarction in individuals with dementia. However, in the recent years, fluorodeoxyglucose (FDG)-PET has been proven to be a valuable assessment method in the diagnosis of Alzheimer's disease. Many studies in the last decade have examined the value of FDG-PET in the diagnosis of dementia. Few studies reported high sensitivity and specificity of FDG-PET in accurately differentiating patients with Alzheimer's dementia from healthy volunteers. The overall value for sensitivity and specificity of this method, based on meta-analysis of all available studies, suggests high sensitivity (91%) and high specificity (86%) for FDG-PET in detecting Alzheimer's dementia, which is higher than the sensitivity and specificity of its clinical diagnosis of Alzheimer's dementia—81% and 70%, respectively.

With advances in understanding pathophysiology of Alzheimer's dementia, it is increasingly recognized that the pathogenic mechanisms start earlier than the clinical manifestations. Also converging lines of evidence from several sources have established the role of β-amyloid accumulation in the pathogenesis of Alzheimer's dementia. Hence, various imaging and neurochemical techniques are targeted at quantifying the β-amyloid deposits in brains of individual patients with dementia. The US Food and Drug Administration (FDA) has approved three tracers for PET imaging—(1) florbetapir, (2) florbetaben and (3) flutemetamol—for use in patients suspected to have dementia. While a positive scan with any of these tracers is not useful, a negative scan reduces the likelihood that index patient's cognitive impairment is due to Alzheimer's dementia. In addition, amyloid imaging scan resulted in a change in the diagnosis of significant percentage of patients of Alzheimer's dementia making it a useful confirmatory diagnostic modality which aids the diagnosis of dementia. With advances in machine learning and advanced computation techniques, the neuroimaging modalities may have an application in aiding the diagnosis of psychiatric disorders in future and may be incorporated into standard diagnostic systems.

FUTURE OF PSYCHIATRY TREATMENT: NOVEL TREATMENT MODALITIES

Utility of brain stimulation techniques namely electroconvulsive therapy (ECT) and repetitive transcranial magnetic stimulation (rTMS) is well established in treatment of psychiatric disorders like depression and schizophrenia. Recent advances in neuromodulation, neurosurgery and virtual reality have resulted in advent of new treatment modalities in psychiatry. These methods are likely to hold promise in the future.

Neuromodulation: A novel and promising areas of immense interest are the novel brain stimulation techniques. Vagus nerve stimulation (VNS) is a novel technique for the treatment of resistant depression. In this, a stimulation generator connected to bipolar electrodes is implanted around the left vagus nerve. Using a remote, handheld computer the parameters for stimulation can be controlled. As significant proportion of vagus afferents terminate in the medulla which in turn is connected to forebrain, stimulation of vagus nerve is associated with widespread functional effects in brain. Many clinical studies have suggested efficacy of VNS in the treatment of resistant depression and this has been approved by the US FDA. While VNS is an efficacious method, the major limitation is invasiveness of the procedure as the electrodes need to be implanted in the body. Hence, many noninvasive brain stimulation techniques are being examined as treatment modalities. Transcranial direct current stimulation (tDCS) is a noninvasive brain stimulation technique of considerable promise. In this technique, direct current is applied via two scalp electrodes overlying the targeted cortical areas. This electric current induces changes in neuronal membrane even after the stimulation is stopped and could have long-lasting effects on synaptic plasticity. Several studies have examined tDCS for the treatment of depression, auditory hallucinations in schizophrenia and negative symptoms of depression with mixed results. In the future, further refining of these physical stimulation methods and application of other novel methods like transcranial alternate current stimulation

(tACS) are likely to result in better treatment of resistant psychiatric conditions. Advances in the field of nanotechnology and targeted drug delivery will also have significant impact in the field of physical treatment of psychiatric disorders.

Advances in psychosurgery: Despite the best available pharmacotherapy and psychotherapy, a considerable proportion of patients remain resistant to these treatments and continue to have symptoms. Many ablative and modulatory approaches are considered for these resistant patients. Though different surgical procedures have been practiced since 60–70 years, it has remained a niche application. With the advent of new technique namely deep brain stimulation (DBS), there is a revival of interest in the application of surgery to treatment of mental disorders. In DBS, electrodes are implanted into subcortical structures via neurosurgical procedure and an extension cable is tunneled under the skin connecting the electrodes with a pacemaker placed below the clavicle in a subcutaneous pocket. After surgery, the pacemaker is programmed to determine the stimulation parameters. DBS has been successfully used for obsessive compulsive disorder and major depression. The indications are likely to expand to other disorders in the future.

Virtual reality-based treatment in psychiatry: This new technology allows one to create analogs of real world and artificial experiences in real time. The rich experience of the virtual reality makes the user to believe that the experience is real and the user is in that situation. The advantage is the degree of control one can exert over the stimulus and the flexibility in regulating the graded exposure to the patient. In the last decade, virtual reality-based treatments have been tested for different psychiatric indications like phobias, social anxiety, obsessive compulsive disorder and schizophrenia. With rapid advances in technology, the virtual reality is likely to take an increasingly important role in treatment of many psychiatric disorders.

INTEGRATED TREATMENTS IN PSYCHIATRY: ROLE OF INDIAN TRADITIONAL MEDICINE IN PSYCHIATRY

The future is likely to witness the integration of traditional medical systems in psychiatric practice. Already numerous well-designed studies have confirmed the benefit from yoga for not only common mental disorders, but also certain severe mental illnesses. Meditation, mindfulness and other healing methods are also important components of behavioral medicine. The Government of India is encouraging use of Ayurveda, Yoga, Unani, Siddha, and Homeopathy in prevention of mental disorders, promotion of mental health and long-term care. Naturopathy and other complementary and alternative medicine systems are also likely to grow further.

WILL HISTORY REPEAT ITSELF IN FUTURE?

Will there be a resurgence of psychodynamics and psychoanalysis in future, this time with evidence from brain psychophysiological and imaging studies? Neuropsychoanalysis is an emerging field which is attempting to build bridges between neuroscience and psychoanalysis. Serendipity has played a big role in the introduction of interventions in psychiatry, which may hopefully come to our help again, may be repeatedly. But, since eyes see only what the mind knows, we have to continue to engage in brainstorming and mindstorming exercises.

CONCLUSION

The developments in the last few decades have paved the way for highly sophisticated and technologically advanced investigations to understand the etiopathogenesis of several psychiatric disorders. Hopefully, this understanding would lead on to safer and more effective interventions. Importance of psychiatry in other medical specialties will continue to keep growing, because there is no health without mental health. It looks promising that psychiatry in future would be more exciting and lead to improvement in the quality of life and sense of well-being of all individuals.

TAKE-HOME MESSAGES

- The importance of psychiatry in future is definitely going to increase, both from a clinical as well as research perspective.
- Psychiatric disorders are frequently comorbid with other medical or psychiatric disorders, which have their own implications and challenges in holistic care.
- Problem-based learning in medical teaching is the way forward to include psychiatry training in medical institutions.
- The humane, social and psychological care, key aspects of clinical practice, make the psychiatrist a core member of multidisciplinary medical teams.
- Rise in mobile-based internet use and associated social consequences will be a major concern and could result in epidemic of behavioral addiction as well as other behavioral problems.
- Recent advances in understanding mental illness and advances in neuroscience research have led to the new area of cognitive neuroscience which will possibly result in newer diagnostic tools and novel treatments.

Index

Page numbers followed by *b* refer to box, *f* refer to figure, *fc* refer to flowchart, and *t* refer to table.